Plagues in World History

Exploring World History

Series Editors

John McNeill, Georgetown University
Jerry Bentley, University of Hawai'i

As the world grows ever more closely linked, students and general readers alike are appreciating the need to become internationally aware. World history offers the crucial connection to understanding past global links and how they influence the present. The series will expand that awareness by offering clear, concise supplemental texts for the undergraduate classroom as well as trade books that advance world history scholarship.

The series will be open to books taking a thematic approach—exploring commodities such as sugar, cotton, and petroleum; technologies; diseases and the like; or regional—for example, Islam in Southeast Asia or east Africa, the Indian Ocean, or the Ottoman Empire. The series sees regions not simply as fixed geographical entities but also as evolving spatial frameworks that have reflected and shaped the movement of people, ideas, goods, capital, institutions, and information. Thus, regional books would move beyond traditional borders to consider the flows that have characterized the global system.

Edited by two of the leading historians in the field, this series will work to synthesize world history for students, engage general readers, and expand the boundaries for scholars.

Plagues in World History
by John Aberth

Smuggling: Contraband and Corruption in World History
by Alan L. Karras

The First World War: A Concise Global History
by William Kelleher Storey

*Insatiable Appetite: The United States and the Ecological
Degradation of the Tropical World*
by Richard P. Tucker

Plagues in World History

John Aberth

ROWMAN & LITTLEFIELD PUBLISHERS, INC.
Lanham • Boulder • New York • Toronto • Plymouth, UK

Published by Rowman & Littlefield Publishers, Inc.
A wholly owned subsidiary of The Rowman & Littlefield Publishing Group, Inc.
4501 Forbes Boulevard, Suite 200, Lanham, Maryland 20706
http://www.rowmanlittlefield.com

Estover Road, Plymouth PL6 7PY, United Kingdom

British Library Cataloguing in Publication Information Available

Library of Congress Cataloging-in-Publication Data

Aberth, John, 1963–
  Plagues in world history / John Aberth.
  p. cm. — (Exploring world history)
  Includes bibliographical references and index.
  ISBN 978-0-7425-5705-5 (cloth : alk. paper) — ISBN 978-1-4422-0796-7 (electronic)
  1. Epidemics—History. 2. Communicable diseases—History. I. Title.
  RA649.A24 2011
  614.4—dc22   2010029028

∞™ The paper used in this publication meets the minimum requirements of American
National Standard for Information Sciences—Permanence of Paper for Printed Library
Materials, ANSI/NISO Z39.48-1992.

Printed in the United States of America

Contents

Introduction

Why study disease? It's not a very pleasant subject to contemplate. The pages of its history are full of suffering and death. Its comings and goings often seem arbitrary and simply inexplicable, the bane of most historians. There is no happy ending.

And yet . . . there is something about plagues that fascinates. For those with morbid minds, the spectacle of mass death is mesmerizing in its capacity to inspire fear, panic, viciousness, and cruelty. But for those of us who hold out some hope for humanity, there is also to be found—even in a time of plague—kindness, generosity, courage, and heroism. Truly, an epidemic tempers a society, subjecting it to trials either to which it must succumb or over which it must triumph. There is no middle ground with plague. It is the litmus test of civilizations.

Obviously, for our purposes, plagues and disease will be used interchangeably. Even though "plague" does refer to a specific disease,[1] which will be a main focus of this book, the origins of the term can be traced back to the Latin word *plaga*, meaning a "blow" or "wound."[2] While in the classical context of the Latin language plague might be associated with a misfortune or disaster of some kind, it was not necessarily associated with disease; this only seems to have emerged during the late Roman Empire, when the Church issued a definitive Latin "Vulgate" edition of the Old and New Testaments, largely through the labors of St. Jerome, by 405 C.E. In this new context, plague naturally came to mean a "blow" from on high, such as when the Hebrew God struck down every firstborn male in Egypt, as recounted in the Book of Exodus. But this idea, if not the term, for plague was a common inheritance from the ancients, all of whom viewed disease as naturally emanating from the gods. Like the Hebrews, the Greeks could conceive of disease as a punishment or test for humans, with perhaps the most famous example being Apollo using his silver bow to rain down plague upon the Greeks, after Agamemnon had insulted his priest, Chryses, in the opening pages of Homer's epic poem *The Iliad*. But in older Egyptian and Mesopotamian cultures, the reasons for the gods sending down disease could also be rather mysterious and unfathomable.

The history of disease, of course, is very old. It goes right back to the very beginnings of humanity, when men and women first became aware of the pain and suffering caused by abnormal conditions, such as the invasion of their bodies by other organisms. Ever since they evolved from apes, humans were infected by the same diseases that afflicted their primate ancestors and that were caused by microbes that originated and adapted to their hosts millions of years ago. Some of these "heirloom" infections include herpes, hepatitis, and yellow fever, all caused by viruses, as well as malaria, caused by a plasmodium. Later, when humans became hunters, other diseases passed to them from animals when they ate raw or partially cooked meats. For instance, Paleolithic man may have suffered from a variety of bacterial diseases, including anthrax, brucellosis, tularemia, and glanders, as a result of the microbes being present in the wild game they hunted.[3]

However, the opportunities for disease causation and spread are thought to have increased dramatically with the advent of settled agriculture at the dawn of the Neolithic period in c. 8000 B.C.E. Maintaining close and regular contact with domesticated animals, not to mention with other humans, as well as creating stagnant reservoir pools such as irrigation ditches and accumulating large amounts of human waste, perhaps within contaminating distance of drinking supplies, opened a new chapter in the disease history of humankind by allowing illnesses to become endemic, or perpetually present, in the artificial microbe pools thus created. Chronic diseases that could thrive even in small populations and that were associated with the new, man-made environments include tuberculosis, schistosomiasis, and typhoid fever. However, some "density-dependent" diseases, such as measles or smallpox, that may have originated in Neolithic man's newfound relationship with domesticated animals nonetheless had to wait until human populations became large enough to sustain them, which could not have happened much before 3000 B.C.E. Other ills that are caused by dietary deficiencies also increased at this time, despite the fact that more and steadier supplies of food were now available, since this was offset by a decline in the variety of foods that had formerly been consumed under more nomadic circumstances.[4]

Eventually, trade, war, migrations, and other activities that brought distant human populations together were also to add to this disease environment, of which illnesses like plague and influenza were to be the primary beneficiaries. Early humans also made efforts to counteract or compensate for disease-ridden conditions by designing sewer systems, imposing unclean food taboos, or setting up social barriers between disparate populations or "castes," such as were distinctive features of ancient civilizations in India and Palestine (Hebrew culture). Yet, such efforts may have had mixed success. For example, the impressive sewer systems uncovered in the urban environments of Mohenjo-Daro and Harappa, part of the Indus River valley civilization in India dating to around 2600 B.C.E., even boasts individual household latrines connecting to the underground drains. It would seem obvious that this was part of an effort to contain waste contamination and protect freshwater drinking supplies, but one should not discount the possibility that it was equally motivated by a desire to efficiently collect waste for use as fertilizer, in which case the likelihood of contracting disease would only increase.[5]

Toward the end of the Neolithic period, we begin to accumulate other evidence of the impact of disease upon human societies aside from the archaeological. Our most valuable sources now become the written records that first make their appearance around 3000 B.C.E. Perhaps the earliest descriptions of and references to disease can be found in ancient Mesopotamian literature. The epic poem *Gilgamesh*, written down around 2000 B.C.E. but recounting events that apparently occurred several centuries earlier, tells of how the hero's friend, Enkidu, contracts a debilitating illness that confines him to his bed for twelve days until he dies. The identity of the disease that kills Enkidu is never made clear, for its symptoms are not described; we know only that it causes Enkidu great pain and that he ascribes it to the curse of the gods in retribution for slaying the Bull of Heaven. However, further details as to what this illness may have entailed are supplied by the "Poem of the Righteous Sufferer," part of the Mesopotamian wisdom literature dating to the Babylonian period during the first half of the third millennium B.C.E. Like Enkidu, the "Babylonian Job" lies prostrate in his bed, although his condition is more fully described: He has become deaf, blind, and dumb; a stiffness has taken over his limbs; and his flesh has become emaciated and inflamed. All this is accompanied by a headache, intestinal distress, and discharge of phlegm; at its worst, the disease forces the patient to spend "the night in my dung like an ox" and wallow "in my excrement like a sheep." If the disease has come from the gods, the sufferer remains mystified as to why, since he has performed all of the usual rituals, libations, prayers, and other observances in honor of his deities. Like the later biblical Job, however, the sufferer is eventually redeemed by the Babylonian god Marduk, who restores him to his former health and happiness.

From the almost equally ancient Egyptian culture comes the first recorded medical literature in history, the medical or surgical papyri, the oldest of which perhaps dates to the time of Imhotep in the 2600s B.C.E., even though the manuscript itself was not written down until about a thousand years later. In these medical papyri, Egyptian physicians describe both the medical conditions they are trying to treat—which as often as not are trauma instead of disease related—and their remedies, which include both magical incantations and more "rational" techniques such as surgery and herbal recipes. Interpretation of these texts, however, is hampered by the still inexact knowledge of hieroglyphics and by the fact that the ancient Egyptian mind-set was quite unlike our modern outlook.[6] In addition, Egyptian art, despite its often stylized representations, sometimes depicts spinal or limb abnormalities in statuary and relief carvings of its subjects, deformities that were possibly caused by disease. Finally, on occasion we are fortunate enough to have the physical evidence of the diseased body itself, preserved in mummified form with even the skin still intact, a unique contribution of ancient Egyptian culture. This has allowed scholars to detect diseases even when they did not penetrate to the bone, such as the smallpox lesions evident on the lower face, neck, and shoulders of the pharaoh, Ramses V, who died in c. 1145 B.C.E.[7] In addition to smallpox, Egyptian mummies have also pointed to the presence of tuberculosis, schistosomiasis, and poliomyelitis.

Before leaving the second millennium, we should not omit the oracle bones dating from the Shang dynasty in China between c. 1500 and 1050 B.C.E. These contain, for their time, some quite remarkable conceptions of disease, centering around the *chi*, a logographic symbol depicting a man lying on a bed pierced by the arrow of disease. This obviously anticipates biblical and classical Greek references to "plague" in the sense of a blow sent down upon humans from on high, but in ancient Chinese culture, the notion of any higher power being responsible for disease seems to be absent, as the Chinese preferred to explain the origins of their civilization in purely humanistic terms going back to mighty ancestors. Instead, the disease agent is more rationally explained as due to a worm or insect of some kind, as in the *li* and *ku* symbols, perhaps referring to schistosomiasis. The ancient Chinese also identified diseases with fever or rash-like symptoms, such as malaria or scabies, and made more amorphous references to sensory, intestinal, and reproductive illnesses.[8]

In the last millennium before Christ, humankind entered a new era in writing about disease. References to disease epidemics multiply in the Bible, but its use of generalized terms such as "plague" make identification of specific illnesses difficult.[9] Fully half of the references to plague in the Bible occur in the first five books of the Old Testament, known collectively as the Torah or Pentateuch, which were composed over the course of half a millennium from the tenth to the fifth centuries B.C.E. In Leviticus and Deuteronomy, which contain approximately sixty mentions of the term, plague is associated with a skin disease that may have been leprosy.[10] While the sixth plague that afflicted the Egyptians in Exodus 9:10 and the plague that struck down the Philistines in 1 Samuel 4:6 are traditionally associated with true plague due to references to "boils" and "tumors," it remains inconclusive whether the original Hebrew supports such an interpretation.[11]

Moreover, the Bible perpetuates older conceptions of disease causation, namely, that the source of illnesses is to be attributed to a higher power. At roughly the same time, however, alternative explanations of disease began to emerge in other cultures in India, China, and Greece. Remarkably, all three proposed similar systems that located diseases' origins in humankind's natural environment and defined the disease condition within the body as resulting from an imbalance of its core elements. This was undoubtedly the beginning of a truly rational approach to disease and medicine, which used dietary and other health regimens to prevent illness and natural compounds, bleeding, and other, human-inspired techniques to cure it. But it is important to remember that these same ancient societies by no means abandoned religious or supernatural methods of healing, such as prayers and magical incantations, since desperate patients would have been willing to try any remedy that might work, and the two realms of religion and medicine were not seen as incompatible.[12]

Most influential for the West, of course, was the Greek medical tradition founded by Hippocrates of Cos (c. 460–377 B.C.E.). Along with the body of works attributed to him, known collectively as the "Hippocratic corpus," Hippocrates and his circle of physicians advocated the humoral theory as an explanation of disease occurrences in the body, namely, that any given illness resulted when the four humors of the body—blood, phlegm, yellow bile (*cholera*), and black bile (*melancholia*)—were in a state of imbalance, a condition the Greeks called *dyscrasia*, literally, "bad mixture." But readers should know that very similar systems had also been proposed in ancient Indian and Chinese medicine. The Ayurvedic tradition, compiled around the sixth century B.C.E. as one of India's sacred Veda texts, states that human health is connected to the three *dosas*, or humors: these include *Vayu*, a dynamic, kinetic principle associated with air; *Pitta*, a thermal, explosive force identified with the sun; and *Kapha*, a cohesive principle that binds everything together. Balance of the *dosas* is to be maintained not only by diet and personal habits but also by mental attitudes and even social taboos that must be observed in accordance with the Hindu caste system.[13]

Likewise, ancient Chinese medicine, culminating in the *Huangdi Nei Jing* (*The Yellow Emperor's Classic of Medicine*), dating to the first century B.C.E., proposed a sixfold classification system of diagnosis that, in its crudest, most simplified form, attempts to strike a balance between the two opposing yin-yang qualities of the body and explained illnesses as resulting from an imbalance in the body's *qi*, a nearly untranslatable term that seems to encompass everything that maintains life. Chinese medical tradition, going back to the Chou dynasty (1050–256 B.C.E.), also relates the advent of diseases to the four seasons and to any abnormalities in their cycle (such as cool spring weather in the summer or hot summer weather in the autumn). This is very similar to how works in the Hippocratic corpus, such as *On Airs, Waters, and Places*, explain disease. Like the Greeks, the Chinese also related the advent of disease to other factors including changes in the air and other aspects of the environment, excessive emotional states, and what the Greeks called bad regimen, such as overexertion, poor diet and hygiene, immoral behaviors such as drunkenness and sexual indulgence, and so on. But while the Greek miasmatic theory of bad air (the original *malaria*) allowed for the concept of contagion, or the direct spread of disease from person to person through the passing of the miasma, this never seems to have entered the classical Chinese medical tradition. And while the Greeks related their humors to four basic elements of the universe, namely, air, water, earth, and fire, the Chinese tradition lists five: wood, fire, earth, metal, and water.[14] Altogether, this ancient heritage identifies an impressive galaxy of diseases; judging from the symptoms described, the ancients likely suffered from cholera, malaria, mumps, measles, leprosy, erysipelas, dysentery, epilepsy, diphtheria, smallpox, tuberculosis, typhoid fever, cancer, influenza, beriberi, rickets, pneumonia, cirrhosis, asthma, arthritis . . . the list goes on and on.[15]

Nonetheless, the real history of disease could be said to have begun in 430–426 B.C.E., when a plague struck the city of Athens at the very start of the Peloponnesian War with its rival, Sparta. For it was the Plague of Athens that inspired the famous account of it by the Greek historian Thucydides as part of his *History of the Peloponnesian War*. Many would regard Thucydides' brief but compelling narrative of the plague as the first example of historical writing about disease. This should be attributed to not only the rational, "enlightened" approach that he takes to disease (a path that was being concurrently blazed by the Hippocratics) but also the comprehensive way in which he discusses the plague's impact, which he sees as affecting the entire body politic and not just the individual patient's body.

Significantly, Thucydides states at the outset that he is eschewing all speculation about the plague's origin or causes, perhaps because he has no wish to bring the gods into the discussion, as most other ancient authors would have been tempted to do. This rigorously scientific approach, while paralleling that in contemporary Hippocratic medicine, was probably an entirely unrelated and independent phenomenon.[16] Above all, Thucydides' preoccupation with disease could be described as quintessentially historical: to describe it in such a way that could prove useful to successive generations of his readers. Consequently, Thucydides' first order of business is to enumerate the characteristic symptoms of the disease, by means of which it can be readily identified by future sufferers; it is a task for which Thucydides was uniquely qualified, as he himself had contracted the disease and survived to tell the tale. These symptoms include a burning fever, inflammation of the throat and tongue, small pustules or ulcers on the skin, nauseating diarrhea and other discharges, and gangrene of the extremities, which, if they killed the victim, did so in about a week. Yet, despite this painstaking description, modern historians have endlessly debated exactly what kind of disease afflicted Athenians during the plague. While it assuredly was not the disease known as bubonic plague, since the characteristic symptom of the bubo is not present in Thucydides' account, consensus opinion seems to have coalesced around smallpox, although other candidates, including typhus, typhoid fever, measles, and anthrax, also have been proposed.[17]

But what elevates Thucydides' narrative to far above the ordinary is his ensuing discussion of the social effects of the plague. In a profoundly perceptive analysis, Thucydides notes how the plague overturned the conventions of his society, whether these be in terms of funerary rites, religious observances, respect for the laws and morals, or even the obligations of family members to care for sick loved ones. It was Thucydides who first advanced the idea that people typically respond to the threat of mass death from disease with a "live for the moment" attitude as they await the imminent prospect of their own potential demise. As he puts it in a justly famous passage,

> Men now coolly ventured on what they had formerly done in a corner and not just where they pleased, seeing the rapid transitions produced by persons in prosperity suddenly dying and those who before had nothing succeeding to their property. So they resolved to spend quickly and enjoy themselves, regarding their lives and riches as alike things of a day. Perseverance in what men called honor was popular with none, it was so uncertain whether they would be spared to attain the object; but it was settled that present enjoyment, and all that contributed to it, was both honorable and useful. Fear of gods or law of man there was none to restrain them. As for the first, they judged it to be just the same whether they worshipped them or not, as they saw all alike perishing; and for the last, no one expected to live to be brought to trial for his offences, but each felt that a far severer sentence had been already passed upon them all and hung ever over their heads, and before this fell it was only reasonable to enjoy life a little.[18]

However, it should be noted here that other Greek sources also record a more conservative reaction to the plague, one that reaffirmed the role of the gods in terms of being able to both cause and cure disease, as evidenced by the rising popularity of the healing cult of Asclepius, son of Apollo, in the decades following the Plague of Athens. Not surprisingly, this reactionary attitude receives almost no mention from Thucydides.[19]

Perhaps the greatest contribution of Thucydides to the history of disease is his implied notion that a disease not only infects individuals but also makes all of society, an entire community, its victim. For a disease, he makes clear, not only affects people's health and well-being but also can determine the fate of large-scale events and situations, even if only in an indirect way. Although he doesn't say so explicitly, Thucydides does seem to suggest that the Plague of Athens altered the whole course of the Peloponnesian War, as indicated by his insertion of the narrative of the disease directly following his account of the funeral oration of Pericles that laid out Athenians' justification for fighting the war.[20] Whether the plague had longer-term effects, however, that resulted in the decline and ultimate fall of the Athenian empire by the end of the war in 404 is a subject that continues to be debated by historians.[21]

Somewhat later in his account, Thucydides does say that nothing did as much harm to the Athenian war effort as the plague: in purely military terms, the disease wiped out 4,400 hoplites and 300 cavalrymen, who most likely represented roughly a third of available forces. Although Thucydides asserts that the plague's decimations among the general population are undiscoverable, modern calculations—assuming a death rate commensurate with that among the army—yield figures in the tens of thousands.[22] With its manpower thus sharply curtailed, Athens was severely hampered in terms of the scope of both land and sea operations; it was not until more than a decade later, in 415, that the Athenians felt capable of launching the ill-fated Sicilian expedition.

But beyond mere numbers, the plague may also have affected how the Athenians fought the entire rest of the war, even though the disease occurred so early in the conflict.[23] Thucydides seems to credit the plague with inculcating a moral failing, or "lawlessness," in the Athenian character, which was to show up later in the war in the form of ruthless and ultimately self-destructive policies, such as its brutal conduct toward the neutral island of Melos in 416, which in Thucydides' famous "dialogue" foreshadows inhumane treatment of Athens' own soldiers when taken prisoner at Syracuse. Yet, it's hard to know if this is really the case, since Athens already revealed a ruthless streak early in its empire when it refused to allow the island of Naxos to secede from the Delian League in 467. Thucydides also notes that the plague was worldwide in its scope; for example, he states that it started in Ethiopia in sub-Saharan Africa and progressed from there northward and westward to Egypt and Libya and eastward to the Persian Empire. Therefore, in so many ways, Thucydides' history of the Plague of Athens provides a model for all other histories of disease that were to follow.[24]

If we now shift our focus to modern historical writing about disease, it quickly becomes apparent that we have expanded considerably upon Thucydides' revolutionary rationality. In terms of the scope, importance, complexity, diversity, and a host of other factors to consider about disease, we have gone well beyond Thucydides' original speculations, even when following the basic lines of his thought. In the first place, whole books have now been devoted to the role that disease played in history, instead of the subject occupying but a minor part in the broader historical narrative. The traditional approach (sometimes also called the "positivist" or "biological" school) of modern historical writing is to follow most ancient authors in treating disease as a discretely defined, exogenous, or foreign variable (now a microorganism rather than an arrow from on high) that suddenly invades a population and wreaks havoc upon it. Taking their cue from Thucydides, who emphasizes how the death from plague of one man, Pericles, altered Athens' subsequent fortunes in the Peloponnesian War, these writers stress the almost whimsical role that disease has played in dramatically changing the lives and course of historical personalities and events.[25] Aligned with this approach are those historians who chronicle humans' heroic struggle to medically "conquer" the biological enemy represented by disease, a war that mankind, until recently, seemed to be winning as history progressed.[26]

Then along came William McNeill's *Plagues and Peoples* in 1976, which some would consider as bringing about a seismic shift in historical studies of disease. McNeill himself claimed to be writing a new chapter in disease history, ascribing to epidemics an importance not previously found in historical surveys. Even though McNeill did pay homage to "antiquarians," such as Hans Zinsser, for pointing out isolated disease incidents such as the Black Death that briefly commanded the historical stage, such acknowledgments, he claimed, were rare and made historians uncomfortable because they did not fit in with their orderly views of the past.[27]

By contrast, McNeill, a world historian who emphasizes cultural fusions among different civilizations that eventually led to Western dominance of the globe,[28] adapts this approach to disease in order to accord it a central place in world events. This is especially the case when new technologies or cultural developments enable a disease to become "pandemic," that is, to be communicated to distant lands far from its epicenter and thus have a dramatic impact on "virgin soil" populations with no prior exposure or immunity to it. McNeill's classic example of this, and the one that actually inspired his book, is the introduction of smallpox to the Americas in the early sixteenth century and the resulting horrific mortalities among Native American populations there; according to McNeill, smallpox by itself is sufficient to explain how conquistadors such as Hernán Cortés and Francisco Pizarro overcame overwhelming odds to swiftly conquer the once-mighty Aztec and Inca empires in Mexico and Peru.[29] In addition to such "transoceanic exchanges," McNeill devotes another chapter to the role played by the Mongol Empire during the late Middle Ages in the dissemination of the Black Death, both east and west. His concluding chapter is perhaps his most conventional, tracing the now familiar success stories of modern medical science in conquering disease from the eighteenth to the twentieth centuries.

So far, nothing that McNeill has to say is exactly new; as a matter of fact, most of what is mentioned above could be fairly said to have been anticipated by the ancient historian Thucydides. For it was Thucydides who first pointed to the world scope of disease, to its devastating impact upon a population unprepared for it, and even to the central role disease could play in history. But I believe that McNeill has made two contributions to the history of disease that are important and unique.

In the first place, McNeill introduces the idea that disease can be a relative construct, not just a discrete biological entity. Although McNeill uses "macroparasitism" to refer to one class of human beings living off the productive capacity of another class, one can also conceive of it in environmental terms, in which humans through their variegated behaviors alter their disease environment, which in turn adapts to their modifications, and so on in an unending war of mutual attrition; in many respects, this is comparable to how microparasites have adapted to their human and animal hosts, selectively evolving to neither kill them outright nor in turn be eliminated completely. In this way then, human beings can, in effect, create their own sense of just what is a disease. McNeill fully realizes that this can change "the very concept of disease," making it entirely dependent on social and historical circumstances. As an example, nearsightedness and a "dull sense of smell" may be considered perfectly normal in today's society, but they would have been crippling debilities—indeed a disease—among Paleolithic hunters struggling to survive. However, McNeill rejects a completely relativist approach to disease, preferring to hold onto "a firm and universal nucleus to the concept of disease," one in which "bodily disorder" mainly arises from "parasitic organisms."[30]

Despite McNeill's reservations, the relativist, or "social constructionist," approach, which increasingly viewed disease as an endogenous phenomenon arising solely out of factors intrinsic to the society or culture in which it occurs, became more popular among historians, particularly during the 1980s; for it was at that time that the emerging AIDS pandemic seemed to be a perfect illustration of how a disease can be a function of socially risky behaviors.[31] Indeed, one historian in this school goes so far as to suggest, perhaps facetiously, that one day harmless skin freckles may be deemed unsightly enough to be classified as a disease, complete with a "National Institute of Freckle Research" devoted to eradicating them.[32] However, if one goes to extremes with such an argument, one wonders what historical statements, if any, can be made about disease, if the very definition of the term is subject to such speculation. It seems that McNeill was right to insist upon a commonsense foundation from which to start a discussion.

McNeill's other contribution comes at the end of his book, where he speculates about the future of disease history. Despite the fact that *Plagues and Peoples* came out at the very same time that the World Health Organization was successfully eradicating smallpox, and in stark contrast to traditional views of medical historians that foresaw an "end to epidemics," McNeill concludes that infectious disease will remain an inseparable part of the history of humanity, indeed, for as long as humanity itself continues to exist. Ironically, he sees the very success of medical treatments of disease as only contributing to its perpetuation. A good example is the rash of polio infections that broke out among even the higher classes of American society in the mid-twentieth century, a circumstance attributable, McNeill insists, to the higher standards of hygiene that wiped out minor infections among children, which earlier had conferred some immunity to more serious, full-blown infections.[33] In a new preface written in 1997 to take account of the current AIDS pandemic, McNeill maintained his pessimistic view of humankind's ability to "conquer" disease, citing the worldwide AIDS crisis as just one more example of how the global transmission of disease was only accelerating the biological evolution and adaptation of microorganisms to their hosts.[34] The efforts of humanity—the "macroparasite"—to wipe out disease were upsetting the natural balance and, as recent disease history made clear, was only making things worse, not better. This gloomy perspective has been taken up by a host of far less restrained authors who peddle an alarmist, even apocalyptic, scenario where disease in the end conquers humankind, not the other way around.[35]

On a very basic level, one can both agree and disagree with McNeill's thesis that disease has played a central role in human history. It seems an intuitive fact that most people who die a "natural death" do so as the result of some disease or other, rather than being blessed with the good fortune of dying of extreme old age, when the cells of the body simply cease to divide and function. In this regard, disease is almost as ubiquitous as death in terms of its presence and importance in our everyday lives. Yet, one could also argue that the very fact that populations around the globe are increasing in number, and have done so at varying rates of propagation throughout history, prove that human fortunes are rarely dictated or limited by disease and its consequent mortality. Instead, one might counter that it is restrictions on reproductive capacity (aside from disease) that have played the greater role in the course of human development, such as the availability of food and other material resources that, from a Malthusian point of view, are forever locked with population in a struggle to achieve equilibrium or balance.[36] In a way, McNeill has sidestepped this whole conundrum by only focusing on large-scale, global pandemics of disease, whose mortalities posed extraordinary challenges to civilizations. His example, by necessity, will be followed in this book.

Nonetheless, even within McNeill's more specialized construct, his thesis has been attacked on two other fronts by revisionist scholars of disease. One group has made the case that disease does not act on its own when impacting human history; rather, it wreaks its devastation only in conjunction with other historical forces, such as the oppressive policies of colonialist/imperialist powers that intensify disease's morbidity and mortality.[37] This is true despite the fact that in some cases colonial powers believed they were acting in the best interests of their native subjects, such as by imposing Western standards of hygiene and medicine upon long-standing traditions of healing and customary responses to disease. Native resistance to high-handed health measures—such as hospitalization, isolation of contacts, disinfection, and quarantine—could effectively blunt their intended benefits. Given that, in some places, such as the Americas or the Pacific Islands, the sheer mortalities of imported diseases assuredly outweighed any medical blessings imperialism supposedly bestowed upon a conquered people, even when the benefits of modern medicine had material effect, imperialism could still amplify disease's impact since these same benefits also allowed Western soldiers and colonists to intrude longer and more deeply into previously inhospitable areas.[38] All this implies that McNeill had accorded an overmighty role to disease on the stage of history, which now should give way to a more nuanced, complex interplay with other factors.

Yet another contingent of historians besieged McNeill's edifice on the grounds that he was too consistently negative about the impacts of disease upon its victims. Instead, it could be argued that disease brought some benefits for certain elements of society, who might even welcome its arrival among them. This debate has been played out especially with respect to the Black Death in Europe during the late Middle Ages. McNeill claimed that the ravages of the Black Death, whose mortality in Europe during its first outbreak in the mid-fourteenth century was as high as 50 percent on average, instilled a "fatalistic" or even "suicidal" mentality upon the collective consciousness of Europeans.[39] But more recent scholars of the Black Death have argued that it set in train necessary "transformations" in many areas of medieval society, including ushering in a more capitalistic-based economic system, new technologies such as the caravel and the printing press, a more empirical approach to science and medicine, and even the Renaissance and Reformation with their greater emphasis on individual portraiture and piety.[40] Not even McNeill's classic case study of "virgin soil" American populations wiped out during the colonial period was immune from this argument, for some native groups, such as the Tlaxcala people of Mexico, actually benefited from the decimation of their rivals and overlords, chiefly the Mexica, on Lake Texcoco.

To take a more modern example of "always looking on the bright side" of disease, at least from a certain perspective, the ongoing AIDS pandemic is seen to have brought about a decline in risky social behaviors, such as sexual promiscuity, that are believed to be major contributing factors to propagation and incidence of the disease. But inducing greater morality in human society is traditionally seen to be the exact opposite of disease's usual impact, going back to Thucydides.[41] On a more prosaic level, AIDS has been a boon to Western pharmaceutical companies, which have been able to profit from antiretroviral drugs and "protease inhibitors" that inhibit full-blown symptoms of the disease almost indefinitely. AIDS has thus created a stable pool of captive customers for "Big Pharma's" products, which will remain the case for as long as a vaccine or cure for the disease remains elusive. Meanwhile, the disease has also created a very large and cheap pool of human "guinea pigs" for trial treatments for AIDS, since the expense of such treatments would otherwise be prohibitive to the vast majority of victims throughout the third world, which is now bearing the brunt of the global AIDS pandemic.

This brings us back to the question with which we opened this chapter: why study disease? Nearly every writer on the topic since Thucydides has clearly demonstrated that disease has had a big impact on human history, and—McNeill is surely right here—it will continue to do so for the foreseeable future. But what about the reverse—the impact that humans can have on disease? For I would argue not only that disease has shaped the history of our predecessors but also that humans have been able to redirect its course and meaning in history. I am particularly fascinated by those moments when civilizations around the world were severely impacted by a disease's mortality and morbidity, such that their very continued existence was in the balance. For it is at times such as these that human responses to disease assume their greatest importance. Yet, neither can such trials that test or temper a society occur without a very real biological disaster occurring among human populations and very often among the animals that live with them as well. While tribulations of the requisite magnitude or global scale may be relatively rare, they nonetheless will form the focus of this book. I hope to demonstrate from all this that humans can alter the extent to which they suffer from disease, even when this calamity seems to come, as the ancients truly believed, like a bolt from the blue. While some historians may not like studying disease for this very reason, in actual fact its course throughout human history has been far from arbitrary. Indeed, this is what makes disease such a fascinating topic of study. Unlike some other themes in history that have become trendy these days, such as the effects of climate change,[42] disease has allowed humans to change their fate at its hands, instead of simply being subject to it. Even without the awesome power of modern technologies, men and women could have a relationship with disease that was not all one way. Humans have thus made their own history of disease even while it was also happening *to* them.

I thereby aim in this book to make a unique contribution to the study of disease, by explaining how humans have had the power to change how disease affects them simply through how they view disease. Although my approach does take a page from the relativist school of disease historians, I am not talking here merely about efforts to redefine the concept of disease but rather about the very practical effects that cultural attitudes toward disease can have in allowing a society to either succumb to or triumph over disease epidemics. These cultural responses to disease are even more important now that modern society has come to realize its limitations in terms of being able to medically cure or thwart challenging new pandemics, such as AIDS. I also will seek in the following pages to go beyond the more obvious impacts humans can have on disease incidence, such as through medicine, imperialism, or bioterrorism, even though these inevitably will be part of the story.[43]

By no means do I claim to be opening up unheard of or unprecedented vistas in the history of disease. After all, it was Thucydides who first noticed how humans themselves could alter the course of a plague, such as by succumbing to despair at the very idea of getting the disease or by neglecting to nurse patients, thus hastening or assuring their demise, even if he did not realize the larger implications of these observations.[44] We all know, instinctively, that psychosomatic disorders can happen, willing ourselves into suffering simply by dwelling upon it. (Medieval doctors rather poetically diagnosed psychosomatic disorders as "accidents of the soul.") But I do claim to be expanding considerably upon this idea of humans' impact upon disease and to be addressing it in a more comprehensive way than ever before. Readers may also find that I am rather more hopeful than other recent writers about disease with regard to humankind's future in fighting epidemics.

Obviously, then, how a society or civilization perceives disease determines how it will respond to it, whether this be at the popular level or at the level of authoritative elites, and in terms of all the manifestations of the various social, economic, political, religious, or artistic aspects of this response. But at the same time, I also believe that what the disease is matters, in terms of establishing a clearly recognizable, biomedical identity.[45] Yet, the complexities of the historical evidence are such that some throw up their hands in despair of ever definitively identifying the epidemics of the past. Certain historians of disease now take the position that it is futile or even wrong to attempt to match up a historical epidemic with a modern definition of a particular illness, on the grounds that the present "laboratory" understanding of disease based on the germ theory is so different from how our distant ancestors approached their own, elusive "plagues."[46]

To my mind, this is nothing less than an intellectual cop-out, or perhaps defeatism, that is hardly justified by any supposed lack of concordance of symptoms. On the contrary, in some cases, particularly as the evidence becomes much fuller beginning with the Black Death of the late Middle Ages, premodern doctors and other authorities writing on the subject are able to give quite convincing diagnoses of a given disease. The Moorish physician Ibn Khātima, who authored a plague treatise in February 1349, gives an impressive symptomology, complete with case studies, of the three forms of bubonic, pneumonic, and septicemic plague, while his predecessor, the ninth-century Persian doctor Muhammad ibn Zakariyā al-Rāzī (known as Rhazes in the West), is able to clearly differentiate between smallpox and measles through a detailed analysis of their respective symptoms. And it was the sixteenth-century Venetian physician, Girolamo Fracastoro, who was the first to name and identify syphilis, as well as typhus. But even when premodern observers describe symptoms that are fantastic or that little accord with the "scientific" diagnoses of nowadays, having an "objective" or "ontological" definition of disease may still be helpful in understanding how our ancestors approached the plagues of the past. For example, some medieval doctors describe the lymphatic swellings of bubonic plague as being red, yellow, green, or black in color, which they said signified the severity of the illness; the fact that modern observers of plague fail to notice this same phenomenon may indicate to some that medieval people were suffering from an entirely different disease.[47] But a detailed reading of medieval plague treatises reveals that actually what this tells us is that medieval doctors were here relying on ancient authority, in this case, the *Prognostics* of Hippocrates, rather than on their own, firsthand observations in order to make a prognosis of the disease. The lesson to take away from all this is not that the Black Death was a different disease from modern plague but rather that medieval doctors had radically different notions of how to diagnose and treat symptoms than their counterparts of today.

Completely abandoning the positivist or ontological definition would thus needlessly deprive us of a valuable tool in our effort to write the history of disease. It may be obvious to say that each disease is unique, but what is less evident is that each disease has its own social/cultural dynamic in terms of how a society or civilization perceives and responds to it. This is no less a part of the "social construction" of disease than the relative values and norms of the culture upon whom the disease is acting. Together, both these forces could intersect to create some quite dramatic impacts in the course of the history of a pandemic. A good instance of this is how many late medieval doctors conceived of plague as a kind of "poison," which seemed a product of both contemporary perceptions of the disease's progress in individual victims, as well as populations at large, and preconceived notions that were inherited from the ancients. Combined with the unprecedented mortality of the disease, this rather unique conceptualization of plague undoubtedly contributed to scapegoating tendencies that attributed the Black Death to a human cause, whereby Jews, witches, the poor, and other perceived enemies of society were believed to be deliberately spreading or prolonging an epidemic for their own nefarious purposes. To take a more modern example, AIDS was initially seen in the mid-1980s as a "gay plague" spread mainly by abrasive anal intercourse (gay-related immunodeficiency disease, or GRID), which led to homophobic responses in the workplace, among health insurers, and elsewhere. (At the present time, AIDS is primarily prevalent in sub-Saharan Africa, where it is spread overwhelmingly by *heterosexual* contact.) In both cases, we now know that these respective views of plague and AIDS were wrong, but this does not change the tragedy of their historical responses.

Likewise, a modern "laboratory" identification of a historical disease or pandemic, even if only speculative, may help illuminate some of the outstanding questions and conundrums posed by it. Identifying the Black Death with plague, for instance, while still controversial, would explain why many late medieval outbreaks were associated by contemporaries particularly with women, children, or the poor, since these demographic groups were more likely to live in domestic conditions that ensured close contact with rats and fleas. It would also help us to understand the importance of trade to medieval society, since this is the medium through which plague is usually spread. Moreover, recent advances in biomolecular archaeology—which attempts to recover the genetic material of disease pathogens in human remains that have been preserved under optimal conditions, such as encapsulated dental pulp—seem to hold out some promise for positively identifying epidemics of the past in the laboratory just as definitively as modern occurrences of disease.[48]

Readers should take note here that, as a consequence of all the above considerations, I deal in this book only with a "positivist" panoply of diseases, namely, those caused by the invasion of the human body by a known, identified microorganism. I therefore leave out a host of noninfectious diseases, such as those caused by vitamin deficiencies or psychological disorders, that may appear in other surveys. I do this because, even though the latter diseases are certainly impacted by human behavior, at the same time, they lack some of the essential criteria for studying human responses to disease, such as, most obviously, the nature of being infectious. In general, I have adopted three standards by which I have selected the diseases that are addressed in the chapters that follow: first, the disease must be, or at least must have been in the past, fatal for large numbers of victims, for there is nothing like the fear of death for eliciting a response from people. Second, the disease must have been, or still is, worldwide in its scope, in order to afford the opportunity to study contrasting responses to it among different cultures and societies. Third, the disease must have been exerting its virulence for a lengthy period of time, to observe evolving attitudes toward it.

In many ways, the topic of disease is ideally suited for a globally oriented world history textbook such as this one. Comparing how different civilizations throughout space and time have reacted to disease is perhaps the best means of recovering the lessons that disease has to teach. And these lessons have not always been learned or passed on, even by the best historians.[49] But by exploring the complex interactions, primarily in cultural terms, between disease and humans, a "new history" of disease that combines and integrates the positivist and relativist approaches may be written, for which some historians have been calling.[50]

I believe that understanding the many ways in which we, as humans with our almost infinite variations of societies and cultures, have coped with disease (or not, as the case may be) is one of the most important lessons of history. This is no mere academic exercise. It is nothing less than a matter of life or death.

CHAPTER 1

Plague

The disease known as "plague" may seem obscure to most people nowadays, but plague has been called the deadliest of all diseases,[1] one that was responsible for perhaps the most lethal pandemic in all of history. And it is a disease that is still very much with us, even in a modern, developed country such as the United States, as John Tull and Lucinda Marker, a couple living in Santa Fe, New Mexico, found out in November of 2002. While Lucinda quickly recovered from her bout with plague, her husband, John, came down with a case of the disease that was so severe he was immediately put into a drug-induced coma that was to last for the next two and a half months, at the end of which John woke up to find both his legs amputated below the knee. John did survive plague, but barely; at one point, all his close family members were rushed to his bedside to pay what were thought to be their final respects. As John tells his tale, it's clear that he'll never forget his near-death experience with plague.[2]

Plague is a specific disease, which should not be confused with its other, more general meaning in which it refers to disease in the abstract. It occurs in three forms, depending on how the microorganism that causes the disease in all cases, a bacterium known as *Yersinia pestis*, invades and spreads within the body. Plague is fairly unique among diseases in that it can be spread by both an insect vector, a trait it shares in common with malaria and typhus, for example, and also by direct, human-to-human transmission, which likewise happens in cases of influenza, tuberculosis, and smallpox.

Bubonic plague is the most common and widely known form of this disease, in which fleas are responsible for infecting hosts when they bite and attempt to feed on their host's blood yet are unable to do so because their stomachs are already "blocked" by a proliferating mass of bacteria, which they must regurgitate along with the blood meal back into the bloodstream of their victims.[3] As its name implies, the rat flea (*Nosopsyllus fasciatus* in Europe and *Xenopsylla cheopsis* in Asia) typically spreads plague among fur-bearing rodents, such as the black rat (*Rattus rattus*), which are highly susceptible to the disease, but once its animal hosts are dead and cold, the fleas will then jump onto any nearby hosts available, including humans. Keeping in mind that up to twenty-five thousand bacteria are injected into a host with each bite of a blocked flea, which can bite repeatedly as it ravenously attempts to feed; that each rat may host up to one hundred fleas on its body, all ready to seek a new host when necessary; and that hundreds if not thousands of fleas have been shown to be present in a home infested with rats, one can see how in some cases victims had so many bacteria introduced into their bloodstreams that they developed the far more virulent form of septicemic plague.[4] As a matter of fact, Tull, who claims to be the only person in recorded history to have survived septicemic plague, was bitten by the same type of flea that had given a typical case of bubonic plague to his wife. Yet, in John's case, the bubo on his groin was hardly noticeable and, instead of the bacteria becoming concentrated in the lymph glands, they seem to have turned inward and invaded nearly every organ in his body.[5] How an individual body reacts to *Yersinia pestis* in terms of being able to isolate the bacteria within its lymphatic system may also determine whether one develops a case of bubonic or septicemic plague.

In pneumonic plague, the bacteria enter the lungs after being breathed in, which typically occurs as the result of exposure to the expectorate, or airborne droplets, that have been coughed or sneezed out by an infected person. Therefore, direct human-to-human contagion is the norm in pneumonic plague, where no other animal intermediary is necessary, even though a pneumonic plague outbreak seems to start out as a secondary symptom of the bubonic form and tends to be localized, owing to the narrow window of time in which this form of the disease can be spread by the symptom of an infective cough. However, since the patient is usually well enough to travel during the incubation period, which in pneumonic plague can last up to three or four days (but in bubonic plague can last up to a week), it is possible that an outbreak of the disease in one locality then gives rise to another at a considerable distance away.[6]

The initial symptoms of all forms of plague are not all that different from other diseases: These include high fever, violent headaches, and body stiffness, chills, or pains. They may also be accompanied by nausea and vomiting, constipation, sensitivity to light, bloodshot eyes and a coated tongue, restlessness and an inability to sleep, delirium or stupor and loss of motor control, and, in general, a vague but unmistakable feeling of anxiety, dread, and fear.[7] But, of course, the distinguishing symptom of plague, at least in its bubonic form, is the bubo, a lymphatic swelling caused by bacterial accumulation at the nodular point closest to where the flea has bitten the victim. This will then usually occur on the groin, armpits, or neck area, where the lymph nodes are located. (Medieval doctors referred to these as the "emunctories" and thought they drained poisonous materials or humors from, respectively, the liver, heart, and brain.) Observers of the Third Pandemic of plague at the turn of the twentieth century noted that inguinal buboes were the most frequent, which makes sense if fleas mostly have access to their human victims on the ground and jump onto them as they walk around the house during the day. Next in frequency were axillary buboes followed lastly by cervical ones, which presumably occurred as a result of patients being bitten on the torso or above by fleas in their bedding as they lay asleep. However, it should be remembered that cervical buboes can also occur in "tonsillar" plague, a sort of intermediary form of the disease that is caused by interhuman transmission, when airborne droplets are breathed in and collect in the throat but do not travel all the way down to the lungs, which results in bubonic symptoms and not pneumonic ones. This may help explain why some medieval observers of the Second Pandemic, the Black Death, seem to attest to a greater frequency of cervical buboes than during the Third Pandemic.[8] It is also not unknown for buboes to form on other places aside from the lymph nodes, such as on the inside of the elbow or on the back of the knee, and medical chroniclers of the Third Pandemic likewise noted other skin manifestations of bubonic plague, such as pustules or carbuncles, that could appear almost anywhere on the body.[9]

The bubo is considered by most medical experts—whether medieval or modern—to be the defining symptom for a conclusive diagnosis of bubonic plague, even when the case is so mild that it can barely be distinguished from other diseases.[10] It is also the symptom that has allowed historians to make a positive identification of the first plague pandemic in history, owing to the description by Procopius of Caesarea and John of Ephesus of the swelling that occurred in the "boubon," the Greek word for groin, that accompanied the disease's appearance in Constantinople in 542 C.E.[11] In both modern and medieval cases, it has been noted that the bubo getting larger in size (approaching the dimensions of a walnut) is actually a good sign for a prognosis of recovery, even as it remains tender or painful to the touch.[12] After about a week of living with these symptoms, recovery is marked by spontaneous suppuration, or bursting open, of the bubo, releasing its pus;[13] in the Middle Ages, the maturing or "ripening" of the boil was typically aided by a poultice or specially prepared plaster, cutting or scarification, cupping (applying a heated glass vessel to the area to create a vacuum suction), or cautery, either using inflammatory compounds or the more direct heat from a red-hot branding iron. Without the timely intervention of modern-day antibiotics, death occurs in 60 to 90 percent of bubonic plague cases, usually three to six days after the onset of symptoms.

In the case of pneumonic plague, the characteristic symptom is the coughing up of bloody sputum, accompanied by rapid and painful breathing, although this can also occur in pneumonia, tuberculosis, and influenza. What seems to ultimately confirm the presence of plague is that in the pneumonic form it is 100 percent fatal and death ensues quite quickly, usually within two days. Unless they die suddenly from heart failure, pneumonic plague patients can be cursed with a horrible death, gasping for hours from "air hunger."[14]

By contrast, septicemic plague has almost no distinguishing symptoms beyond those characterizing the general onset of the disease, since it usually kills the patient too quickly—sometimes in twenty-four hours or less—to allow more marked outward signs such as the bubo to manifest themselves. However, for those who do live a little longer, before they invariably die, some very odd symptoms can emerge, such as spontaneous bleeding from the nose and eyes, blood present in the urine and stool, and subcutaneous bleeding all over the body resulting in dark, purplish spots, called in medical parlance "petechiae" or "disseminated intravascular coagulation" (DIC).[15] Tull still bears the purpuric spots on his skin from his bout with septicemic plague to this day. Interestingly enough, these same symptoms of petechiae or DIC also seem to have been noted by medieval observers of the plague.

As noted earlier, some disease epidemics that are called plagues were not true plague, as is the case of the "Plague of Athens" of 430–426 B.C.E., or the "Antonine Plague" that struck the Roman Empire in 164–180 C.E.; both these ills were probably smallpox (to be discussed in chapter 2). Yet, plague was probably present in endemic form in the Mediterranean and the Near East in ancient times, even if it never seems to have broken out beyond localized epidemics. Its symptoms, especially the occurrence of *bubones* or bubonic swellings, are discussed extensively in the *Epidemics* attributed to the Hippocratic corpus at the end of the fifth and first half of the fourth centuries B.C.E. and by the Greek physician Rufus of Ephesus who practiced during the reign of the Roman emperor Trajan (98–117 C.E.) but who was quoting earlier works dating back to the third and first century B.C.E.[16] Possibly because plague was a newly evolved disease and because populations in the ancient world did not have the requisite densities, it was not until the sixth century C.E. that the first worldwide outbreak, or pandemic, of plague occurred.[17]

In terms of the historical occurrence of the disease, plague is therefore reserved for one of three pandemics: the First Pandemic, sometimes also known as the "Plague of Justinian," that struck the Mediterranean world between 541 and 750 C.E.; the Second Pandemic, more commonly referred to as the "Black

Death," that struck Europe and the Middle East beginning in 1347–1348 and persisted periodically right down to the eighteenth and nineteenth centuries; and the Third Pandemic, which struck Asia at the turn of the twentieth century, beginning with Hong Kong in 1894 and Bombay, India, in 1896, and that lasted down to the 1940s in India and Senegal, the 1950s in Thailand, and the 1960s in Vietnam. Indeed, the presence of plague to this day in the western United States stems from this last pandemic of the disease, when it first arrived in San Francisco in 1900. Each of these pandemics will now be discussed in turn.

A theme running through all three pandemics is that plague inspired some dramatic responses among the populations affected that had enduring consequences for cultural identity and survival. Not all of these responses, perhaps, are unique to plague, but they are usually associated with the disease because of both its unique nature and how it was perceived. As we have already noted, plague is a particularly deadly disease, killing in all of its forms an average of 70 to 80 percent of its victims, as well as striking with a very high morbidity, or incidence among the population at large, even if not all of them succumb to its mortality. (During the Second Pandemic in Europe, the high average mortality rate of 50 percent means that morbidity had to be well above that number.) But plague was also seen, and quite rightly, as an especially horrible disease to die from: either patients suffered a prolonged illness accompanied by distinctively nauseating symptoms, as in the case of bubonic plague, or they could die quite suddenly and unexpectedly, with little warning or opportunity to prepare for death, as in the case of pneumonic or septicemic plague. Plague thus made a great impression on all concerned, whether they came down with the disease or not, and they reacted accordingly.

The First Pandemic of plague is important above all for setting the pattern of various societal responses to the disease, which were to recur during the Second and even Third Pandemics centuries later. Otherwise, its historical impact, both relative to the other pandemics and in the contemporary context of the early Middle Ages when it occurred, is still very much open to debate. Perhaps the most neglected of the three pandemics, the First Pandemic is only now starting to get some of the scholarly attention that it deserves.[18]

The First Pandemic seems to have originated in Upper Egypt, arrived at the eastern end of the Nile delta during the summer of 541, and spread eastward from there into the hinterland of southern Palestine.[19] Alexandria was struck in the autumn of that year, followed by Jerusalem at the beginning of 542. By the following spring, the plague had come to Constantinople, the capital of the Byzantine Empire, from where it probably spread to Asia Minor, northern Palestine, Syria, and Persia. The plague persisted in the capital until August and then by the end of the year had reached North Africa and possibly Sicily and

Spain. In 543 the disease spread to Italy, the Balkans, Spain, and France, and it reached Ireland in 544 but does not seem to have been known in England until a century later. There is further speculation that it may have struck Scandinavia and Poland at some point, but this is based entirely on interpreting the evidence of mass grave sites. After this first outbreak, plague seems to have returned to various parts of primarily the Mediterranean region in recurring waves, striking, with few exceptions, almost once a decade throughout the second half of the sixth, the whole of the seventh, and the first half of the eighth centuries. The last outbreak apparently encompassed Syria, Mesopotamia, Sicily, Rome, and Constantinople between 744 and 750.[20]

Obviously, it was the first outbreak of 541–544 that became the most famous disease incident of this pandemic and has had the most historical impact. This is partly due to the attention it received from the Byzantine court historian, Procopius of Caesarea. But it is often overlooked that other sixth-century writers also recorded the pandemic, the most important of which was John of Ephesus, a churchman who witnessed the plague firsthand in his travels to Alexandria, Palestine, Mesopotamia, and Syria. Procopius, for his part, gives us an invaluable perspective from the capital, Constantinople, where he remained throughout the course of the epidemic. Based on the descriptions of these authors and others, there is little disputing that the disease that struck in 541–542 featured bubonic plague: both Procopius and John of Ephesus mention the *bubones*, or swellings in the groin, that became a signature symptom of the pandemic.[21] A third eyewitness, Evagrius Scholasticus, adds the authority of his own personal experience to this identification, for he says that he himself came down with buboes during this first outbreak when he was a boy and later watched his wife, children, and several other members of his family and servants succumb to the same symptoms in later recurrences of the disease.[22] For sources in Syriac and Arabic, special terms evolved that denoted the bubonic swellings and that were used to specifically distinguish plague from more general references to "mortality" or "pestilence."[23] Elsewhere, the occurrence of this symptom in the historical record is practically our only sure record of the disease: For example, Bede's mention that St. Cuthbert received a "tumor" on his thigh is our first evidence that plague struck England in 664.[24]

How did Byzantine society and culture react to the First Pandemic? As would be expected, attributions of the plague to the marvelous and the divine figure large in contemporary accounts. Procopius reports visions "of supernatural beings in human guise" and dream portents accompanying the advent of the plague in Constantinople.[25] This is very reminiscent of the cult of Asclepius from ancient Greece, and it should be no surprise that similar responses make their reappearance in a society imbued with Greek culture. "Terrifying phantoms" or specters were likewise cited by John of Ephesus as heralding the arrival of plague in southern Palestine, in the form of "headless black people" appearing on the sea off the coast in shining copper boats, a testament, perhaps, to the importance of maritime trade in spreading the disease. Otherwise, John of Ephesus employs a common rhetorical trope toward the beginning of his account in an attempt to convey the stupefying scale of the catastrophe: even if words could be found to describe it, a task that the author claims to find almost excessively daunting, who would be left alive to read them when the world is about to end, a sentiment summed up by the memorable phrase "for whom does the writer write?" These are the kinds of literary flourishes we encounter again during the Second Pandemic, or Black Death. John's only answer to his own question is that perhaps future generations will learn from his contemporaries' punishment for their transgressions and so avoid their fate, a supremely ironic observation in light of the even more catastrophic Black Death some six centuries later.[26]

John's theme of the plague being a punishment for people's sins is, of course, greatly amplified by his ample quotations from the Old Testament, which provides numerous examples of how disasters such as the plague were just instruments of God's wrath.[27] But one must remember that, at this same time, the concept of original sin was being promulgated and developed by the Christian Church, largely through its leading thinkers such as St. Augustine (354–430 C.E.). Deriving its theology ultimately from the New Testament rather than the Old, original sin imposed an individual need for repentance upon the believer as the descendant of Adam, as opposed to the collective sense of guilt of an entire people when punished by Yahweh. It is striking, for example, how the plague apparently persuaded people to amend their lives, especially when they feared an immediate death, even though they would backslide once again as soon as the threat had passed. Here, Procopius is reporting a response that is almost the exact opposite of what had been chronicled by Thucydides.[28] Both authors concur, however, that many people who could have been saved from the disease instead died from sheer neglect, although Procopius excuses this un-Christian response with the exhausting effort that was required to attend plague patients.[29] John of Ephesus, on the other hand, tells a couple of stories of how people who sought to profit from the plague by seizing valuables of the dead were then immediately struck down as punishment for their greed.[30]

Perhaps the most distinct impression of all that was made by the plague upon its chroniclers is the disposal of the ever-mounting corpses of its victims. The daunting and distressing prospect of what to do with all the dead had already been briefly noted by Thucydides, who reports that Athenian citizens resorted to mass cremation.[31] Since this method of disposal was proscribed to Christian authorities, the challenge was what to physically do with perhaps thousands of bodies dying each day. It seems this was the most important and urgent brief for the imperial government during the crisis, dictated by both Christian duty and medical necessity, and both Procopius and John of Ephesus report that Justinian's court responded with impressive alacrity and efficiency, something that is not always evident even in a modern, developed society of today.[32] Mass burial pits were dug or improvised in existing buildings on Galata across the Bosphorous straits from the city, and corpse-bearers were drafted from among the soldiery, bribed with money from the imperial treasury, or simply forthcoming out of a sense of charity.[33] A memorable detail, supplied by John of Ephesus, tells of how gravediggers piled up and pressed down layers of bodies "as a man might heap up hay in a stack" or trod on them with their feet "like spoiled grapes," while the trampled bodies sank and were immersed in the pus of five- to ten-day-old rotting corpses below.[34] This is just one of any number of John's anecdotes that stick in the mind: litters bearing dead bodies bumping into each other on their way down to the docks; pus and viscera bursting out of rotting, bloated bodies and flowing down to the sea; noble families abandoned by their servants, including even the royal household, now reduced to a miserable handful huddled together in an empty palace; a house full of twenty forgotten victims whose bodies were so decayed worms were crawling through them; and infants still suckling from the breasts of their mothers even though they had died.[35] One can't help but wonder if at least some of these searing images were directly inspired by what the author himself had witnessed.

The sheer enormity of the mortality—which meant that all the usual rites of Christian burial had to be set aside and the dead treated like beasts—is what seems to have shocked observers the most. Allied to this was John of Ephesus' observation that people of all ranks, ages, and conditions were jumbled together into a degrading, meaningless muddle by the "wine press" of mass burial.[36] This is a theme that will crop up later during the Black Death and perhaps inspire the Dance of Death, one of the most powerful and popular artistic genres in the later Middle Ages. The fear of dying a nameless death was such that people took to going out with identification tags hung on their arms or necks.[37] The business of making wills and providing for inheritance was thrown into chaos, and both chroniclers report that all traffic and commerce came to a complete halt in the capital, which was mirrored in the countryside with domestic animals wandering about wild in the pastures and stands of grain ripening unharvested in the fields.[38] Aside from performing autopsies to investigate the source of bubonic swellings, physicians were alleged to be markedly ineffective in prognosis and treatment of the disease.[39]

What is strikingly absent from contemporary descriptions is any role or presence of the Church during the crisis; instead, people resorted to their own prayers or superstitions in an attempt to ward off the plague, such as hurling pitchers from their windows, which John of Ephesus claims was started by some mad "foolish women" inspired by demons. Indeed, monks and priests were apparently viewed as messengers of death and shunned with personal invocations of protection whenever they were encountered in the street.[40] There is even evidence of Christian backsliding in the face of the disaster, which is perhaps not unsurprising at this early stage of Christianity. In the border regions of Palestine, inhabitants began worshipping a bronze pagan idol, while even a good Christian like Evagrius might wonder how God could take away his whole family and yet leave the children of his pagan neighbors untouched.[41] Pagans and homosexuals seem to be the only candidates for scapegoats during the crisis, even though measures were taken against them only after the danger had passed.[42] While guilt could certainly be collective as an explanation for why God allowed plague to happen, authorities also made it clear that the extraordinary sin of certain groups provoked divine displeasure and therefore were in urgent need of correction.[43] This provided an important precedent that would help justify later pogroms, such as against the Jews during the Black Death.

It is probably fair to say that the First Pandemic of plague helped prevent the *renovatio imperii*, or "restoration of the empire," that had been the life's ambition of the Byzantine emperor Justinian (527–565).[44] By 554, Justinian had completed the reconquest of North Africa, Italy, and part of Spain, thus re-creating in large part the Mediterranean sphere of influence that had once been the glory of ancient Rome. The empire's failure to hang on to these conquests as the sixth century came to a close has been attributed to a number of other factors besides the plague.[45] But the massive mortality occasioned by the First Pandemic undoubtedly played its part, largely by sapping the empire of the manpower it needed to defend its newly won territory. This was particularly true as the plague kept striking again and again after its first arrival on the scene in 541–542: plague's returns to Constantinople in 558 and 573–574, for example, were especially ill timed due to incursions by a new enemy, the Avars, in the Balkans.[46] Moreover, the plague seems to have engendered a sense of weariness, and perhaps even guilt, over what otherwise should have been much celebrated accomplishments of the reign. In his *Secret History*, for example, Procopius confesses what he really thought of his emperor, whom he blamed for the death of no less than a trillion people. Most of these lives, we are informed, were lost in Justinian's unending series of wars, for which the emperor was directly responsible. However, Procopius also believed that Justinian was, quite literally, a "demon in human form," whose very presence goaded God to allow natural catastrophes to occur, one of which was, of course, the plague of 542.[47] Perhaps no writer in history has been so abashed of his civilization's success.

Before we take our leave of the First Pandemic, we should note some other, later outbreaks of the disease and responses to them that were to have important implications for the Second Pandemic of the late Middle Ages. In 590, an outbreak of bubonic plague struck Rome that, according to the chronicler Gregory of Tours, inspired the new pope, Gregory the Great, to preach a sermon calling for a procession of all the churchmen and inhabitants of the city. Like John of Ephesus, Pope Gregory amply quotes from the Old Testament to show how plague is an expression of God's anger in retribution for people's wickedness and sin; the difference, of course, is that Gregory now holds out the promise of reprieve from God's punishment if the faithful but show their repentance. Despite the fact that eighty people fell dead in their midst, the procession continued.[48] Later legend supplied by Jacob of Voragine in the thirteenth century credited the procession with ending the plague when Gregory had a vision of an angel atop the Tomb of Hadrian sheathing his sword, indicating that the divine displeasure had finally been appeased. (By the ninth century, the tomb had been renamed the Castel Sant'Angelo to commemorate the event.) Yet, even this later medieval fiction had its Old Testament prototype, namely, the story told in the first book of Chronicles of how King David persuaded God to spare Jerusalem from a pestilence that had already killed seventy thousand Israelites.[49] Thus was established a precedent for prayers and processions, including perhaps the Flagellant movement, that were to play such a central role in how medieval society responded to the Black Death.

By the seventh century, sermon cycles were being compiled to be recited on a regular basis whenever plague struck a region as part of the Church's now standard response to urge its flock to repent in the face of God's wrathful chastisement; this at least is the overarching theme of four homilies composed at this time in Toledo, Spain, which, as expected, are replete with quotations from the Old Testament.[50] Yet, one sermon, the third in the series, adopts a strikingly different tone by employing the carrot rather than the stick (although even the sermons that dwell on God's anger and chastisement hold out the hope of forgiveness and abatement of the plague if hearers will only repent). In a remarkable passage, one that seems to be inspired by the New Testament, in particular the letters of St. Paul, the preacher now dangles the promise of immortality during the Christian afterlife or resurrection in order to help his listeners conquer their fear of imminent death from the "groin disease":

> But what should we say? You who take fright at this blow (not because you fear the uncertainty of slavery, but because you fear death, that is, you show yourselves to be terrified), oh that you would be able to change life into something better, and not only that you could not be frightened by approaching death, but rather that you

would desire to come to death. When we die, we are carried by death to immortality. Eternal life cannot approach unless one passes away from here. Death is not an end, but a transition from this temporary life to eternal life. Who would not hurry to go to better things? Who would not long to be changed more quickly and reformed into the likeness of Christ and the dignity of celestial grace? Who would not long to cross over to rest, and see the face of his king, whom he had honored in life, in glory? And if Christ our king now summons us to see him, why do we not embrace death, through which we are carried to the eternal shrine? For unless we have made the passage through death, we cannot see the face of Christ our king.[51]

A very similar kind of response was developed concurrently in the Muslim world, as we will shortly see.

The last major outbreak to mention is the first to occur in the Islamic tradition, the so-called Plague of 'Amwâs (named after the town in Palestine where Islamic troops first contracted the disease), which struck Syria and Mesopotamia in 638–639.[52] This was an epidemic of bubonic plague that hit hardest in Syria and Palestine, including the capital, Damascus, beginning in the spring of 638 and not burning itself out until the autumn of 639. By taking out a whole generation of Muslim leaders, the plague seems to have paved the way for the rise of Mu'awiya, the founder of the Umayyad dynasty of caliphs (661–680). In 640, after the death of several Companions of the Prophet, which included his own brother, Mu'awiya was made governor of Syria, a position from which he was able to claim the caliphate after the assassinations of Uthman (644–655) and Ali (656–661). By extension, then, the plague also had a hand in the eventual splintering of Islam between the Shi'ites (followers of Ali) and the Sunnis, who followed Mu'awiya.

But for our purposes, the most important outcome of the Plague of 'Amwâs was the germination of the Muslim tradition that flight to or from a plague-infested area was prohibited to believers. This tradition only fully emerged later, by the eighth century; all that can be known for certain from a historical point of view is that Caliph Umar ibn al-Khattâb (r. 634–644) attempted to make a journey from Arabia to Syria in c. 638 but turned back upon hearing of a "pestilence" there. Embellishments over the course of the next century and more added much drama to this story: how Umar, upon reaching the way station of Sargh on the border between Arabia and Syria, was met by the commander of his forces in Syria, Abū 'Ubayda, who warned him that plague was raging in the region; how a debate then ensued among the caliph's advisers about what to do, some urging him to keep going and not turn back and others urging him to not expose himself and other leaders, including the Companions of the Prophet, to the plague; how after Umar decided upon retreat 'Ubayda (who was to die from the plague in Syria) taunted him with the words "fleeing from the decree of

God?"; how Umar then employed the parable of grazing camels on a lush slope rather than the opposite, barren slope to explain how they were "fleeing from the decree of God to the decree of God"; and how the debate was ended when one of the Companions belatedly arrived on the scene to quote Muhammad's precedent, "If you hear of it [the plague] in a land, do not approach it; but if it breaks out in a land and you are already there, then do not leave in flight from it." On this basis, Umar finally turned back to Medina. On historical grounds, the "Umar at Sargh" story has an air of inconsistency about it: why would 'Ubayda, for example, both warn Umar against the plague and rebuke him for trying to avoid it? But in terms of the Prophetic tradition of Islam, it both satisfied a recurring theme in the Qur'an that resists any flight from adversity and deferred to a practical need to avoid unnecessary risks to the lives of the faithful. It was also a way to quarantine Arabia, which as yet was untouched by the plague, and to redeem the reputation of one of Sunni Islam's most revered leaders, who was otherwise known as a fearless campaigner against the Byzantine and Persian Empires that he conquered.[53] This issue, along with two other alleged tenets of Islam concerning the plague—that the disease was a mercy and martyrdom for believers and that there was no contagion of plague since it came directly from the will of God—were to assume a very important and highly contested role in the religious/legal/medical communities of the Islamic world when the Second Pandemic, or Black Death, struck in 1348–1349. But for now, it is unclear what guidance was available to believers about how to respond to plague; it should be noted that, throughout the Near East during the First Pandemic, settled populations seem to have fled the disease in large numbers.[54]

How did such concerns play out in the Christian West? We have already noted how a sort of martyrdom that promised a spiritual communion with Christ was proffered to the faithful who died of plague in a Toledo sermon from the seventh century. By and large, however, the Christian tradition seemed to emphasize punishment rather than reward in its religious interpretation of plague, in contrast to the Muslim approach.[55] Perhaps this has something to do with the influence of the Old Testament and the Hebrew legacy upon Christianity. But I also think it very much ties in with Augustine's theology of original sin, which would naturally endorse a more flagellating attitude. It is significant that the second Toledo sermon urging repentance in the face of plague bases itself on and quotes generously from Augustine's own sermon on the threatened destruction of the city of Constantinople, which was narrowly averted by communal procession and prayer (*De excidio urbis*).[56]

On the other hand, Christian tolerance for flight from the plague (which during the Black Death was arguably far more pronounced and universal than in Islam, whose greater emphasis was on one's duty to stay and tend the sick) seems to be traceable back to pagan Greek influences upon Christianity, specifically the *Quaestiones et Responsiones* (*Questions and Answers*) of Anastasius of Sinai, a Greek monk writing toward the end of the seventh century. In Question 114, Anastasius offers a compromise between the religious and rational responses on the issue of whether one can escape the plague by fleeing from it: If the plague comes from God's will, then flight is useless, an answer that accords quite well with Islamic beliefs, except for the interpretation that the disease is a form of divine punishment. But if the plague originates from corrupt air, then fleeing to a healthier location is efficacious, which obviously owes much to the Hippocratic corpus (which also will form the basis of the Arabic medical tradition). Since Anastasius was both a Greek and a Christian, he seems here to be trying to reconcile the two sides of his heritage, a struggle that was quite a common one for the apologists in the early days of Christianity.[57] Although flight was to become a perfectly acceptable response for Europeans, even if they were churchmen, by the time of the Black Death, this by no means precluded that plague ultimately came from God's design, a widely held notion even among late medieval doctors. As it did for Islam at this time, the plague therefore posed something of a conundrum for Christians in terms of how to respond to it based on competing traditions, which was not to be resolved until the Second Pandemic centuries later.

Yet another literary tradition emerged during the First Pandemic that likewise evinced ambivalent attitudes toward the flight response to plague, but this time primarily from a social, rather than religious, point of view. Paul the Deacon, in his eighth-century *History of the Lombards*, recalls how, during a plague in Italy in 565, even close family members abandoned each other, as allegedly "sons fled, leaving the corpses of their parents unburied; parents forgetful of their duty abandoned their children in raging fever." This might seem to be a clear condemnation of those who abrogated their social obligations in order to save their own skins, yet the moral of Paul's story is rather ambiguous, since he also tells us that even those who stayed behind out of "longstanding affection" to bury relatives were themselves unburied and unmourned. What is incontestable is that people believed plague was contagious and therefore were faced with a stark choice, to either run away or face death. This, at least, seems to have been the general consensus of the population according to Paul, for "common report had it that those who fled would avoid the plague," with the result that "dwellings were left deserted by their inhabitants, and the dogs only kept house."[58]

Paul was not the only one who observed the fragile social fabric in the face of plague; the East Syrian Orthodox monk John bar Penkāyē alleged that, during a plague in North Mesopotamia in 686–687, "No brother had any pity on his brother, or father on his son; a mother's compassion for her children was cut off." John certainly disapproved of this behavior, for he noted that, when Christians failed to bury their dead and simply fled, their behavior descended to the level of pagans (in this case the Persian Zoroastrians) or else of "dogs and wild animals." Further proof of their ungodliness was how they responded if reminded that "no one can escape from God, except by means of repentance and conversion to Him." According to John, they replied with blasphemous rebukes such as, "Get out; we know very well that escape is much more profitable to us than supplication." This indicates that the rational response noted by Anastasius of Sinai was alive and well among the population at large. If not pursued by the plague itself, such sinful refugees were "harvested" by looters or dogs and wild animals. A more practical consideration was that abandoned exposed corpses, strewn about like "manure on the earth," then contaminated water sources such as springs and rivers, which would only help perpetuate the disease.[59] On both moral and medical grounds, John informs us, flight had its drawbacks, even if it seemed to be dictated by self-preservation. These issues will necessarily be raised again during the Second Pandemic.

Scholarly consensus is inclined to be cautious in assessing the long-term impact of the First Pandemic of plague. There seems to be a desire to attribute neither too much impact to the disease nor too little.[60] This is in contrast to the cataclysmic upheaval almost universally accorded to the Black Death of the late Middle Ages. Yet, the case has been made that the First Pandemic of plague did no less than usher in the Middle Ages by sweeping away classical civilizations in Byzantium and Persia, thus clearing the way for the rise of peoples formerly on the periphery of the empire, such as the northern "barbarians" of Europe or the nomadic tribesmen in Arabia, both of whom allegedly suffered far less from the plague's ravages.[61] This thesis is easily refuted if one but remembers that the Roman Empire, at least in the West, declined and fell well before the plague first struck in 541, or that Muslim armies had to contend with plague, particularly in their conquest of Syria, no less than Byzantine or Persian ones. In fact, the Umayyad dynasty was to reach its greatest extent at the very time when its power base in Syria was heavily targeted by plague, buffeting it with depopulations, agricultural contraction, and urban and rural dislocations; curiously, however, the dynasty came to an end at the very moment when the First Pandemic also reached its demise.[62] And it was not until the dawn of the ninth century, when a generation or more of Europeans had lived with no need to fear of plague, that the northern barbarian kingdoms under the leadership of Charlemagne were finally able to achieve recognition as equals from rivals in Constantinople and Baghdad. If plague did indeed play a role in such momentous events as the rise and fall of empires or the emergence of Europe, then surely it was only in conjunction with other forces that crashed in on the late classical or early medieval world: the mass migrations of Germanic tribes, for instance, or the birth of a dynamic, new religion—Islam—that was to become the great rival of Christianity. Instead, I believe that the varied and intangible cultural responses to plague outlined above, both with respect to Christian and Muslim communities in Europe and the Middle East, comprised the most enduring legacy of the First Pandemic: as already indicated, they helped set the stage for what was to come during the Second Pandemic centuries later.

Six centuries, to be exact, were to pass before another major outbreak of plague was to arrive in Europe and the Middle East. Since trade had played an instrumental role in spreading the plague in the Mediterranean at the beginning of the First Pandemic, particularly so as Egypt was the grain basket of the empire, the steady decline of international commerce through to at least the eighth century was probably responsible for the disappearance of the disease. Much new evidence has come to light—including distribution of pottery shards, shipwrecks, and even traces of ancient pollution trapped in ice cores or peat bogs (indicating the relative strength of the metal smelting industry)—that points to the contraction of the Mediterranean economy and its shipping traffic, both on the sea and inland along rivers, which would thereby impose a virtual quarantine on the increasingly isolated port cities, first in the West and then later in the East.[63] Over time, the process also probably snowballed due to the fact that plague and the economy were undoubtedly intertwined: the more population declined due to disease, so too inevitably did demand for goods from abroad.[64] Indeed, the repeated occurrences of plague about once a decade throughout the First Pandemic ironically contributed to the very circumstances of the plague's demise. For instance, we now know that it was the plague, and not the irruption of Islam, that caused so much upheaval to the urban environments and settled regions of the Near East.[65] Other factors aside from plague assuredly played their role in disrupting Mediterranean trade and commerce and thus breaking the chain of infection of the disease; in turn, other possibilities besides trade, such as unintentional quarantine as people fled or avoided the already declining population centers of the Mediterranean once they became infected and changes due to genetic mutation or contamination in the virulence of *Yersinia pestis*, may have contributed to the decline of plague.[66]

Plague returned to the world in a Second Pandemic that is traditionally seen to have begun in the 1330s from an endemic center in Central Asia. Evidence for this includes the archaeological discovery of three Nestorian Christian headstones from the region of Lake Issyk Kul in present-day Kyrgyzstan, which record ten victims as dying from "pestilence" in 1338–1339.[67] Meanwhile, our most informed contemporary source, the Muslim author Ibn al-Wardī, writing in 1348 from Aleppo in northern Syria, a hub of trade for routes further east, states that the plague "began in the land of darkness" fifteen years earlier and then

spread eastward from there to China and India and westward to the land of the
Uzbeks, Transoxiana, Persia, the land of the Khitai (perhaps Turkestan), and finally, Crimea and the Byzantine Empire.[68] (According to the fourteenth-century
Muslim traveler Ibn Battūta, the "land of darkness" was an unexplored region
lying beyond the Volga Bulgar state in present-day Tartarstan.) Modern-day research has confirmed that the Central Asian steppes are an ancient reservoir of
plague, containing perhaps the oldest strains of *Yersinia pestis* based on the genetic mapping of its DNA.[69]

Some scholars, however, propose southern Russia as an alternative origin to
the Second Pandemic in place of Central Asia, arguing that references to "pestilence" and "land of darkness" are too vague to indicate a specific disease or
geographical location, that the overland trade route across Central Asia presented
insurmountable obstacles and would have taken too long to spread the plague
from its endemic center to the West, and, finally, that the Mongol Khanates of
the Golden Horde, Persia, and Turkestan all converted to Islam by 1326, which
ensured a disruption of trade to both China and Europe.[70] If so, then this would
imply that the Second Pandemic, like the first, was confined to Europe and the
Middle East. Yet, Mongol efforts to expel the Genoese trading presence at Tana
and Caffa during the 1340s were actually motivated more by the ongoing commercial rivalry between Genoa and Venice, the latter allying itself with the Kipchak Khanate of the Golden Horde, and were therefore not designed to eliminate all Christian merchants from Mongol trade, let alone Muslim merchants
who served as al-Wardī's informants.[71] And although the various references to
disease outbreaks in the East may be too vague to positively identify them as
plague, neither do they rule it out. In addition to the Nestorian headstones at
Issyk Kul, native Chinese annals do record a major epidemic in Hopei province
in 1331 and epidemics in other regions beginning in 1345–1346, while Battūta
mentions a disease epidemic in Madurai in southern India in 1344, from which
he himself suffered. Both the Mongols in China and the Delhi Sultanate in India
were in trade contact with Central Asia at this time, and there is a catastrophic
drop in China's population recorded at the end of the fourteenth century that
needs to be explained. If the Black Death was indeed a worldwide pandemic,
affecting both East and West, then a Central Asian origin, at the crossroads of
trade, is by far the most logical choice. Moreover, since Chinese annals report a
series of other natural disasters—including floods, famines, droughts, and
earthquakes—that coincided with its epidemics during the 1330s, this provides
a powerful ecological explanation for why plague at this time should have suddenly erupted out of its endemic centers to become pandemic.[72] The sudden
advent of a wetter and more unpredictable climate—part of a "Little Ice Age"
that began in the early fourteenth century—may have forced rodents carrying

the plague out of their remote habitats and into closer contact with humans.[73] It is also likely that the bad weather created famine conditions—as it did in northern Europe between 1315 and 1322—that compelled natives to hunt and eat marmots in greater numbers and more indiscriminately.

Wherever the plague began, there seems little disputing that the disease's entry point into Europe came at the Crimea, along the north coast of the Black Sea in southern Russia. Muslim and Christian merchants traveling back from this region, which served as the westernmost terminus of the Mongol trade routes, carried reports back to the chroniclers al-Wardī and Gabriele de Mussis of Piacenza that the plague was rampant here in 1346. The Muslim source claims to have counted eighty-five thousand dead in the Crimea in that year, while Mussis tells his famous story of how Genoese merchants besieged in their trading factory at Caffa by the Mongol forces of the Kipchak Khan, Janibeg, were given the plague in an early form of biological warfare when the Mongols decided to catapult their dead into the town once they began to be decimated by the disease.[74] In reality, it is far more likely that plague was communicated via rats making their own, unobtrusive siege of the town or else by means of fleas hitching a ride on animal furs, which was the most important export product of southern Russia. However it came about, it is significant that plague first appeared outside Central Asia in the Crimea, rather than, say, in Iraq (1349) or Yemen (1351). This argues strongly for an overland dissemination route rather than by sea from the Indian Ocean and up through the Persian Gulf or the Red Sea.

From the Crimea, plague next commenced its march through the Middle East and Europe. It invaded the Byzantine capital of Constantinople by the late spring or summer of 1347 and then reached Sicily and Alexandria in Egypt around the same time, by the autumn of that year. At the end of 1347, plague may also have established bridgeheads at other strategic places in the Mediterranean, including the island of Mallorca off the eastern coast of Spain, the port of Marseilles in southern France, and the trading cities of Genoa, Pisa, and Venice in Italy. In 1348, plague spread along the coast of North Africa and northward from Egypt through Palestine and Syria, hitting Gaza, Ascalon, Acre, Jerusalem, Beirut, Damascus, Aleppo, and Antioch. In Europe, the plague in that year spread through Italy, the Balkans, much of France, and Spain and invaded Austria, Switzerland, southern England, and perhaps Ireland, Norway, and Denmark. By 1349 and 1350, plague completed its conquest of North Africa, Spain, France, Austria, Switzerland, England, Ireland, Denmark, and Norway, and in addition it had come to Iraq, Germany, Belgium, the Netherlands, Sweden, Wales, Scotland, Poland, Bohemia, Hungary, Romania, and the Baltic States of Estonia, Latvia, and Lithuania. It was not until 1351 to 1353 that plague seems to have spread throughout eastern Germany, Poland, and Russia north of the

Caucasus. Based on all the available sources, which now include more than just chronicle accounts, it seems that the only large areas bypassed by the plague were Iceland and Finland, perhaps due to their isolation and sparse inhabitation.[75]

Before we go any further, we should say a word about the controversy over whether the Black Death of the late Middle Ages was actually another pandemic of the disease known as plague. It is curious that no such debate exists for the First Pandemic, even though theoretically the same objections ought to apply, but perhaps this is a function of far less surviving material available to pore through and dissect.[76] Recent research, including the emerging field of biomolecular archaeology, is fast rendering this debate obsolete: a tired, stale old chestnut that, to my mind at least, has now been definitely settled in favor of identifying the Black Death as plague. Indeed, so convincing is the accumulating evidence in plague's corner that I would contend that those who still insist on holding out against it are simply being ornery or, at worst, hypocritical, since by rights they ought to make the same case for contesting the identity of the First Pandemic but so far have utterly failed to do so.[77] Such revisionist histories of the Black Death also seem to find it easier, and perhaps more attention grabbing, to make a negative case against plague than a positive one for any other disease.[78] In fact, a very positive case can now be made for identifying the Black Death with plague, based on the recovery of *Yersinia pestis* DNA from human dental pulp found on centuries-old victims of plague. This was first achieved a decade ago when late medieval and Early Modern mass graves were excavated at Montpellier, France. Although challenged as an isolated and unreliable result, it has now been duplicated in London and Germany for victims from the First Pandemic of plague.[79] Provided that such positive identifications continue, biomolecular archaeology will thus soon definitively settle the matter.

One other bone of contention needs to be addressed here with regard to the medieval Black Death: its demographic impact. How many people in the Middle Ages were killed off by the disease? The numerical percentages are important, because they determine how much of an impact the Black Death may have had upon late medieval society. A nearly universal mantra among both past and present histories of the Black Death is that it killed off roughly a third of the population, on average, in its first outbreak in Europe and the Middle East between 1347 and 1350, with progressively lower mortalities rates thereafter when the plague returned throughout the second half of the fourteenth and throughout the fifteenth centuries. Such an assertion made it quite easy for past scholars of the plague to downplay even its initial impact, claiming that this was nothing out of the ordinary within the context of periodic Malthusian declines that are predestined to occur throughout history.[80]

However, in recent years, a veritable tidal wave of data has been painstakingly extracted from various sources mainly in England, Spain, Italy, and France, all of which points to an *average* mortality of 50–60 percent during the first outbreak of the Black Death in 1347–1350. This figure can probably be applied to all of Europe and the Middle East, even where comparable records are not available, since what records we do have give a fair enough representation of different patterns of human settlement (i.e., both urban and rural populations), as well as class members of society (i.e., peasantry, priests, professionals, etc.). This is an astonishingly high number that is undoubtedly the highest mortality percentage ever recorded for a single disease outbreak, and best estimates are that it represents a loss of as much as fifty million people throughout Europe in just a few years.[81] No such loss can be sustained without very dramatic social, economic, and psychological impacts upon a society.

As in the First Pandemic, plague was to return to Europe about once a decade throughout the later Middle Ages, striking on average every eleven years in fifteen recorded outbreaks between 1360–1361 and c. 1500. (This almost exactly matches the average of 11.6 years for the eighteen outbreaks recorded between 541 and 750 C.E.)[82] Although the virulence of these recurrences of plague seems to have gradually declined, based on testamentary and other evidence, the cumulative impact of even low mortalities could take their toll. Thereafter, plague recurred slightly less frequently during the Early Modern period, averaging an outbreak every 13.4 years between 1535 and 1683. However, plague continued to have the reputation of being the most lethal disease: Indeed, one of the ways in which seventeenth-century Italian doctors distinguished plague from other fever-type diseases such as malaria or typhus was whether or not the epidemic carried off the majority of the town's population.[83] Spectacular eruptions of the disease continued to occur, such as the Plague of Naples in 1656 that killed half of the city's roughly three hundred thousand inhabitants, or the Great Plague of London of 1665 that carried off one hundred thousand victims, representing 20 percent of the city's population. By 1670, plague is thought to have virtually ceased in Western Europe, but it continued to strike in Eastern Europe and Russia down through the eighteenth century. In the Balkans, North Africa, and Southwest Asia, plague was endemic up until the first half of the nineteenth century. The last major outbreak in Europe, in 1720 at Marseilles in southern France, came from a cargo ship originating in Syria.

The varied impact of plague's ravages upon late medieval society—medical, religious, social, and economic—will now be examined in a comparative way between Europe and the Middle East. First to be considered is the medical response to the Black Death. In terms of the first outbreak of 1348–1350, doctors in both Europe and the Middle East had a remarkably similar set of answers to the all-important questions of what caused the disease, how was it to be prevented, and how was it to be cured? These framed the structure of almost all medical treatises on the plague down to the end of the Middle Ages and beyond. Such consistency owes largely to the common inheritance that both Christian and Muslim cultures shared from the ancient world, namely, the Greek and Roman medical traditions of Hippocrates and Galen, as mediated by Arabic physicians of the early and high Middle Ages, especially Ibn Sina or Avicenna (980–1037). This meant that both Christian and Islamic physicians explained the plague as caused by a miasma, or substantial corruption of the air, either from a higher source (i.e., the planets) or a lower one (swamps, rotting corpses, earthquakes, etc.). Both subscribed to the six "nonnaturals" as a means of prevention—regulating intake of air, diet, exercise, sleep, repletion and evacuation, and "accidents of the soul," or mental states—in order to avoid predisposing the body to the disease. And both prescribed surgical intervention and special medicines in their "cures" of plague. Although both acknowledged that the Second Pandemic of plague presented an unprecedented and overwhelming challenge (both in terms of its virulence and its geographical extent) that was virtually unknown to ancient authors, this did not invalidate, in their minds, the age-old theoretical underpinnings of their profession. After all, plenty of explanations, such as the predisposition of an individual's "complexion" to the disease, could be brought forward to explain failures of treatment. Indeed, the typical contemporary response to the plague was to do what their predecessors had done, only to do it more intensely and more urgently, such as by bleeding in greater amounts and as soon as possible, with little regard to the usual constraints and cautions surrounding the procedure. Likewise, theriacs, pestilential pills, and other medicinal compounds, whose recipes were handed down since ancient times, were now prescribed in greater variety and number. Rather than any real evolution in medical attitudes or approaches to plague over the course of the later Middle Ages and down into Early Modern times, it seems that whatever empirical observation and experience doctors obtained of plague was used to actually reinforce the traditional assumptions, or "paradigm," they had inherited from past authorities.[84] If ancient doctors had never had to face a disease like the Black Death, then this simply meant that they never had the chance to apply and test their medical expertise in the crucible of plague, as doctors were now doing. That a First Pandemic had equally challenged the medical profession was either unknown or conveniently forgotten.[85]

In terms of other communal responses to the Black Death, three "religiolegal principles" are assumed to distinguish medieval Muslim communities in the Middle East and Spain as compared to those in the Christian West: these include that plague is a mercy and martyrdom for believers; that one should not flee from or enter into a plague-infected region; and that plague comes directly from God and through no other agency, such as person-to-person contagion.[86] In actual fact, the differences between the respective communities along these lines are much more nuanced than have been previously portrayed, as are the nature of the beliefs held within each community itself.[87]

Contrary to popular perception, the Prophetic tradition of Islam was not universally hostile to the concept of contagion. Since Islam embraced, and indeed passed down to the West, much of the intellectual heritage of ancient Greece and Rome, it should come as no surprise that Galen's theory of contagion as the "seeds of disease" passing from person to person in the form of a localized miasma should be taken up by doctors in the Muslim world during the ninth and tenth centuries, who applied it especially to leprosy and who interpreted it as no different from an infection that spread from a sick person to a healthy one. Pre-Islamic societies in Arabia also subscribed to contagion, expressed as the "stinging of the *jinn*" or demonic spirits, a concept that Muhammad according to the hadith is said to have explicitly endorsed, along with another tradition in which the Prophet allegedly commanded, "Flee from the leper as you would flee from a lion." Contagion was also instinctively understood from the spread of mange disease among the Arabs' camel herds, even though the hadith has Muhammad counter with the reply "And who caused the mange in the first one?" as a way of drawing the ultimate chain of causation back to God. A contradictory attitude is likewise evinced to the *jinn* during the Plague of 'Amwâs in the seventh century, when one of the Companions of the Prophet reportedly spread this belief among the rank and file of the Arab army in Syria, until he was sharply rebuked and contradicted by a more pious superior, who asserted that the plague was a "chastisement" (evidently not yet the "martyrdom" for believers of later tradition) sent down from God as he had done earlier to the Israelites. But by the fourteenth century, on the eve of the Black Death, even the "medicine of the Prophet," which claimed to be rooted in the religious canons of Muhammad, accepted the Greek humoral theory of disease causation and listed contagion as one of the possible secondary causes of plague that was not incompatible with God as its ultimate source.[88]

The famous plague treatises of the Moorish physicians and scholars, Ibn al-Khatīb and Ibn Khātima, who wrote at the time of the first outbreak of the Black Death in 1349, were not therefore rationalist exceptions to the Islamic tradition just because they endorsed contagion with empirical arguments. Even though they took diametrically opposite views on the relationship that religion should have with medicine, both Khatīb and Khātima cite concrete "proofs" for person-to-person transmission of the plague, such as through the infected breath or bodily vapors of the sick or through their personal belongings, including clothing, furnishings, utensils, and even a single earring! But of course, this is not an accurate depiction of the epidemiological realities of bubonic plague, so one can question whether it is indeed a rational or empirical response to the disease at all (except for cases of pneumonic plague, which Khātima does seem to provide).[89]

Furthermore, both Khātima and Khatīb do attempt to demonstrate that their "empirical" observations of plague's contagion are not incompatible with the Prophetic tradition of Islam. This is far more pronounced in the case of Khātima, who devotes the last four chapters of his treatise solely to the Prophetic tradition itself (thus being concerned with religious rather than medical matters) in an effort to reconcile and smooth over what seems like a jarring contradiction on the subject of contagion, especially as stated briefly under the heading of "infection" in an earlier chapter. While subscribing to a very orthodox position that God is the sole author of disease, Khātima also advances the idea that contagion is a secondary (but not independent) cause. He thus follows in the footsteps of a long tradition dating back to at least the ninth century, which included not only the adherents of Prophetic medicine but also certain commentators on the hadith who were concerned with maintaining its integrity in the face of the challenging conundrum posed by contagion. But even Khatīb takes a (very brief and seemingly halfhearted) stab at trying to harmonize contagion with Islamic law, drawing on both selective quotations from the hadith that seemed to support his position and the principle of *maslaha*, or the privileging of what was for the good of the Muslim community over specific *fatwas* that might do it harm (such as not to flee the plague). In the end, however, Khatīb prefers to abruptly end the discussion by stating simply that it "is not among the duties of medicine," in contrast to the way his colleague, Khātima, extensively grapples with the issue.[90]

The real innovation of Khatīb, and the one that stood most in contrast to the writings of Khātima and that has made him such an attractive figure to modern skeptics of the Prophetic tradition in both the Middle East and the West, is his insistence on a separation of the two realms of religion and science (in this case, medicine) should the interests and agendas of the two intersect and conflict. Particularly important is his notion that, in a matter of science, that is, where the public health as threatened by the plague is concerned, empirical observation and proof should be privileged over religious authority. While this may not be entirely unprecedented, it is prescient in that it foreshadows one of the founding principles of the Scientific Revolution centuries later. It is also a very controversial position, one that would have raised eyebrows among contemporaries in both Islamic and Christian contexts. Toward the close of his short treatise, for example, Khatīb states the following: "One principle that cannot be ignored is that if the senses and observation oppose a revealed indication, the latter needs to be interpreted, and the correct course in this case is to interpret it according to what a group of those who affirm contagion say."[91] This is not so different, after all, from what Galileo Galilei was saying in the seventeenth century, which resulted in his condemnation as a heretic before the Roman Inquisition in 1633. By contrast, Khatīb's trial, which ended with his death at the hands of a lynch mob in his prison at Fez in 1374, seems to have been primarily a politically motivated one relating to his time as vizier of Grenada during the 1350s and 1360s. However, one of the accusations at his trial, that Khatīb followed "the doctrines of the classical philosophers in questions of faith," may be quite relevant to his views on contagion. Although what exactly his offense was in this matter is not entirely clear, if it was seen that Khatīb was privileging Greek rationalism where it conflicted with faith, then this would be quite similar in principle to what he expressed in his plague treatise.[92]

The difference between Muslim and Christian commentators on contagion was therefore not a straightforwardly simple one, in which one society or culture accepted the concept and the other did not, but rather one of degrees in terms of this acceptance. In this sense, Christian Europe was an unabashed subscriber to contagion, with little to no reservations, compared to the Islamic world. Out of the hundreds of plague treatises I have consulted from fourteenth- and fifteenth-century Europe, there are none that I know of that deny contagion, on religious or any other grounds. (This also applies to the two Hebrew treatises of Rabbi Isaac Ben Todros and Abraham Kashlari.) When European plague doctors specifically discuss contagion, they do so largely in a theoretical way that almost seems to take the concept for granted and that precludes disagreement or challenge. For example, the famous Perugian physician, Gentile da Foligno, explains contagion in his *Long Consilium* of 1348 as "poisonous vapors" that can pass "not only from man to man but also from region to region" by means of being breathed in or else absorbed through the pores of the body, which then generate a "poisonous matter" in the region of the heart and lungs. Rather than cite his own observation or contemporary empirical evidence, Foligno quotes the unimpeachable source of Galen and his theory of the "seeds of pestilence" from *De Differentiis Febrium* (Concerning Different Types of Fevers), and he asserts, again on the authority of Galen, that anyone who stays in a neighborhood infected with plague and who converses with those "covered with sores" or "whose breath is putrid" will be sure to get the disease "just as if they were cast into an oven like bread dough."[93] To justify plague contagion by sight (what the Muslims termed the "evil eye"), an anonymous practitioner from Montpellier in 1349 quoted at length from Euclid's theory of optics, but he also referred to legendary tales of the basilisk and of the "venomous virgin," both of whom could kill by look alone, that would nonetheless be just as convincing to his readers since one could find them in respectable sources such as medieval bestiaries and the *Secretum Secretorum* (Book of the Secret of Secrets) attributed to Aristotle.[94] On occasion, Christian plague doctors do cite empirical evidence and observation in support of contagion, just like their Muslim colleagues: the author of an anonymous German treatise from the fifteenth century testifies that he saw two boys touch a dead woman's bedding that had been thrown out into the street to dry in the sun, after which they both straightaway died of the disease.[95] This is exactly analogous to Khātima's witnessing the deaths of people who used to traffic "in the clothes of the dead and their furnishings" at the old-clothes market in Almería, Spain.[96]

In contrast with the Christian West, the concept of contagion was a highly contested one in the Islamic world. While Khātima and Khatīb vigorously defended contagion, other contemporary authorities explicitly denied it. Chief among these was the fourteenth-century Granadan jurist, Ibn Lubb, who rejected contagion on a number of grounds, including theological objections (backed by a long line of commentators on the hadith) as well as claiming that it conflicted with the social and moral obligations of Muslims. He was joined by a number of other fourteenth-century authors from North Africa and al-Andalus, including the famous Ibn Khaldun, who seemed to deny any role for secondary causes in the plague, and therefore of contagion. In the fifteenth century, the enormously influential plague treatise of the Egyptian scholar Ibn Hajar al-'Asqalānī apparently turned the tide of majority Muslim opinion against contagion, largely by refusing to rely solely on the Prophetic tradition to make his case. Hajar claimed that plague had to have a nonnatural (i.e., noncontagious) cause because in his own times he observed that some people, even those within the same household as a plague victim, did not contract the disease and because doctors still hadn't found a cure, which only God could ordain. (In response to both observations, most Christian physicians would probably have pointed to the individual complexions of patients that differentially predisposed them to disease and to the need to start a cure almost immediately, at most within twelve hours of the onset of symptoms, for it to be successful.) Hajar's preferred explanation was the *jinn*, for which, incredibly to modern readers, he likewise advanced sure proofs in the form of testimony from no less a personage than the Egyptian sultan's private secretary, who related how he had overhead two invisible demons arguing behind his back over whether to "pierce" him with the plague or not; in the end, they decided to strike out the eye of a horse instead. This is really not so different from the Montpellier physician's appeal to the basilisk and the venomous virgin in support of contagion by sight. Hajar thus provided a potent counterargument to those who would defend contagion, particularly as it marshaled doctors' favorite weapon, empirical evidence and observation, against them. His writings and opinions changed the whole terms of the debate over contagion in subsequent plague treatises written in North Africa down to the nineteenth century. By contrast, plague treatises in the Christian West showed remarkable consistency: their theoretical underpinnings were to remain essentially unchanged throughout Europe's late medieval and Early Modern experience with the disease.

If there was debate or disagreement among Christian plague doctors, it was in terms of the role that God played in causing the disease, specifically as a punishment for human wickedness or sin. In their *Consultation* penned for the king of France in October 1348, the Paris medical faculty included a formulaic nod from medicine to religion along the lines of "an epidemic always proceeds from the divine will" and that "God alone heals the sick," although they also did not "neglect to mention" that their profession was sanctioned by God and that prayer did not preclude consulting doctors, which was a paraphrase of the "honor the physician" passage from one of the apocrypha, Ecclesiasticus 38:1–14, attributed to Jesus ben Sirach. Earlier that year, the Lérida physician Jacme d'Agramont declared that, "if the corruption and putrefaction of the air has come because of our sins, [then] the remedies of the medical art are of little value, for only He who binds can unbind."[97] In 1448, the Apulian doctor Saladin Ferro de Esculo listed as his first cause of plague God's desire "to punish the sins of men," which he would not elaborate on because it was incapable of doubt.[98] Yet, even these deferential doctors were making the point that God was only one of many possible causes of plague; more usually, Christian commentators preferred to argue over whether the disease came from a higher natural cause (such as planetary conjunctions) or a more local one (such as the stench arising from swamps, rotting corpses, earthquakes, etc.).

However, a significant handful of Christian Europeans resisted the notion that God had anything at all to do with the disease. The German science writer (and priest), Konrad of Megenberg, in a treatise of c. 1350 on "whether the mortality of these years comes from divine vengeance on account of the iniquities of men, or from a certain natural course [of events]," came down in favor of the latter conclusion on two grounds: first, if God "made this plague for the correction of men" then he did so "to no purpose" (which is not to be admitted), because "experience teaches us that His people have in no way amended themselves of any vice"; second, God in his vengeance "would have struck down all mortal sinners," but again, experience shows this not to be true. He then goes on to make a positive case for his preferred, natural explanation of the plague, earthquakes.[99] Around this same time, the Naples doctor Giovanni della Penna urged his colleagues to investigate "natural causes" for plague, "since [only] unskilled and ignorant physicians say that it proceeds from God or from the heavens."[100] A century later, an anonymous Bohemian treatise of c. 1450 complained that patients often gave in to a sense of despair and lost hope during a plague because they believed "that it's God's vengeance or anger over them" and this belief engendered a fatal sense of guilt over their sins. This was one of six "contributory causes" of plague that defied the doctor's best efforts to help people avoid or cure the disease.[101] All this skepticism about God's role in the plague finds no parallel in the medieval Islamic world.

Closely related to the issue of contagion was whether to flee or avoid persons and places infected with plague. On this question, Christianity and Islam emerged on opposite sides by the end of the Middle Ages even more clearly than in the case of contagion. From the very beginning, Islam seems to have decided firmly against sanctioning flight from a plague-infected region, dating back to at least the eighth-century rendition of the Plague of 'Amwâs during the First Pandemic. As we have seen, this established a rule, said to have come from the mouth of the Prophet himself, that if a plague is "in a land, do not approach it; but if it breaks out in a land and you are already there, then do not leave in flight from it." At the same time, in the Christian tradition, Anastasius of Sinai hedged on this issue, allowing for flight if the disease originated from corrupt air instead of directly from God's will. However, in one Muslim interpretation of the 'Amwâs incident from the twelfth century, that of the Moorish jurist Ibn Rushd al-Jadd (grandfather to the more famous Averroes), the Prophet's dictum against flight was to be interpreted not as a blanket prohibition but rather as "humane guidance and advice," so that it was permissible (if not preferable) to enter or leave a plague-infected region so long as "one's intention is correct and one relies on God."[102] But this interpretation seems to have been a unique one that was not widely accepted in the Islamic world. It could be said that Khatīb also advocated flight from the plague in his treatise of c. 1349, but this is by inference only (since he so strongly espouses the concept of contagion); nowhere does he actually come out and *say* that people should flee. The examples he gives of those who successfully avoided the plague are those who quarantined themselves rather than availed of the option of flight: one Ibn Abū Madyan of the city of Salé, who walled himself up along with his whole family after hoarding enough food to live on, and the thousands incarcerated in the prisons of Seville who also miraculously survived.[103] Khatīb's advocacy of flight was therefore rather ambiguous, even as he condemned those who would deny Muslims this course of action.

On the other hand, fourteenth-century Islamic Spain also witnessed a highly influential *fatwa* that was issued in no uncertain terms *against* any kind of seeking of refuge from the plague. This came from the quill of the jurist Lubb, who was a contemporary of Khatīb and who like him was based in Grenada, Spain. In fact, it is quite likely that it was Lubb's two *fatwas* on the plague that Khatīb had in mind when he famously wrote, "And amidst the horrible afflictions that the plague has imposed upon the people, God has afflicted the people with some learned religious scholars who issue *fatwas*, so that the quills with which the scholars wrote these *fatwas* were like swords upon which the Muslims died."[104] Khatīb then goes on to cite approvingly the example of "a group of pious people in North Africa" who nonetheless renounced their previous *fatwas* on the plague "in order to avoid being in the posion of declaring it permissible for people to engage in suicidal behavior."[105] One can easily imagine that Lubb himself did not see things quite this way.

It was in his second *fatwa* that Lubb responded to an enquiry as to whether it was permissible for a Muslim to flee a plague epidemic once one saw it afflicting his religious brethren. Given that his first *fatwa* emphatically denied plague contagion, it should come as no surprise that Lubb also denied to Muslims any right to flee the plague under any circumstances, citing a series of precedents from the Prophetic tradition culminating with that of the Plague of 'Amwâs. As Lubb movingly recites, "A Muslim is a brother to a Muslim, he does not forsake or oppress him." As he did in the first *fatwa*, Lubb did not just rely on religious arguments to make his case; he also appealed to the social and moral duty of a Muslim not to abandon a fellow believer when sick with the plague. To do otherwise would be to threaten the integrity of the whole fabric of the *umma*, or Islamic community.[106] Thus, in evident contrast to Khatīb, who seems focused on saving individual lives, for Lubb the greater cruelty was *to* allow a Muslim to flee and forsake his obligations to others: one must never forget that one is part of a whole. This argument against flight as a "moral failing" was to persist in Muslim plague treatises down through the fifteenth century and beyond. The only exception comes in a fifteenth-century poem or *maqāma* attributed to 'Umar of Málaga, who urged the sultan of Granada to flee to Málaga to save his life during a plague in 1441, on the grounds that the Prophet's injunction not to flee was not an absolute decree, along the lines earlier laid out by Rushd.[107] But his was a lone voice in the wilderness.

On the Christian side, there was an equally strong tradition *in favor* of fleeing the plague. It was nearly ubiquitous advice in European plague treatises to advise readers that, as soon as there was word that plague was coming to town, "to start early, go far, and return late," a turn of phrase apparently derived ultimately from Galen.[108] Yet, some doctors also recognized that patients who were left unattended were more likely to succumb to the plague: the fifteenth-century German doctor John of Saxony listed "a lack of faithful servants to assist the sick man," particularly in performing his "operations of nature," as one of the contributory causes to why people died of the disease, and an anonymous Bohemian treatise of c. 1450 said basically the same thing. But if doctors were advising people to flee the plague because they believed it was contagious, then they really only had themselves to blame if sick patients were left unattended.

John of Saxony can hardly have been surprised, for example, when he observed that even "parents during this plague also fear to draw near to their children and other beloved relatives," an observation that was echoed in many chronicles of the Black Death.[109] Moreover, the plague regulations passed by some Italian cities, such as Milan in 1374, actually penalized those who attended the sick by quarantining them from the rest of society for a period of days.[110] In a sense, this paradoxical dilemma distantly reflects the early history of Christianity itself, when Jesus' followers saw it as their duty to both succor the sick and the poor *and* flee from the world with all its dangers and temptations (as the desert fathers did in a very literal sense).

To square this circle, doctors did not so much advise people not to flee as provide preventative measures so family members and servants might safely stay and nurse the sick: precautions such as fumigation or ventilation of the air around the patient or keeping one's distance from the patient, all the while inhaling aromatics, taking pills, and evacuating one's excess humors by means of bloodletting—all intended to "fortify" the body against the plague. The dilemma doctors faced in terms of these competing agendas can be seen in the various *consilia* on the plague written by Foligno. We have already seen how in his *Long Consilium* written early in 1348 Foligno fully endorsed plague contagion on the basis of Galen, and on these grounds he advised that "it is of the highest importance that one flee from [bad] air" before the plague spread inexorably "from man to man, household to household, neighborhood to neighborhood, and city to city."[111] But in a shorter *Consilium* written later that year, Foligno changed his tune, stating that it was important for the healthy to take preventative measures, "in order that those who attend the sick may be able to be by their side more securely [and] in order that those who become sick are not neglected beyond all inhumanity and abandoned in such a miserable way as hitherto and in a manner that is usually accorded to brute beasts."[112] The anonymous physician from Montpellier who championed contagion by sight in a treatise of 1349 warned that attendants of plague patients were in especial danger, particularly if they look "at the sick man in his death throes." But any visitor, whether he is "a doctor or priest or friend," could easily remedy this situation by blindfolding the patient.[113] (So much for the medieval bedside manner!) Over a century later, another anonymous treatise, dated to 1481, gave six special medicines to be taken by anyone having to stay with a sick person; even though it also advised fleeing the ill, this was to happen particularly when patients were in their last death throes, by which time it was understood that there was not much to be done for them anyway.

In addition to these medical misgivings, some Christian Europeans also had social and moral reservations against flight. Giovanni Boccaccio, for example, in his introduction to the *Decameron* that describes the impact of plague in his native city of Florence, famously writes that, during the Black Death of 1348, "this scourge had implanted so great a terror in the hearts of men and women that brothers abandoned brothers, uncles their nephews, sisters their brothers, and in many cases wives deserted their husbands. But even worse, and almost incredible, was the fact that fathers and mothers refused to nurse and assist their own children, as though they did not belong to them."[114] As we have seen, some such observation had already been made during the First Pandemic by Paul the Deacon and John bar Penkāyē. However, the plaint of abandonment received much wider circulation during the Black Death: it was repeated by no less than nine other Italian chroniclers; three writers from Avignon, including the surgeon Gui de Chauliac; and by two French poets, Simon of Corvino and Guillaume de Machaut. Either all these various authors were borrowing from Paul, or each other, or else at least some of them were recording genuine historical incidents, which seems more likely given that plague doctors *were* advising their clients to flee the plague.

It is even argued by one historian that Boccaccio's entire introduction is designed as a "strong, moral critique" of doctors and their medical advice, which he saw as a threat to society's obligations to have compassion and take care of the sick.[115] At one point, Boccaccio writes,

> Some people, pursuing what was possibly the safer alternative, callously maintained that there was no better or more efficacious remedy against a plague than to run away from it. Swayed by this argument, and sparing no thought for anyone but themselves, large numbers of men and women abandoned their city, their homes, their relatives, their estates and their belongings, and headed for the countryside, either in Florentine territory or, better still, abroad. It was as though they imagined that the wrath of God would not unleash this plague against men for their iniquities irrespective of where they happened to be, but would only be aroused against those who found themselves within the city walls; or possibly they assumed that the whole of the population would be exterminated and that the city's last hour had come.[116]

This kind of behavior had real consequences and was in effect a self-fulfilling prophecy of doom for the city's remaining inhabitants, since as a result of being abandoned "a great many people died who would perhaps have survived had they received some assistance."[117] All this is quite similar to what Lubb was saying in his *fatwas* on the plague in Islamic Spain.

At the same time, however, Boccaccio and others who seemed to disapprove of flight freely admitted that plague was contagious, which Boccaccio illustrated with his own eyewitness testimony of how two pigs fell down dead after mauling the rags of a pauper who had died of the disease. If plague could transfer itself not only from sick to healthy people but even through inanimate objects like clothing, it was no wonder that it spread "with the speed of a fire racing through dry or oily substances that happened to be placed within its reach."[118] Could anyone then be blamed for seeking to save his life by fleeing? Is this not what Boccaccio's ten protagonists do, who while away their time in voluntary exile from Florence by each telling a story on each of ten days (something that plague doctors also recommended in order to take the mind off the plague, as it could be spread by what was called "accidents of the soul")? So long as he admitted contagion, Boccaccio could not very well come out and explicitly forbid people to flee, as Lubb did; the most he could do was shame them into staying.

Toward the end of the Middle Ages, in fact, the Church finally issued a kind of pronouncement on the morality of flight, which definitively settled the matter in favor of the right of everyone, including priests, to flee the plague. This comes in a little-known treatise residing in the Vatican Archives in Rome entitled *Quod liceat pestilentiam fugere* ("That it should be permitted to flee the pestilence"), by the Italian bishop of Brescia, Dominico Amanti, who wrote it at the request of the papal cardinal of St. Grisogono, James of Pavia.[119] Thus it has the unmistakable stamp of authority, written apparently in order to settle "some matter of doubt" or debate among "learned and eminent men" on the question of flight, which had evidently existed ever since Boccaccio raised the issue in the *Decameron*. Although the treatise is undated, it was penned between 1464 and 1477 when Amanti was bishop and James was cardinal, and it represents the fullest and most direct treatment of the subject in the medieval Christian West.

It is in the last third of his treatise that Amanti addresses Boccaccio's objection that flight from the plague "is contrary to [Christian] charity, prayers, and good works." Amanti concedes that, in his day, "a father abandons his son, and brother abandons brother, and a servant abandons his fellow servant: there is no one who [is left] to console a poor soul" and that this moral failing is perhaps why "pestilences rage more frequently [now] than in former times." However, Amanti refuses to conclude from this that flight from the plague will lead to a breakdown of society, since that would impose an impossibly burdensome communal duty upon each individual, such that everyone would need to be a tiller of the land or a builder of houses, because we all need food and shelter to live; by the same logic, even "all of us clerics should get married, because marriage is necessary for the [propagation of the] human race." Amanti goes so far as to turn the charity argument on its head, pointing out that for a prelate "it would be against charity to not flee [the plague]," since "his death would do great damage to God's Church." He also quotes St. Augustine's *De Doctrina Christiana* (On Christian Doctrine) for claiming that the order of charity decrees that care of one's own body take precedence over that of one's neighbor. The only exception Amanti allows that would prohibit flight is if a pastor would thereby provide a "pernicious example" to his flock, who would then abandon sick neighbors to their death and despair. But since churchmen can usually arrange for a substitute to do their duties in their absence, this is largely a moot point. In any case, Amanti concludes that the act of flight from the plague is, by its very nature (*ex genere*), intrinsically good; only the end or circumstance surrounding it can make it bad. What this is, however, must be up to the individual, for the conditions can vary "in terms of place, time, person and many other circumstances."

In the earlier part of his treatise, Amanti responds to another objection that one also finds in Boccaccio and that is reflected in the Prophetic tradition of Islam, namely, that flight is an attempt "to alter God's design" that had brought the plague in the first place. Here, Amanti is in remarkable sympathy with medical doctors and their theories about the plague. Quoting Avicenna, who taught men "how to recognize pestilential air from its qualities" so that they could then "apply the most preferable remedy, namely flight," he notes that animals such as kites and storks are accustomed to flee before the "corrupt air" (a very common observation in European plague treatises), so that to deny to humans what is done instinctively by beasts is to set oneself up as "an enemy of nature." In the same way, "if you refuse anyone the right to flee, it is also necessary that you refuse to allow anyone to send for a physician or to seek medications, which is absurd." On the contrary, medicine is sanctioned by the Bible, and here Amanti quotes from the same "honor the physician" passage from Ecclesiasticus 38:1–14 that was also used by the Paris medical faculty in their *Consultation* of 1348 to the king of France.

But Amanti also posits a theological response to the objection, in that he turns it into a discussion of predestination and free will. Those who would fatally resign themselves to facing the plague by not fleeing what had been allegedly decreed by God as a just punishment are like those who deny good works as having any role in human salvation or who are convinced prematurely of their own damnation: just as God may have "decided to save you in this way, namely by your doing good works," so does God save you when "He has decided to deliver you from the pestilence. . . . He has decided that you might be delivered in this way, namely by fleeing." Therefore, to deny the option of flight is to deny to humankind the use of his God-given reason, which recognizes "that corrupt air harms a man and that the disease of the pestilence is contagious"; viewed in this way, flight is simply one means by which he chooses to save himself, "since the means by which he ought to do this is his choice, just as if these should be ordained by God." By implication, then, Amanti accuses those who would resist flight from the plague as guilty of a kind of proto-Protestant heresy. Not only that, they are simpletons and fools, akin to those who in their "silliness" interpret their religion so literally that they take that part of the Lord's prayer, "Give us this day our daily bread," as meaning they should not work but simply "sit unprepared at table [and wait] for the Lord to send down bread through his angels!"

Finally, there is the last Islamic tenet on the plague to consider that is perhaps best summed up by a writer from Aleppo in northern Palestine who himself succumbed to the Black Death in 1349, al-Wardī:

> This plague is for the Muslims a martyrdom and a reward, and for the disbelievers a punishment and a rebuke. When the Muslim endures misfortune, then patience is his worship. It has been established by our Prophet, God bless him and give him peace, that the plague-stricken are martyrs. This noble tradition is true and assures martyrdom. And this secret should be pleasing to the true believer.[120]

Al-Wardī goes on to refute contagion, citing the Prophet's response to the pagan Bedouin (who believed in contagion): "Who infected the first?" In other words, Muhammad was bypassing intermediary causes to ask who infected the first mangy camel, which must have come directly from God. It was also "devotion to noble tradition," al-Wardī assures us, that "prevented us from running away from the plague," for which he apparently paid with his life. But al-Wardī ends his "Essay on the Report of the Pestilence" with a series of supplications to God that certainly sounds like he would much rather not be blessed with martyrdom from plague at all, which he describes as an "evil and torture." This impression is buttressed by the contemporary chronicle of Ibn Kathīr from Damascus, who records plague processions and prayers that the crowd hoped and expected would take away the plague, something that one more usually associates with the Christian response to placate an angry God who had sent the plague down as a punishment, for believers and infidels alike.[121] Other fourteenth-century Muslim writers who discuss the Prophetic tradition of plague as a mercy and martyrdom do so in a distinctly ambivalent way. Ibn al-Qayyim, for example, begins his chapter on the plague in his treatise on Prophetic medicine with a standard statement that plague is a martyrdom for every Muslim, but he then goes on to endorse contagion as a secondary cause of plague much in line with Galenic theories of the spread of disease. Likewise, Lubb only mentions the martyrdom interpretation of the plague in a halfhearted way at the very end of his first *fatwa*, which otherwise could have cleared up much of the contradictions in the Prophetic tradition regarding contagion that he addresses in earlier sections. It is only with Hajar's plague treatise of the mid-fifteenth century, which was to influence nearly all other treatises that came after it, that we get a strong, unreserved endorsement of the tradition that plague is a martyrdom for believers, to which Hajar devotes an entire chapter.[122]

According to one scholar, the interpretation that plague was a mercy and martyrdom was "a major theological innovation of Islam" and unique to it, being akin to the promise of paradise for those who waged jihad, or Muslim holy war.[123] This is not quite accurate, however. We have already seen how in seventh-century Spain, the promise of the resurrection was held out to those who died of plague in one sermon composed during the First Pandemic, which is somewhat akin to Muslims' positive spin on the plague. An even closer parallel is to be found in the German physician John of Saxony's treatise from the fifteenth century, in which he states that one of his impediments for treating people with plague was their morbid resignation to death, either due to their belief that "a fixed term of life and death has been established for each individual" or else, even worse, they had "a disposition and desire to die" because "they hoped to go immediately to heaven, which is why they did not seek out doctors to prolong their life." John recalled how during "a certain great pestilence in Montpellier" this happened when "many men chose to die because the pope gave absolution to those dying [from the plague] for their penance and their sins."[124]

Otherwise, some Christians challenged the notion that plague was always a punishment from God that had to be feared. Petrarch first questioned this in a letter to his friend, Louis Sanctus, in May 1349, when he mused almost blasphemously as to whether "could it be perhaps that certain great truths are to be held suspect, that God does not care for mortal men," since he chooses to punish the current generation in a much harsher way through the plague than our forebears who had sinned equally as much?[125] Over a century later, Amanti attempted to resolve this conundrum, such as that Job or the children of the sinners of Sodom and Gomorrah were punished even though they were innocent, by pointing to a silver lining to disasters like the plague: For some, he claimed, the disease was a blessing "in that they don't wallow in their sin, for in their wisdom, one is carried off by the plague in order that no evil quality might change their soul." For others, it inspires them to turn to prayer and penitence that God might save them from the plague, which he does by inspiring his elect to flee![126] In a rather innovative theological twist, a Lübeck doctor speculated in 1411 that, since pestilences "cannot be altered by cures, prayers, or other offerings," it was not a punishment from God but rather his way of gathering "unto Himself those pleasing to Him, that is, young boys and other good people, so that His host with its great numbers may be able to overpower the host of the devil."[127] The late medieval English mystic, Julian of Norwich, also came up with an alternative theology to explain why a merciful and loving God would allow evils such as disease: for her it is simply part of God's plan for the ultimate salvation and redemption of the human race, or as she famously puts it, "Synne is behovely [necessary], but alle shalle be wele, and alle shalle be wele, and alle maner of thynge shalle be wele."[128]

Two other responses to the Black Death, this time exclusively on the part of the Christian community, have also been seen as emblematic of a religious or cultural divide between Christianity and Islam. One is the Flagellant movement, which spread from Austria and Hungary in 1348 westward through Bohemia, central and southern Germany, and Strasbourg before finally ending up in Flanders by the late summer and early autumn of 1349. This movement consisted of processions sometimes hundreds strong that would come to town to engage in ritualistic whipping ceremonies that, according to one observer, Heinrich of Herford, might spatter the walls nearby with the Flagellants' blood and move the spectators to tears.[129]

Traditionally, the Flagellants have been viewed by historians as an apocalyptic or millenarian movement with a radical heretical taint.[130] One scholar uses this as a pretext for noting a major difference between Christian and Muslim responses to the Black Death: according to Michael Dols, there is no apocalyptic ideology in "orthodox" or Sunni Islam that would have given birth to a Flagellant movement.[131] (Shi'ia Islam, however, does have some millenarian tendencies, and to this day flagellation does figure in some Shi'ite commemorations to Husayn ibn Ali during Muharram, the first month of the Islamic calendar.) But in fact, a closer look at the evidence reveals very little support for Christian Flagellants being any more motivated than Muslims would have been by beliefs in an impending apocalypse—nor do I think that guilt over sin played a major role in why the Flagellant movement arose in Europe and not in the Middle East or Spain. According to Dols, "There is no doctrine of original sin and of man's insuperable guilt in Islamic theology," as there is in Christianity.[132] Regardless of the truth of this statement, I see it as irrelevant to the raison d'être behind the Flagellants. For even though the "Christian belief in plague as a divine punishment for men's sins" certainly underlay why flagellation was chosen as the means by which the Flagellants were to achieve their ends, atonement in and of itself does not satisfactorily explain why the Flagellants were performing their whipping ceremonies nor why these were so popular, at least among their supporters.[133]

As for why Muslims did not also flagellate themselves during the Black Death, the answer may be found not in some esoteric difference in theology but rather in a more eminently practical explanation. The Flagellants participated in an itinerant-based movement that depended on an infusion of fresh recruits as they traveled from town to town. This was simply impractical for Muslim communities if they were to abide by the long-standing Prophetic tradition to not flee to or from a plague-infested area. For all we know, isolated flagellant demonstrations may in fact have taken place in the course of Muslim processions against the plague but did not attract the attention of chroniclers because they were not part of a broad-based, wide-ranging movement as in Christian Europe.[134]

Another puzzle is why no scapegoats emerged in Islamic countries during the Black Death, such as we typically find in the Jewish pogroms that occurred in over three hundred towns and other communities in primarily German-speaking lands from ·Switzerland, Alsace, and the Low Countries in the west to Poland, Bohemia, and Austria in the east between 1348 and 1351.[135] (Pogroms also occurred in northeastern Spain, southern France, and the Savoy between the spring and autumn of 1348.) It is no longer sufficient to say that Jewish pogroms in Europe were an outgrowth of the Flagellant movement, since the connections between the two are tenuous at best. In terms of timing, Flagellants often arrived in town long *after* a Jewish pogrom occurred, as was the case in Strasbourg, where two thousand Jews were burnt in February 1349, months before the Flagellants arrived later that year in June or July. We must therefore find some other reason for why such a phenomenon occurred, and why it did so among Christians and not Muslims.[136]

Respective attitudes toward the Jews are irrelevant, in my view, toward explaining the pogroms. Like the Flagellants, the Jewish massacres were really about a desperate attempt to end the Black Death, although certainly medieval Christian "anti-Judaism" helps explain why Jews were targeted. Instead of being a religiously based accusation bound up with the victims' Jewishness, the charge of well poisoning that was leveled against the Jews during the Black Death was part of an entirely rational outlook that was grounded in contemporary medical and scientific theories about the disease that likewise viewed it as primarily caused in the human body by some sort of "poisoning." The latter were usually interpreted in terms of a naturally occurring causation, such as a "poisonous vapor" ingested into the body from the surrounding air, but a few Christian doctors, such as the Spanish physician based at the medical school at Montpellier in southern France Alfonso de Córdoba, did admit of plague poisoning by human agency. These theories were then mutually reinforced by trials against Jews and poor men that charged them with poisoning wells or food in order to spread the Black Death among Christians; these trials first took place in the Languedoc, Provençal, Dauphiné, and Savoyard regions of France and Switzerland, all quite close to Córdoba's theater of operations at Montpellier.[137]

If we are right that the poison accusation was primarily about a mistaken hope to end the plague, why then did it not take root in Islamic lands? The answer, I believe, goes back to the Prophetic tradition that plague can only come from the will of God. Even though various authors, such as Khātima, argued for contagion as a secondary natural cause that was not incompatible with this fundamental religious tenet, it would have been another thing entirely to argue that humans themselves could cause the plague by a sheer act of will. This would then place the plague almost entirely out of God's causation, something that no Islamic jurist would stomach. Therefore, it is most unlikely that Muslim jurisprudence would grant the legal imprimatur that had made possible the trials and massacres that we see in Christian Europe. It may be supposed that God could have acted here indirectly by allowing the poisoners to be demonically inspired, as indeed many Christians believed they were, but Muslims usually interpreted the *jinn* or demonic influence as acting *directly* to instill the disease in human beings, not to use them as puppets such as we see alleged during the European witch hunt. A Polish astrologer and physician, Heinrich Ribbeniz, did link an alleged propensity of Jews to poison people with the influence of Saturn during plague that made them more likely to "sin against their gods,"[138] but Muslim authors of plague treatises were far more skeptical of astrological influences, preferring to adhere to a strict Hippocratic interpretation of plague as arising (secondarily) from unnatural changes in the seasons. For Muslims, the role for humans in terms of acting according to the free use of their reason came only *after* plague had been sent down by God: at least, this seems to be the meaning of Umar's parable of grazing camels either on the lush or barren slope of the *wadi*, which he allegedly told to 'Ubayda during the Plague of 'Amwâs of 638–639.

How to sum up a comparison of Christian and Islamic responses to and interpretations of the plague? Any attempt to paint such differences with too broad a brush, as perhaps Dols is guilty of, is criticized these days as failing to take into account the manifold differences of opinions *within* each religious tradition, at both the popular and intellectual level, and the lack of clarity that this then produces for establishing differences *between* the two traditions themselves, since points of overlap or obfuscation can always be found.[139] Certainly, one can uncover authors on both sides who endorsed contagion, who condoned flight from the plague, and who saw the disease as a mercy, or at least somehow beneficial, for its sufferers. But it would also be false to deny that there weren't differences of *emphasis* between the two faiths in terms of how they approached the plague. Christian doctors, for instance, were able to endorse contagion unreservedly, without having to take into account religious objections as did their Muslim colleagues. It was also easier for Christian physicians to advise fleeing the plague, since any moral or ethical objections could be overcome simply by prescribing the appropriate medical precautions to take for those who stayed, whether by choice or necessity, as opposed to having to confront a long cultural tradition that frowned upon such behavior. Finally, Christian commentators on the plague were far more willing to question God's direct agency and entertain alternative explanations of the disease, whether these be purely natural causes or human-directed ones. These still made a difference and had an impact upon each society's experience with the plague, such as why the Flagellant movement or the Jewish pogroms arose in one culture and not in the other.

It also very much mattered *how* each side expressed itself in taking the positions that they did, even if there were similarities or concurrences between them. Dols has been criticized for insisting on making religious interpretations of the plague emblematic of an entire culture's response to the disease, disregarding other influences.[140] But this is precisely the point: religious responses to plague were all too often bound up with medical, social, psychological, and other cultural considerations, in which the manner of the response indicates how these various perspectives interacted with each other and which had significant consequences for each culture's history with the disease. Bishop Amanti's fifteenth-century treatise on flight from the plague is an excellent example of this. I've already noted how much in sympathy Amanti was with the medical agenda of his day, marshaling principles enunciated in medical plague treatises in support of his position that flight is a morally acceptable response to plague; he was even willing to equate the medical necessity of flight with a Christian virtue, while any opposition to it was akin to a wrongheaded religious interpretation or worse, heresy. For Amanti, a priest was not even obligated to seek out plague patients to give them last rites, unless their case was incurable or there was no one left to attend them. (This certainly gives some substance to the criticisms of priests' behavior during the Black Death that was made by chroniclers!) One need only contrast this with the hostile attitude toward medicine and the medical profession evident in the Islamic treatises of al-Qayyim in the fourteenth century and Hajar in the fifteenth. Amanti's treatise also supports Dols's contention that Christians were more concerned with individual priorities over communal interests, especially when this is compared with the works of Lubb or of the sixteenth-century Ottoman jurist Tāshköprüzāde.[141] The parallel anecdotes told by Gilles li Muisis of Tournai and Ibn Battūta from Morocco (the Christian chronicler relating how some pilgrims "left in great haste" once they learned in the morning that their host and his whole family were dead from plague, while Battūta and his companion stay to pray over and bury a *faqir*, or Muslim holy man, who had died in their company during the night) neatly illustrate the differences here as well.[142]

Islamic religious hostility toward medicine almost assuredly had wide-ranging consequences for communities facing plague, if one is to go by Khatīb's complaint "that the quills with which the scholars wrote these *fatwas* were like swords upon which the Muslims died."[143] This is also borne out by the rather less known and studied plague treatise of Khatīb's student and fellow physician in Granada, Muhammad ibn 'Alī ash-Shaqūrī. Although Shaqūrī does not encroach upon the thorny issue of contagion in the manner of his teacher, he does come to the defense of medicine as "a sanctuary provided by God and His mercy," whose practitioners are like "beacons of light in a dark cave" of ignorance and folly.[144] This is rather like Christian doctors who quoted perfunctorily from the "honor the physician" passage in Ecclesiasticus 38:1–14. But Shaqūrī goes further than this in the following passage:

> Many people understand from what is often said that medicine runs counter to God's command, yet there is scarcely anyone more ignorant than the person who makes this claim. The person who violates God's command is the one who hinders a created being in any fashion. Obligatory belief in this regard is that medicine is among God's commands, and it is among the affairs that He entrusted to His emissary [the Prophet Muhammad], God's peace and prayer upon him. It is also among the blessings and the deeds which God has bestowed upon those who worship Him. It is His command, and thus does He wish it. There is no gainsaying His wisdom.[145]

Nestled within this spirited defense of medicine is considerable resentment and indignation at those who would oppose medical practitioners out of a misguided and blind belief that, by opposing, they are doing God's will, which echoes much of the tone of Shaqūrī's teacher, Khatīb. This is important evidence, I think, of the frustration and obstruction late medieval Muslim doctors had to contend with compared to their Christian colleagues, who did not need to justify their profession to nearly the same extent.

On the other hand, the ease and readiness with which Christian authorities such as Amanti proved willing to conform their religious principles to medical priorities is of great significance for the implementation of plague controls around this same time in northern Italy. By the mid-fifteenth century, and even earlier in the case of Milan, permanent health boards were being set up by some Italian cities in order to be able to respond to plague outbreaks with measures such as quarantine, setting up of sanitary cordons, disinfection or outright destruction of the living quarters and belongings of plague patients, isolation of the sick and those deemed contagious in their homes or in *lazarettos* and pesthouses, and so on. Amanti seemed to be signaling that, from his quarter at least, nothing was going to stand in the way of these controls, although mercantile interests in Florence and other Italian republics may have had concerns about their impact on trade.[146] By the seventeenth century, when plague controls were at their height of implementation by health boards across Europe, they began to attract some resistance, even to the point of physical threats made against health board members, due to the intrusiveness, scope, and rigor with which they had been allowed to be imposed, unfettered by any competing cultural considerations except perhaps economic ones. As expected, these protests came largely from the merchant community, who objected to the disruption caused to trade and to the putting-out system of cottage industry, but also from the Church, which, perhaps to its chagrin considering its earlier acquiescence to such controls, now began to be alarmed at restrictions placed upon processions and other religious services during time of plague. Yet, the threat that plague posed to public health was deemed too great, and its controls—directed largely against the poor and other "dangerous" classes at the margins of society—were deemed too effective, to be seriously dislodged; moreover, health boards had much the upper hand over their would-be detractors, backed up as they were by the full force of the law and the power of government apparatuses.[147]

By contrast, when Western-style plague controls were introduced into Muslim countries, such as Tunisia in North Africa, by the eighteenth century, their effectiveness was already limited by opposition from the *ulema*, or religious scholars who spoke on behalf of the Muslim community. This opposition was such that it forced the Tunisian *bey* to rescind some of the more objectionable measures, such as burning the clothes and possessions of those who had died from the plague. Natives also questioned the medical necessity of plague controls when the disease reappeared in spite of them. Although some Islamic traditions, such as that one must not flee to or from a plague-infected area, might be more compatible with other measures like quarantine, Western observers frequently noted how Muslim attitudes, in particular their fatalistic acceptance of the disease as well as native remedies for plague, differed very much from their own.[148] If one accepts that these controls played a role in the demise of the Second Pandemic of plague,[149] then their greater acceptance in the Christian West as opposed to the Muslim Middle East may help explain why plague ended a hundred years earlier in Europe, by the early eighteenth century, as opposed to the early nineteenth century in North Africa and Palestine. On the other hand, these controls did not come without a price, as those who protested them in both Europe and the Middle East knew all too well. Such conflicts during the Black Death set the stage for even greater clashes between European colonial powers and their native subjects when the former attempted to impose similar controls during the Third Pandemic of plague primarily in India at the turn of the twentieth century.

In other respects, both Muslim and Christian responses to the Black Death followed a familiar pattern that had already been set during the First Pandemic of plague. Such high mortality necessitated mass burials and hurried, disordered funerals: the description by al-Maqrīzī of Cairo, of how "funeral processions were so many that they could not file past without bumping into each other" and how the dead were carried to their graves on bare wooden planks or whatever else was to hand, echoes that of John of Ephesus during the plague of 542 in Constantinople.[150] Likewise, Marchionne di Coppo Stefani's vivid analogy of how the dead were layered with dirt in mass graves in Florence "just as one makes lasagna with layers of pasta and cheese" rivals John of Ephesus's imagery of the dead being pressed together like in a winepress.[151] Prayers and processions of supplication to end the plague again took place as they had during the First Pandemic, even in Islamic cities over the objections of some religious scholars that this went against the traditional view of plague as a mercy and martyrdom for the faithful.[152] Just as the tolling of bells ceased in many European cities as a sign of the plague's disruption of everyday life, so too did the call of muezzins to prayer in Cairo or Damascus, although the latter did not go so far as to deliberately constrain or even ban commemorative and religious services in line with medical prescriptions against the plague that we find contained in some European ordinances passed in response to the Black Death. And there were people who found a way to profit from the plague in both Christian and Muslim lands, whether these are the *becchini* who carted away the dead for fat fees in Florence or the readers of the Qur'an who now made ten *dirhams* per funeral in Cairo.[153]

However, there is one area in which I believe Europe had a cultural advantage over the Middle East in terms of addressing plague, aside from its greater propensity for medical plague controls. This relates to each culture's attitudes toward and beliefs in the afterlife. Medieval Europe during the Second Pandemic had a remarkably concrete, palpably tangible conceptualization of the afterlife, one that was quite possibly unique in all of recorded history. One only has to read Dante's *Divine Comedy* from the early fourteenth century, just before the arrival of the great outbreak of plague in 1348, to understand just how fully articulated and profoundly real this conceptualization was to our medieval forebears. Purgatory, in particular, was ideally suited to a "cult of remembrance" of the dead, in which the dead were assured that they would not be forgotten among the living in their prayers and the living were comforted with the promise that death was not the end but just the beginning of their spiritual journey, a journey that would end only with the Last Judgment when bodies ravaged by disease would finally triumph over death by being resurrected whole and sound to rejoin their souls. This cult of remembrance so intimately bound up with the concept of purgatory was bound to be attractive at a time of plague when its mass death threatened to consign all to oblivion in a common grave. Purgatory, which was "invented" by the Western Church in the late twelfth or early thirteenth century and which is described by Dante as a great mountain of nine terraces, was completely foreign to Hebraic and Muslim cultures, even though they too had their versions of final judgment and resurrection. Europe's late medieval cult of remembrance is well attested by the wills proved in central Italy and in Douai in Flanders during the second half of the fourteenth and during the fifteenth centuries, when a greater percentage of them in the aftermath of plague specify some kind of commemoration, such as individual portraiture in tomb sculptures or within larger artistic commissions.[154] Thus, when facing a uniquely mortal disease like plague, which portended for its many victims a swift and sudden demise, Europe's "death-friendly" culture, I would argue, with its detailed topography of purgatory and elaborate preparations for death in this life, was uniquely equipped for the psychological challenge posed by plague compared to the belief systems in place in the Middle East and in other regions around the world.[155]

Finally, there is the differential economic impact of the plague in Europe and the Middle East. This is a question that recent scholars have tried to tease out from the thorny issue of how differences in religious culture between Christianity and Islam played themselves out during the plague, although, as we will see, economic factors cannot be so easily disentangled from other considerations such as the social and political makeup of societies.[156] Mortality during the Black Death is thought to have been at least as severe in the Middle East as in Europe: even though considerably fewer archival resources are available in the former region, enough has been recovered from sources such as cadastral surveys in Egypt to suggest that the two were comparable.[157] Traditionally, the assumption then followed, largely based on chronicle accounts, that the economic trajectory of the Middle East followed that of Europe's in the aftermath of the Black Death, despite the fact that, by the end of the Middle Ages, Europe, and England in particular, had emerged with its economy poised to take full advantage of the benefits of a new, capitalist-based system, while that of the Mamluk dynasty in Egypt, for example, lay in ruins.[158] New research on Egyptian sources such as endowment deeds and chancery manuals that supplement narrative chronicles has greatly revised this comparative picture.[159]

A comparison of England's economic response to the plague with Egypt's over the course of the fourteenth and fifteenth centuries reveals that the two were diametrically opposite: in England, the long-term economic impact of the massive depopulation caused by successive waves of the plague led to growing prosperity in the population at large (with the significant exception of the landholding class), since, in general, wages of laborers rose, prices of agricultural necessities fell, and rents declined, all tending to raise peasant incomes and spelling the end of the oppressive manorial system; however, in Egypt, the reverse was true, with wages falling, grain prices rising, and rents increasing, all leading to the collapse of the economy based on *fellahin* labor. A simple comparison of the agrarian GDP (gross domestic product) in the two countries by the early sixteenth century, after they had started out on roughly equivalent terms before the Black Death during the early fourteenth century, dramatically illustrates the disparity: Egypt's fell by nearly 60 percent during this period, while England's recovered and actually increased by 7 percent, so that England's GDP was by this time double that of Egypt's.[160]

Obviously, a catastrophic mortality from the plague occurred in both countries that triggered these changes but not with the same result since very different social and political circumstances then interacted with and responded to the demographic decline. In Egypt, the Mamluk military elite that ruled the country from Cairo owned the *iqtā'* landholdings in the countryside (which were *not* the same as fiefs in Europe) on a nonhereditary, unstable basis and administered them through an elaborate bureaucracy that discouraged personal supervision and control. Furthermore, the Mamluk caste of soldiery was able to respond to the disruptions caused by the plague as a cohesive, unified body, or "collective bargaining unit," that successfully suppressed any attempts by the *fellahin* to take advantage of greater demands for their labor that was now much more scarce in the aftermath of the Black Death. Additionally, the complex irrigation network that maintained Egypt's agricultural estates along the Nile River valley was a highly labor-intensive system that inevitably suffered from population declines inaugurated by the plague but that was now largely administered by emirs pursuing their private self-interest instead of by the central government of the sultan. This irrigation system also suffered from Bedouin incursions in the outlying districts. Thus, a combination of unique political, social, and geographical circumstances led to the decay in Egypt's agriculture throughout the late Middle Ages in response to the Black Death.[161]

By contrast, in England and elsewhere in Europe, feudalism ensured a decentralized, local control over landholdings such that, despite the aristocracy's best efforts at passing labor legislation in national parliaments, peasant communities were the ones who were able to bargain more effectively as a collective unit by taking advantage of landholders' rivalry and economic competition with each other. Despite the fact that, from the elite's point of view, Egypt's autocratic response was far more preferable, in the long run and with hindsight it was Europe's seemingly chaotic, socially undermining response that held the greatest overall economic benefits for its population, one that set the stage for its rise and dominance over the Middle East in the modern era. The economic winners and losers from plague were therefore determined not just by the disease's mortality itself but also by its interaction with a whole host of factors that were unique to each society, ones not necessarily bound up with its religious culture. These economic benefits and costs were also not necessarily intended or foreseen at the time; in fact, a society or culture may have been straining for exactly the opposite result. There is some question remaining, however, as to whether a comparative case study such as that between Egypt and England can hold true for entire regions or continents, that is, Europe versus the Middle East. Were Egypt's circumstances the same as those in Syria or Iran?[162] Was England's drive toward a renter, capitalistic economy by the fifteenth century mirrored in Spain, Italy, or Eastern Europe? The evidence suggests rather that even within a geographic entity that shared a similar set of cultural values, such as Christian ethics and feudal and manorial landholding systems, variations could still occur in terms of the economic impact of the Black Death. But at least it is clear now that Europe and the Middle East could differ dramatically in terms of their respective responses to plague in more ways than just along the religious divide traditionally demarcated between the two cultures.

A last legacy of the Second Pandemic of plague to consider is how both Christian and Muslim chroniclers personified the disease in their writings, perhaps as an indication of just how feared the plague was by premodern societies. An anonymous doctor writing from Lübeck in Germany in 1411 called plague the "[evil] stepmother of the human race" due to the way it carried off "too many" of his friends and fellow citizens; rather than characterizing the disease as an "illness," he called it simply a "death."[163] He and another fifteenth-century German doctor, Primus of Görlitz, also portrayed plague as an enemy to be fought and hopefully conquered by their regimens; in the former case, the physician's victory over plague apostemes was compared to banners raised on castle turrets to signify surrender.[164] In his more poetic passages, the Muslim Syrian writer al-Wardī compared the Black Death variously to a lion, a silkworm, a storm, a taxpayer, a king who "swayed with power" on his throne, and a lover who poisons her victims as she kisses and embraces them. In another passage, the plague enters a house as if it were the agent of the qadi, or religious judge, announcing that it was there to "arrest" all those within.[165] Clearly for our ancestors, plague had become all too personal and real. Their fear of the disease stemmed not only from its high mortality but also from the horribly painful way in which it killed (at least in the bubonic form) and the sudden swiftness of its grim harvest (particularly in the pneumonic and septicemic forms), which left precious little time for preparation for the afterlife. This literary treatment of the plague set it apart from all other diseases and accorded it a special place in human history.

The Third Pandemic of plague apparently began as early as 1854 in the Yunnan province of southwestern China, spreading from there to other Chinese provinces until it eventually arrived at the ports of Canton and Hong Kong in 1894.[166] Two years later, it called at the port of Bombay in India and then spread particularly to the northern and western regions of the country and decimated approximately twelve million of the native population by 1930, comprising 95 percent of the world's mortality from the pandemic. Another major outbreak in Asia came in Manchuria in northeastern China, where the disease manifested itself as exclusively pneumonic plague and swept away 60,000 inhabitants in 1910–1911 and 8,500 more in 1920–1921. By the turn of the twentieth century, largely through the power of modern steamship transport, plague made its way around the world, infecting and establishing new endemic centers in Madagascar and South Africa, Southeast Asia, South America, Russia, and Australia, often in defiance of local quarantine measures.[167] In 1900, plague called at San Francisco and from there spread throughout the western United States, where it has an endemic presence down to the present day, as shown by the case of Tull and Marker mentioned at the beginning of this chapter. The continued relevance of plague is also demonstrated by recent epidemics in Surat, India, and in Madagascar, where a new, antibiotic-resistant strain of *Yersinia pestis* has emerged.

The Third Pandemic presented microbiologists with an unprecedented, golden opportunity to study plague using the new tools of modern science, in this case, that of bacteriology and the germ theory of disease, as inaugurated earlier in the nineteenth century by such pioneers as Louis Pasteur and Robert Koch. A student of Pasteur's, Alexandre Yersin, is credited with being the first to discover the bacillus that causes plague in both rodents and humans (hence its name, *Yersinia pestis*). The rat-flea nexus that spreads the bacteria in cases of bubonic plague was then explained by another protégé of Pasteur's, the French bacteriologist Paul-Louis Simond. Special research bodies were also set up to study the disease and publish their results, including the Indian Plague Commission, which issued a *Minutes of Evidence* and *Report* in 1900–1901, supplemented by annual articles in the *Journal of Hygiene* between 1906 and 1937, and the North Manchurian Plague Prevention Service, which came out with three *Reports* on the plague in Manchuria between 1914 and 1922. However, it would be a mistake to assume that these "scientific" reports on the Third Pandemic are all entirely trustworthy or characterize the behavior of the plague in all places and at all times. Like any other document, they are a product of their specific historical context, and some of their assertions, such as that plague was communicated through the soles of the feet or that "one of the safest places during an epidemic is the ward of a sanitary plague hospital," were motivated primarily by political or racial considerations and are therefore misleading or outright wrong.

Of more interest to scholars of the Third Pandemic have been the cultural conflicts that emerged between colonial authorities such as Britain who were trying to implement modern, Western-style plague controls and medical ideas in their empires, and the native subjects in India and elsewhere who bore the brunt of this so-called disease imperialism.[168] Some of the issues here also crop up in the British government's handling of other diseases that threatened India, such as smallpox and cholera (chapters 2 and 4), but plague presented a unique concatenation of circumstances: the Third Pandemic proved to be an intriguing intersection of a long history of dealing with plague in both Europe and Asia combined with a new knowledge and awareness of how the disease was actually caused and spread. Imperial powers such as Britain wielded the weapons of modern medical science almost like a club, determined to bludgeon its Indian empire into health on the conviction that it could now finally eradicate an age-old disease. Yet, this newfound and arguably unprecedented determination to collectively cure a nation came up against an equally determined native resistance in India, and to some extent this was also true of the response of Chinese authorities to the pneumonic plague outbreak in Manchuria.[169] While scholars have typically explored the Third Pandemic for its political ramifications in terms of Britain's and Europe's colonial policies, our concern here is more strictly epidemiological: did the modern "scientific" effort against plague work, and if not, why? Somewhat to their surprise, British authorities discovered that their energetic efforts to combat the plague—which initially included compulsory hospitalization of all patients who had come down with plague, segregation of contacts, house-to-house searches and disinfection of all homes where plague occurred, and inspection of plague corpses—could be stymied by the bitter opposition of natives, which was bolstered when a recrudescence of plague occurred during the late summer of 1897 despite the apparent success in temporarily halting the 1896 outbreak. This required a new policy from the British government by 1898–1899 of accommodation to native customs and sensibilities, which proved to be a more effective response to the disease.

Nonetheless, some larger questions remain: Was the British failure to contain the epidemic in 1896–1897 simply a function of insensitive imperialism, or were its policies, which had much in common with those adopted by European health boards during the Second Pandemic, when the disease was understood to be miasmatic rather than microbial in character, truly suited to fight the spread of plague germs? Could native responses, such as evacuation and flight from areas where plague (as well as its oppressive controls) occurred, have actually been more effective in breaking the chain of the flea-rat-human connection that spread bubonic plague? How did this dynamic play out in China, where Western medical approaches were implemented by native ruling elites after 1894 (ostensibly in order to co-opt foreign interference) and where there was a more straightforward, human-to-human contagion of pneumonic plague? Was the native popular resistance to antiplague measures, whether in India or China, motivated by colonial resentment toward a Western imperialist foreign influence, by a traditional distrust of modern innovations, or simply as part of a "generalized panic" in response to a truly horrific disease like plague? And what lessons do all these issues hold for current efforts to fight our own emerging pandemics, such as avian influenza or swine flu?

It is remarkable how, despite all the new advances and information that emerged during the Third Pandemic with respect to identifying the causative microorganism behind plague and explaining its transmission, the actual measures taken by modern medical authorities against the disease in both India and China mirrored those adopted by European health boards during the Second

Pandemic primarily between the fifteenth and seventeenth centuries. As during the late medieval and Early Modern periods, authorities implementing anti-plague measures during the Third Pandemic often felt stymied and frustrated by the perceived ignorance, superstition, and at least passive resistance of the masses they were trying to help. Even in China, where native authorities had better compliance from their subject population than the British medical service had in India, resistance to such measures as hospitalization of victims and isolation of contacts could be significant. Dr. Wu Liande, chief medical officer of the North Manchurian Plague Prevention Service, who was put in charge of all Chinese efforts to contain the pneumonic plague outbreaks in Manchuria and who received his medical training at the University of Cambridge in England, complained that "one of the most difficult problems of plague-prevention in China was this passive opposition of the populace in not reporting cases when alive and then throwing the bodies out when dead." This happened even among "well-to-do and educated persons," and Wu frankly admitted that it hindered his efforts at fighting plague, for "if there had been cooperation between the public and the authorities at the beginning, the epidemic would have been more confined, but the cases were hidden and the families or friends were thus infected." However, Wu also allowed that there was at least a culturally, if not medically, valid reason for why his Chinese subjects refused to cooperate in this regard, which was their fear of isolation from their families, whose importance had been stressed in China going back to the philosopher Confucius during the sixth and fifth centuries B.C.E. "This fear of isolation," Wu wrote, was prevalent throughout the country, "in North and South China alike"[170]—nor can the masses really be blamed for harboring such fears when patients were doomed to spend their last days in the solitary confinement of what even Wu described as stark, "puritan-like" hospital rooms with only a cast-iron bed and spittoon for company, all the while tended by masked and therefore faceless attendants, and when isolation wards for healthy contacts consisted of railway boxcars normally fit only for carrying freight but that were left idle during the quarantine imposed by the plague. When plague hospitals, such as the one at Harbin, are also described as surrounded by barbed wire and posted armed guards to keep their infectious residents from escaping, one can be forgiven for comparing their general atmosphere and conditions to that of prisons for the most hopelessly condemned.[171]

Likewise in India, even the most well-intentioned, well-thought-out precautions against plague could be stonewalled or undone altogether by native resistance, which included substituting healthy people for sick ones in roll calls, hiding corpses in dust heaps, and inducing native doctors to diagnose victims as suffering from asthma or bronchitis instead of plague. Even worse, from the authorities' point of view, was inducing friends or relatives to hide plague victims from their prying eyes, since plague was still deemed to be contagious, even though this is not strictly true in the case of bubonic plague (unless patients develop secondary plague pneumonia). It also must have been most demoralizing for the British Civil Service in India to hear of "plague rumors," not all of which were unjustified and which arguably reflected a very real terror of plague: these included that British medical staff at plague hospitals and segregation camps poisoned native patients, stole their possessions, forcibly carted away healthy persons for extortion purposes or else compelled them to be guinea pigs for inoculation trials, and even that they cut up native bodies and boiled them down to extract a healing balm known as *momiai*.[172] (Manchuria also had its share of these plague rumors during the 1920–1921 outbreak, such as that Wu's staff put poison in people's wells, flour, and other food in order to collect the three-dollar reward for each corpse supposedly dead of plague, and that Wu himself was said to be secretly shooting the sick behind the walls of his plague hospital at Harbin.[173]) The French colony of Senegal in West Africa, where a major epidemic of bubonic plague occurred in 1914, presents a third example of how native resistance to antiplague measures could force a compromise in colonial policies, especially when the mother country faced the simultaneous pressure of just having entered the First World War. Here, the paternalistic medical response of the French government included quarantine and residential segregation, disinfection and burning of affected houses, and mandatory vaccination, while the native resistance, characterized as "the most militant popular opposition" in the colony's history, included mass street protests and general strikes among market sellers of produce.[174]

But since the dynamics of bubonic plague (spread by rats and fleas) are so very different from pneumonic plague (communicated by human-to-human contact), one can question the relative effectiveness of such measures as quarantine and disinfection in India, China, and Senegal. Whereas Wu was able to slash the number of deaths to less than a sixth of their former total after a decade of fighting pneumonic plague in Manchuria, India at least initially had rather less success, since half of all its deaths from bubonic plague occurred during its first ten years of living with the disease from 1898 to 1908. Indeed, the fact that India's antiplague measures were basically unchanged from the Second Pandemic indicates that they were adopted by the British out of long habit and expectation (their "traditional" response in the same way that the natives had theirs), rather than being specifically formulated to meet the new realities of the germ theory and their spread by insect and rodent vectors. This also seems to have been the case in Senegal in 1914, where medical authorities placed very low priority on disrupting flea and rat infestations of straw huts and granaries in both city and countryside.[175] By the same token, this leads one to question whether human attempts to control plague had any role at all in ending the Second Pandemic, or was it rather due to independent biological factors, such as emerging rat immunity to the disease, that had nothing to do with the human response?[176] Disinfecting homes and burning clothes and bedding undoubtedly helped reduce the number of fleas that could communicate bubonic plague, but this may also have unintentionally driven rats to seek the shelter of other dwellings, where they then continued to spread the disease. The only truly effective means of breaking the chain of connection between plague-infected rats and fleas and their potential human hosts, the Indian Plague Commission found, was the long-standing tradition that native Indians already had of evacuating to the surrounding countryside whenever the disease broke out in their villages.

As in China, authorities in India also underestimated the strength of family ties that bitterly resisted any attempt to separate members of a household once plague was discovered there. The broad powers that the British government arrogated to itself by the terms of the Epidemic Diseases Act passed in February 1897 in order to segregate and hospitalize anyone tainted by the plague provoked an outcry of native protest. One native newspaper in Pune, the *Burdwan Sanjivani*, declared that, no matter how justified such measures might be in sacrificing individual needs for the general welfare, "few will desire to live in a country where the wife is separated from the husband, the child from the parent, and the parent from the child. We call this selfishness, and not self-sacrifice."[177] Indeed, according to another native newspaper, the *Vyápári*, "The moral effect of segregation alone, apart from the character of the arrangements at the segregation hospital, is sufficient to retard the recovery of a patient compulsorily removed from among his relations."[178] This contradicted the testimony of some of the British agents who appeared before the Indian Plague Commission, such as Colonel Donald Robertson from the Mysore state and Major G. E. Hyde-Cates of Cutch, who alleged that some natives abandoned their relatives, to the point that mothers even refused to nurse their children, once they were infected with plague.[179] Yet, this is so similar to what European chroniclers were saying of family behavior during the Black Death that it begs the question of whether modern observations (at least those made from a Western point of view) were conditioned by what was known of the earlier Second Pandemic? Or rather, were such cases of abandonment an extreme response, not at all indicative of the behavior of the population at large, that nonetheless drew the attention of many observers during both pandemics? For all the data generated by its modern, scientific approach to the disease, in many ways the Third Pandemic raises more questions, both with respect to its own experience of plague and that of the past, than it answers.

Finally, the Third Pandemic has been portrayed by its historians as a classic example of Western imperialism imposing its concepts of medicine and disease upon the colonial subjects of its empires, but is this really or entirely the case? It has been fairly pointed out that the native Indian response to plague and to the draconian measures imposed by the British government was a complex one that did not always fall along neatly antagonistic lines.[180] Nonetheless, some elements of how the disease played out particularly in India do suggest that resistance to plague was tantamount to resistance to imperialism. Most obvious in this regard was the assassination on June 22, 1897, of the British Civil Service officer, W. C. Rand, who was in charge of enforcing plague-prevention measures in Pune. Rand had, in effect, become a symbol of oppressive, "white bull" British rule in India, for he had a notorious reputation for carrying out measures such as house inspection in a brutally harsh and offensive manner, which contrasted with more enlightened regimes such as that of General W. F. Gatacre in Bombay. (Rand boasted that his efforts to control plague "were perhaps the most drastic that had ever been taken to stamp out an epidemic."[181]) The editors of one native newspaper in Pune, *Dnyán Prakásh*, concluded that Rand's Plague Committee had no other motive for its actions than that they were being done "for tyranny's sake— for no other reason save that the members of that body take a peculiar delight in making the citizens feel their power."[182] Certainly a connection between plague controls and imperialist policies existed in the minds of some British authorities, such as W. L. Reade, the medical officer who eventually succeeded Rand as the man in charge of plague operations at Pune. In a letter to his superiors back in London, Reade frankly confessed that "plague operations, properly undertaken, present one of the best opportunities for riveting our rule in India, as it is not only an opportunity for showing a kindness to the people, but also for showing the superiority of our Western Science, and thoroughness."[183] Clearly for Reade, conquering the plague and the allegiance of native Indians to the British Empire went hand in hand, even though he certainly presented an overly optimistic view of how well plague controls were working and the natives' reception of them for the benefit of the India Office back home, as well as for the sake of his own self-promotion. Some native newspapers also made this connection quite explicit, such as when *Poona Vaibhav*, responding to the passing of the Epidemic Diseases Act in February 1897, stated that, "if [the British] government under such circumstances will oppress people in the shape of plague preventive measures and pass laws giving ample powers to their officers to carry them out, there is every probability that the government and the people will be the bitterest enemies of each other." The paper also issued a thinly veiled warning to British authorities by calling to mind the numerous "examples in Indian history of oppressive regimes being overthrown through agencies sent by God for the deliverance of the oppressed," a reference, perhaps, to the not-so-distant Sepoy Mutiny of 1857; other papers sardonically paraded similar examples of resistance to tyranny from

Britain's own history, such as when the barons of England forced King John to sign Magna Carta in 1215.[184]

However, as Reade's letter makes clear, British imperialist intentions with respect to the plague were inseparable from the supposed technological superiority of modern Western medicine when compared to what was available from native traditional healers, the Hindu *vaids* and Muslim *hakims*. (This in spite of the fact that the British response of plague controls could be considered just as traditional, in the European context of the Second Pandemic, as the Indian one.) In this sense, then, it did not matter who administered the antiplague measures so much as that they were alien to a people's customary way of life and culture. This much is clear from the fact that resistance blossomed even in China, where plague controls were administered by native agents (albeit, in Wu's case, one who had been heavily influenced by Western ideas, as transmitted through his Cambridge training). A revealing anecdote from Wu is when he unfavorably compares his own people to the Japanese, whom he praises for overcoming their fear of plague controls such as isolation due to the fact that the "new universal education of the masses produced its beneficial results." To counter the sometimes violent resistance of the mob, which included gun and knife threats made against members of his staff, Wu authorized the publication of "thousands of circulars," as well as a daily newspaper, giving details of the service's ongoing fight against the epidemic. In addition, Wu's assistants "gave public lectures whenever possible and answered any questions that might be asked them by their audience" as part of his own education offensive in Manchuria.[185] Wu's counterpart in India was Dr. U. L. Desai, a native physician also educated in England posted at the plague hospital in Nasik, who recommended farther reaching measures against the plague than even the British Civil Service was willing to contemplate, to include improvements in sewage systems, better housing, educational schemes to promote hygiene, and compulsory registration of all medical practitioners, aimed particularly at native *vaids* and *hakims*.[186] Some native newspapers also sided with the British government by urging their readers to submit to plague measures, even if they be distasteful, for the greater good of the public health. On the other hand, when newspapers did advance people's objections to such measures, many did so primarily from a cultural, rather than colonial, point of view. The *Bangavasi* of Pune, for example, cited a Hindu fatalism toward disease, somewhat akin to the Muslim one reported in Tunisia, when it rhetorically asked its readers, "Why prevent the helpless and long suffering Hindu from dying in peace? When death summons us we must die. Why disturb and distract us in the name of science?"[187] When *Vyápári* objected to plague measures such as "the limewashing of houses, the destruction of huts, [and] the compulsory segregation of plague patients," which it characterized as "nothing but folly and madness," it likewise did so on the grounds that modern medicine was foreign to native customs and beliefs:

> These may be the most approved means, according to Western sanitary science, of stamping out the plague, but it will be very difficult to persuade an orthodox Native to believe in their efficacy. Our people, who are brought up in the old order of ideas, generally look upon such epidemic diseases as the result of Divine displeasure and so they seek to suppress them by offering oblations to the Deity and so forth.

Since "no one knows anything for certain about the plague and the proper means of suppressing it," the editors felt that the government's efforts as of February 1897 were a laughable "misdirection of energy."[188]

A third view, however, claims that native objections to Western science and medicine as represented by British plague controls in India were not based on an inveterately hostile cultural response, which was never "uniform" or "homogenous" in any case, but rather on the fact that, even though it had now entered a promising new era, the modern medical tradition of the West was too often simply ineffective and incapable of curing or preventing the plague. When accessible and accommodating to native sensibilities, locals could in fact prove themselves quite willing to avail themselves of Western doctors and hospitals. This suggests that the political and cultural dynamics of the Third Pandemic in India were conditioned primarily by the disease of plague itself, which due to its uniquely dramatic history (particularly during the Black Death) and characteristics, set off a "panic" both in the British government and among its native subjects, who had to respond not only to the plague but also to the unusually oppressive measures devised to contain it.[189] If true, such an interpretation would imply a continuity of historical responses to plague, but a possible objection is that native protests to plague controls in India were not exactly comparable to those made in Italy during the Second Pandemic, since the latter were based primarily on economic, rather than medical or cultural, grounds.

Although the case studies in India, China, and Senegal during the Third Pandemic of plague are the most studied and well known, the dynamics of modern efforts to control plague likewise played out at ports of call all around the world. For instance, significant native resistance to plague controls imposed by imperial or Western-leaning governments occurred in the British colony of Hong Kong in 1894; at Rio de Janeiro in Brazil, Honolulu in Hawaii, and San Francisco in the United States in 1900; and at Cape Town in South Africa in 1901. However, at Alexandria in Egypt and Sydney in Australia, plague's impact was minimal, and resistance to antiplague measures was muted in 1899–1900; in the former case, this was perhaps because the native Muslim medical tradition was somewhat compatible with the West's and the government's health policy respected its population's pluralistic culture, while in the latter case, health authorities eventually shifted their focus to controlling the rodent population rather than quarantining the human one, which proved to be a more enlightened approach to combating plague. At Rio de Janeiro, Cape Town, Honolulu, and San Francisco, there was a markedly racial element to authorities' plague measures, which disproportionately targeted native people of color and immigrant Chinese. In Rio, both the government's policies toward plague and popular resistance to them, which ended with the demolition of the Afro-Brazilian district of the city, were influenced by roughly concurrent measures against two other diseases, yellow fever and smallpox. Honolulu's Chinatown was accidentally destroyed by a fire set initially as a "controlled burn" to contain plague and for which the U.S. government never adequately compensated its victims. The forced segregation of black Africans by the British in Cape Town became an important precedent for the later apartheid policy in South Africa. And in both Buenos Aires, Argentina, and in San Francisco, authorities engaged in a counterproductive denial of the existence of plague, with the collusion of the local press.[190]

One of the three general lessons to be learned from all three pandemics of plague, and which we will see apply to other diseases as well, is therefore this one: that throughout the ages and into the foreseeable future, medicine will be limited in terms of its effectiveness in fighting some diseases, like plague. While modern medicine has proven its ability to eradicate certain illnesses, such as smallpox (discussed in the next chapter), a disease like plague is too extensively endemic in too many places around the world to simply disappear from human history. This, of course, is not even counting the fact that newly emerging diseases, like the 2009 swine flu pandemic, will always arise to challenge medicine and that even older diseases like plague and tuberculosis can mutate into drug-resistant strains to elude our cures. But even when medicine was woefully impotent against plague, as it was during the First and Second Pandemics, doctors were still convinced they could make headway against the disease, and who knows, with some measures like self-imposed quarantine and mass evacuation that were adopted by Venice during a plague in 1576, perhaps they did.[191] In turn, modern medicine during the Third Pandemic learned to be humble in the face of plague, when its very response to the disease, even when armed with its new knowledge about germs, provoked a reaction from its would-be patients that proved counterproductive to its efforts. Modern medicine thus needs to strike a balance with diseases like plague, particularly when its "miracle cures," like vaccination or antibiotics, prove ineffective or are not at hand, so that it will be forced to fall back on what are now "traditional" measures, like quarantine. How will modern society react to such outdated methods to control disease when these may seem as culturally foreign and objectionable as the British plague hospitals did to native Indians during the Third Pandemic? Certain implications of plague controls, such as that family members might become separated or that economic livelihoods may be disrupted, probably will always be protested no matter how culturally predisposed a civilization or society is to them. This past year, for example, the Vermont department of health asked my wife and I in a phone survey if we would be willing to quarantine ourselves in our home for a whole month should an untreatable flu outbreak occur. While we have no ideological objections to such a measure, it did raise some eminently practical questions, like how would we stock up on enough food and survive an enforced unemployment for such a lengthy period of time? Our society, and each individual within it, will have to decide how far it is willing to go in order to safeguard itself from a terrifying, "plague-like" disease.

The second lesson of plague is that a disease that can follow in the wake of either animal or human migrations will always be global in scope, insofar as this is defined by the trade and travel patterns of the times. During the First Pandemic, plague was largely delineated by the sea networks of the Mediterranean region; during the Second Pandemic, by the overland trade routes of the Mongol Empire across Eurasia; and during the Third Pandemic and into modern times, there now seems to be no geographical limit to disease, what with the global reach of ship and airplane transport. So what once used to be a localized outbreak in some exotic corner of the globe is now our backyard epidemic. This necessitates, of course, ever greater and more sophisticated vigilance to try to contain pandemics, only to be led by agencies with transnational authority and clout, such as the World Health Organization (WHO). We can only hope they are up to the challenge.

The third and last lesson of plague is how there are always winners and losers to disease, both *within* a given society or culture and *between* rival civilizations. During all three pandemics, some civilizations appeared to benefit from, or at least tried to profit by, the plague: the Islamic Umayyad caliphate rose to power during the First Pandemic; Europe emerged economically and technologically superior to the Middle East by the end of the Second Pandemic; and the British Empire attempted to cement its rule in India during the Third Pandemic. In England during the Black Death, the peasant classes seemed to benefit economically the most from the plague, while the opposite was true in Egypt. Yet, these impacts were, for the most part, entirely unpredictable. When the British Civil Service, for example, intentionally tried to use the Third Pandemic as an opportunity to demonstrate the medical benefits of the empire and so further its influence among its native subjects, what it ended up with was, in the words of one scholar, "the greatest upsurge of public resistance to Western medicine and sanitation that nineteenth-century India had witnessed," such that it represented "a profound crisis for . . . the power of the colonial state."[192] While plague and its controls instilled chaos, terror, and social tensions in towns and villages across India that brought everyday life to a standstill, some disreputable elements were nonetheless able to benefit by means of extortion and crime.[193] By contrast, when the government of medieval England tried and failed to turn the clock back on the economic effects of the Black Death through its labor legislation, it benefited enormously from the economic power unleashed from its eventually liberated peasantry. With such unintended results as these, who indeed would wish to be visited by plague in the hope that somehow they will be the victor by it?

Of one thing we can be certain: plague, the most dramatic of all diseases in terms of its absolute mortality, has also had the most drastic cultural impacts upon the civilization or society that was made to feel, whether for good or ill, its wrath.

CHAPTER 2

Smallpox

Smallpox is an ancient disease, perhaps even older than plague, that seems to have first arisen among the earliest human civilizations with settled populations large enough to sustain its epidemics, such as in Mesopotamia, Egypt, or the Indus River valley. Conclusive evidence of smallpox emerged during the second millennium B.C.E. in Egypt, with the physical evidence of its characteristic pustules on the skin preserved in the mummified remains of certain individuals, such as the Pharaoh Ramses V (reigned c. 1149–1145). Positive identification of the smallpox rash on Ramses' mummy was made in 1979 by the medical specialist and historian of smallpox Donald Hopkins.[1] The contemporary Ebers Papyrus, one of the oldest medical manuscripts in existence, may also confirm the presence of smallpox in ancient Egypt, as it contains a brief reference to a skin ailment.[2] Equally ancient evidence of smallpox seems to come from India, where the Sanskrit medical text, the *Susruta Samhita*, attributed to the Hindu physician Dhanwantari and dating to c. 400 C.E., but perhaps preserving some passages that go as far back as 1500 B.C.E., gives what appears to be a detailed description of the disease, including fever, backache, prostration, and, of course, the telltale inflamed and dimpled pustules.[3]

Smallpox is caused by a virus, a microscopic infectious disease agent that, unlike a bacterium, is an incomplete organism that needs to invade a host cell in order to reproduce and spread within the body. It consists of nucleic acid, either DNA or, more commonly, RNA, surrounded by a protein coat that allows the virus to attach itself to a host cell and then penetrate it in order to use the host cell's biological mechanisms to replicate itself. Some viruses, instead of simply duplicating the viral genome, use their RNA template to manufacture DNA, a process known as reverse transcription; one class of these viruses, known as ret-roviruses, which includes the human immunodeficiency virus (HIV) that causes AIDS (acquired immune deficiency syndrome), are particularly insidious as they incorporate their manufactured DNA into that of the host cell, thus making this "Frankenstein's monster" practically indistinguishable from other, healthy cells. Once assembled, the viral copies are then released when the host cell ruptures and dies, a process called lysis. Viruses are also prone to genetic mutations, called antigenic drift, as well as to recombinations with other viruses, or antigenic shift; it is by such processes that new, often deadly viruses are created, as typically hap-pens with ever-changing influenza strains. This also makes it difficult to treat certain viruses or prevent infection by them. The smallpox or variola virus is an example of a DNA virus.

Smallpox probably originated as a virus prevalent in an animal reservoir that then made the jump to humans following the domestication of animals some eleven or twelve thousand years ago. It is a member of the orthopoxvirus family, which includes viruses that also affect monkeys, rodents, cats, camels, elephants, and water buffalo and cattle; the last is probably the most likely contender as the vector that passed the smallpox virus from animals to humans.[4] Even today, cowpox and buffalopox viruses can cause mild infections in human victims, typically by milking infected udders. There are two main types of the smallpox virus, *Variola major* and *Variola minor*, with the former being the more com-monly occurring in human history and also the more deadly, killing on average about a third of its victims. Infection with *Variola minor* was almost a godsend, as it killed just 1 percent or less of those who contracted it, yet it conferred life-long immunity to the disease, even in its more severe form. The virus itself was not physically seen and identified with an electron microscope until the 1940s, even though awareness of viruses as organisms distinct from bacteria, which was achieved through special, fine filters that could separate the two, was achieved by the end of the nineteenth century. The Latin term, *variola*, which in the Middle Ages came to mean "pox" and was probably derived from the Latin word for "spotted" (*varius*) or "pimple" (*varus*), was first used in connection with the disease during the sixth century C.E. It was at the very end of the Middle Ages, in around 1494, that smallpox acquired its name in order to distinguish it from a new disease to Europe that struck the soldiers of the French king, Charles VIII, as they were besieging Naples in that year; *la grosse vérole*, or "great pox," also known as the "French disease," was a venereal-type illness that some identify with syphilis just imported from the New World in the wake of Columbus's voy-ages, while the older disease producing pustule symptoms was now called *la pe-tite vérole*, or "small pox."

Smallpox's symptoms were intimately bound up with how the disease was spread. After an incubation period of nine to twelve days, the victim typically experienced a violent fever accompanied by chills, nausea, aches and pains, and sometimes convulsions and delirium. Then a rash of small reddish spots appeared on the mucous membranes of the mouth, tongue, upper palate, and throat, which quickly enlarged and ruptured, releasing millions of viruses into the saliva, making the disease highly contagious at this stage from person to person by means of droplet infection. Next, the virus invaded the outer skin cells, forming raised pimples and then broader pustules filled with fluid (not pus) that became opaque and then slowly leaked out until the lesions dried up, scabbed over, and flaked off, which happened two to three weeks later. Scarring and sometimes blindness occurred, leaving the characteristic pockmarks that forever signaled to the world a victim of smallpox. Since the pustules formed heaviest on the face and the extremities, smallpox was a very visible disease, practically impossible to hide, so that even though the victim was infectious for as long as he or she exhibited its symptoms, it was also abundantly clear who had the disease and thus who should have been avoided.

Nevertheless, the scabs and liquid "matter" of smallpox victims present in their clothing or bedding (what the sixteenth-century physician Girolamo Fracastoro called the "fomites" or seeds of disease) could still have infected others even when no direct contact was made with the victims themselves; usually, however, smallpox contagion occurred through close, direct contact with victims, such as often happened among members of the same household, and when victims were in the most infectious stage of the disease during the first week of the rash appearing on their bodies. Some types of smallpox were invariably fatal, such as the "malignant" variety—whereby the pustules were slower to mature and remained flush with the skin (hence the name "flat smallpox"); fulminating or hemorrhagic smallpox—characterized by massive bleeding internally and into the skin, forming petechiae that made the skin appear black and turned the eyes red but with little to no pustules; and confluent smallpox, in which the pustules ran into each other and formed single, extensive sheets that peeled off to expose the inner epidermis and tissue that easily became infected, so that the victims died of secondary or opportunistic bacterial diseases rather than from the smallpox itself. Milder versions of smallpox included the less frequent *Variola minor* variety where scarring was less likely to occur, even though it had the same type of symptoms and method of transmission as the ordinary version, and "modified" smallpox, often confused with chickenpox, which typically appeared in people previously vaccinated for the disease but in whom the vaccine was no longer effective.

The history of smallpox is mainly characterized by the differential way in which it strikes its victims, both within a given society or culture and between sometimes competing civilizations. Smallpox in this respect is therefore quite different from plague, which confers no compensating immunity upon those who are made to suffer its ravages and which during the time of the Black Death in late medieval Europe had a notorious reputation, even if this was not borne out in fact, of equitably harvesting its victims, as evidenced by the popular Dance of Death artistic motif that was frequently associated with plague, in which various members of the social hierarchy, in descending order from pope and emperor on down to hermit and poor man, must all dance a reel with death.[5] Smallpox then had a very different dynamic from plague, in which its impact was felt not so much through any massive mortality on the scale of the Black Death but instead through the simple reality that not everyone was killed off or even affected by the disease. There was thus a kind of disease "favoritism" at work with smallpox, which could be quite vindicating for those fortunate enough to be immune, but rather demoralizing, to say the least, for those who were disproportionately impacted by it. This also meant that smallpox was much more disposed to interacting with other sociological and cultural factors besides disease, such as colonialism and imperialism, than plague, which tended to be more autonomous due to its overwhelming mortality and morbidity. In addition, one should keep in mind that smallpox is now an extinct disease, one that was uniquely conquered by modern medicine, which is quite a different experience from that of more intractable diseases that still plague us to this day, including tuberculosis, influenza, and, yes, plague.

The major epidemics of smallpox around the world and throughout history amply reveal its distinguishing, differential characteristic. Perhaps the first outbreak to receive the attention of ancient historians of disease was the Plague of Athens of 430–426 B.C.E., as chronicled by Thucydides. We have already explored in the introduction the issues of identifying the Plague of Athens with smallpox and its long-term impacts upon Athens' conduct of the Peloponnesian War. Smallpox accords well not only with Thucydides' description of symptoms but also with his account of its rapid spread; although the disease seems to have died down after 426, giving the Athenian population a chance to recover its former numbers, its early timing may well have set the stage for the city's conduct during the rest of the war by supposedly undermining its celebrated veneer as a civilized, moral standard-bearer for Greece—or, to borrow Thucydides' phrase as put into the mouth of Pericles, as the "school of Hellas"—that was used to justify the war in the first place.

But for our purposes here, the main thing to be noted about the Plague of Athens is how it coincided with war and at the same time with a lopsided mortality and morbidity that affected only one side in the conflict, a fact that was duly noted by Thucydides. This naturally suggested to the Athenians that their enemies, the Spartans, who seemed immune to the disease, must have deliberately planted the epidemic among them as part of a campaign of biological warfare; this was all the more easy to believe as the Athenians themselves had apparently employed this tactic during their siege of Cirrha in the sixth century, when they poisoned a stream supplying water to the city. Rationally speaking, however, observers like Thucydides recognized that overcrowding in the city, as refugees poured in at the start of the war to take cover behind the "long walls" from the Peloponnesian army that was ravaging the countryside, was really at the root of the outbreak. Athenian trade and its cosmopolitan openness to foreigners, which was so celebrated by Pericles in his "Funeral Oration" to honor the first Athenian dead in the war, as reported by Thucydides, must have also played a role in bringing the disease to Athens, just as the closed-door policy of Sparta ensured its virtual quarantine. Psychologically speaking, this differential quality to the Plague of Athens had its demoralizing effect on the populace, a factor that nonetheless the Spartans failed to exploit due to their own fears of contracting the illness.[6] As we will see, however, the later history of smallpox was to prove not so forgiving.

The next major outbreak of smallpox to be recorded in history is believed to be the Plague of the Antonines, which struck the Roman Empire beginning in 165 C.E., during the reign of the last of the Five Good Emperors, Marcus Aurelius Antoninus (161–180), who seems to have died of the disease, and extending perhaps into that of his son, Lucius Aurelius Commodus Antoninus (180–192). While no hard mortality statistics are available for this epidemic, best estimates are that it carried off 10 percent of the empire's population, which would be enough to make an impact, certainly, but not so much that a relatively swift recovery could not be made. Nonetheless, it has been argued that, once again, smallpox was ill timed to coincide with war, when the empire began facing challenges from the Parthian Empire in the east and from the Germans to the north; the loss of manpower to disease at such a critical time may have made a difference in Rome's future ability to fight off the "Barbarian" threat and compelled it to recruit soldiers from among the Germans themselves in order to make up the numbers, a policy that would have grave implications later by the end of the empire in the fifth century.[7]

The Middle Ages saw an important breakthrough in medical diagnosis and treatment of smallpox when the Persian physician, Muhammad ibn Zakariyā al-Rāzī (865–925), known simply as Rhazes in the West, composed his *Treatise on the Small-pox and Measles* based on his experience treating patients as head of the hospital at Baghdad, the capital of the Abbasid caliphs. Rhazes provided the first definitive symptomatology of smallpox, distinguishing it from measles primarily by the presence of severe backache, but he also noticed that smallpox was characterized by a "continuous fever," a "stinging pain in the whole body," a "violent redness of the cheeks and eyes," as well as a "pain in the throat and breast," all of which were also noted by Thucydides during the Plague of Athens. Rhazes also supplied the important evidence that smallpox was primarily a childhood disease in his time, which indicates that it had by now become endemic to the Eurasian continent as a regularly occurring disease.[8]

By far the most controversial, notorious, and studied outbreak of smallpox in human history seems to be that which occurred in the American hemisphere—Mexico, the Caribbean, and Central, South, and North America— beginning in the early sixteenth century and raging through to the next century and beyond. This has been called nothing less than an American "Holocaust" or "Apocalypse" of mortality among the native populations of these regions, but it must be remembered that it took at least a century for such demographic losses to be registered in what records we have; what is more, a panoply of diseases besides smallpox helped bring about the catastrophe, including other directly contagious ills like measles, influenza, pneumonic plague, and mumps, as well as those spread by other means such as an insect vector or contaminated water supplies, which would include typhus, bubonic plague, yellow fever, malaria, and cholera. Smallpox, however, was among the earliest and apparently most deadly diseases to strike the Americas, making landfall first on the island of Hispaniola (modern-day Dominican Republic and Haiti) in 1518 and then the mainland of Mexico in 1520 in the wake of the expedition of Hernán Cortés that culminated with the conquest of the Aztec Empire. Around the same time, during the 1520s, smallpox also arrived in Guatemala, Panama, and Ecuador in Central and South America. Throughout the rest of the century, smallpox reappeared somewhere in the western hemisphere on a regular basis almost every other decade; it finally appeared in Brazil in 1562, and by the end of the century it was the turn of the natives in North America to also feel its wrath. Smallpox seems to have arrived first in the southwestern United States and northern Mexico during the 1580s and 1590s, then the northeastern region in the second or fourth decade of the seventeenth century, followed by Florida and the southeast in 1655, and finally the Pacific Northwest and Great Plains during the 1780s. In the latter two regions, smallpox continued its ravages even into the first half of the nineteenth century, before federal vaccination efforts took effect. Even though Old World diseases came later to Brazil and North America compared to the rest of the hemisphere, and native populations there were more dispersed than in the population centers of the Aztec and Inca empires, declines are estimated to be just as great as anywhere else, especially since Brazil and North America became just as much, if not more, active in the slave trade from Africa, which was another source of disease introduction to the New World.[9]

Much debate still exists as to the exact numbers of victims who succumbed at this time: mainly the issue centers around pre-Columbian estimates of population, which must rely on inexact measures such as anecdotal testimonial evidence, archaeological artifacts, and educated guesses as to the "carrying capacity" of the land. Mexico, for example, may have had a total native population in 1519 ranging from three to fifty-eight million, which would put its decline by 1605 at anywhere from 67 to 98 percent; the Andes region in South America may have numbered from two to thirty-seven million in 1532, making its decline by 1620 somewhere between 70 and 98 percent.[10] But even when opting for the lowest estimates of population loss, the Native American die-off was enormous, prompting one historian, David Noble Cook, to dub it the "greatest human catastrophe in history."[11]

For an older generation of historians, led initially by John Duffy, Alfred Crosby, and William McNeill, disease was assigned an almost monocausal role in the American Holocaust, even when other factors besides the introduction of germs, such as the importation from Europe of new plants and animals to the Americas, were invoked to explain how disease was able to wreak its havoc.[12] Disease was able to reach such tragic proportions in the Americas supposedly because it took root in the "virgin soil" of a population that had no prior exposure to Europe's epidemics, even though Native Americans did have their own, pre-Columbian illnesses, including dysentery and other gastrointestinal diseases, tuberculosis, fungal and streptococcal infections, bacterial pneumonia, and possibly malaria, yellow fever, typhus, and influenza. They also had some form of venereal disease, such as syphilis, that may have been their "gift" back the other way to the Europeans. Yet, the successive waves of ever-changing epidemic disease crashing in on American shores with each new generation of settlers or slaves arriving from Europe and Africa never gave natives a chance to recover their numbers from any single outbreak; even in the case of those who survived a bout with smallpox or measles and thus developed immunity to it, there was always the specter of some new illness on the horizon to claim its share of victims. For example, after Mexico's disastrous encounter with smallpox during the 1520s, measles struck Mexico and Central America during the 1530s, then it was the turn of typhus and possibly pneumonic plague in the 1540s, followed by a lethal combination of smallpox, influenza, and measles in Guatemala and the Andes during the 1550s and 1560s, with typhus added to the mix during the 1570s, 1580s, and early 1590s.[13]

For some scholars, no other explanation aside from disease need be considered in order to account for the precipitous decline in numbers and, by implication, in cultural vitality, of Native American populations during the century or more following Columbus's first contact in 1492. Thomas Whitmore, for instance, declares that the "presumption of disease mortality as the overwhelming cause of Amerindian population decline throughout the New World seems virtually irrefutable," since "the principle of Occam's razor [that the simplest explanation is best] suggests that it is not necessary to assume that there were other important causes of death."[14] Others, drawing on the older positions of disease historians like Hans Zinnser and Henry Sigerist, also place some emphasis on the mercurial nature of disease to mow down the "great actors" of history, such as the Aztec leader Cuitláhuac and the Inca emperor Huayna Capac, both of whom succumbed to smallpox, in sealing the fate of American civilizations.[15] But did disease really act alone to deal out all this damage? More recent scholars of the New World Holocaust seem not so satisfied with this answer.

Instead, the latest consensus has coalesced around the idea that disease must interact with other cultural factors, in this case primarily colonial or imperialistic oppression, in order to satisfactorily explain the collapse of Native American societies. Perhaps the most persuasive argument to be made for this position is a comparative one, in which the smallpox epidemic in the Americas is analyzed alongside the outbreak of plague in Europe during the late Middle Ages, which we just explored in the previous chapter. Why did Europe recover, both culturally and in demographic terms, from its bout with deadly epidemic disease at the dawn of the Early Modern period whereas at this very same time American civilizations were about to embark on a completely different trajectory with the arrival of their own plagues? Keep in mind that the Black Death, no less than smallpox in the Americas, behaved as if it were rampaging on virgin soil in Europe, given the extremely high mortalities achieved in just a few years. Also remember that plague kept coming back to decimate European populations in successive waves in succeeding decades, just as smallpox did in the New World, and that it likewise did so in conjunction with other illnesses, albeit ones perhaps not as deadly as each new disease was in the Americas.[16] One study based on the obituary lists for Christ Church Priory in Kent throughout the fifteenth century reveals that plague, a killer in a third of all disease outbreaks among the monks, was accompanied by tuberculosis, the "sweat" (a mysterious deadly disease characterized by chills, fever, and profuse sweating that first broke out in England in 1485), dropsy or edema, and strangury (a painful inability to urinate).[17] A doctor writing from Avignon in 1382, Raymond Chalin de Vinario, also pointed to the "great variety of epidemic diseases" that were appearing in his time, including ulcerous scabies (a skin itch or rash), intestinal worms, and "semi-tertian fevers" (malaria).[18]

The obvious answer to this comparative conundrum seems to be that Europe hadn't had to face an invasion by another civilization bent on its conquest at the same time that it was being conquered by disease, a civilization that was not only ruthless and in some ways technologically superior but also, most significantly, seemingly immune to the very diseases before which the natives were so helpless. Imagine if, during the Black Death, Europe also faced a massive onslaught from the Mongol Empire, in which the invading Mongol armies were indifferent to the plague, rather than being just as susceptible to it as the Europeans, and indeed seemed to use the disease as their ally. Would Europe as we know it have survived? This scenario is not so very far-fetched as it might seem; just a century earlier the armies of the Great Khan had reached the gates of Vienna before the death of their leader called them back east, and we have already seen how in 1346 the Mongols at Caffa communicated the plague to some Genoese merchants through a form a biological warfare, even as their own ranks were falling to the Black Death.

It has recently been argued that the Mesoamerican experience with disease during the sixteenth and seventeenth centuries in many ways mirrored that of the Europeans and other cultures during their own epidemic crises, such as the Black Death. This similarity extends to the severity of each disease outbreak, which in both Europe and the Americas supposedly averaged between 25 and 50 percent; the circumstances surrounding epidemics in both regions were likewise comparable, being caused and spread primarily by trade contacts and networks and accompanied by exacerbating factors such as warfare. Human responses to disease among Native Americans could also strike similar chords in other cultures, such as their attribution of outbreaks to a combination of divine or supernatural causes and natural ones, and their explanation of the occurrence of disease in humans as owing to an imbalance that needed to be corrected if prevention or cure was to be effected. For example, Andean healers believed in the three fluids of life of air, blood, and fat that correspond to the Indian Ayurvedic *dosas* or the Greek humoral system, while the Aztecs subscribed to a cosmic dualism that has parallels with the yin-yang concept in China.[19] As in Europe and the Middle East, the Aztecs also usually attributed disease to a higher power such as their gods, whom they believed they had offended in some fashion, and they treated illnesses through a familiar combination of prayer, bloodletting, diet (expressed in opposites of hot and cold), and herbal remedies, in which they were known to be particularly expert.[20]

The disease Holocaust in the New World should therefore not be taken as the exception to the human experience with epidemics that it has traditionally been thought but rather needs to be fully integrated into the overall history of disease. At the same time, however, even the proponents of this view will admit there are some aspects of the American experience with disease that are uniquely tragic and catastrophic. One difference is the confluence of "virgin soil" diseases that struck the Americas almost simultaneously compared to the rest of the world, especially since Europe, Africa, China, and India were all interconnected epidemically by ancient trade patterns that made them part of one "disease pool," with the result that European colonialism within this pool did not enjoy the same demographic advantages as it did in the New World. Of far greater impact, however, was the simultaneous occurrence of colonial oppression, popularly known as the "Black Legend," that was chronicled by propagandists even among the Spanish themselves, such as the Dominican friar Bartolomé de las Casas, which augmented and sometimes exacerbated the massive population losses to disease. Here, untold thousands succumbed to a combination of outright military conquest, slavery, and forced labor and migration. Although these losses have long been known to scholars, and indeed have lately been discounted somewhat as the product of propaganda exaggeration, until now the implications of their interconnectedness with the concurrent die-offs due to disease have not been fully realized.[21]

It is true that in Europe, too, disease often coincided with warfare, sometimes with deliberate timing, as when Florence launched attacks on its rivals on the Italian peninsula to coincide with outbreaks of plague during the late fourteenth and early fifteenth centuries.[22] But there is probably nothing to compare with the concerted assault from European colonial powers upon the disease-ridden New World, an assault that, unlike the wars in Europe, came from an entirely alien culture that, as already mentioned, was largely immune to the epidemics decimating its rival civilizations. In the territories administered by Spain, Portugal, and France, it can confidently be asserted that the native die-off from disease was unintentional, since these countries relied on indigenous labor and contacts in order to exploit their colonies for their benefit. In the English colonies of North America, however, the settlers' hunger for land was entirely inimical to the natives' presence, and so the latter's epidemiological misfortunes were actually celebrated or even deliberately planned, as in the famous incident of Jeffrey Amherst, British commander at Fort Pitt in present-day Pennsylvania, ordering the distribution of smallpox-infected blankets among the Ottawa tribe during the Pontiac rebellion of 1763 as a form of biological warfare. But even among those whose treatment of the natives could be said to be the least detrimental to their survival, such as the Catholic missionaries in New Spain and New France, their policies of resettlement or *reducciónes* of Native American populations, whereby whole tribes were herded together into missions for the purposes of conversion, unwittingly helped spread crowd diseases like smallpox much faster and more effectively than if their charges were simply left alone.

I also believe that, aside from the numbers directly killed by its impact, European colonialism interacted in a synergistic way with disease to greatly augment population losses during epidemics, in that colonial policies helped to drastically lower native cultural abilities to resist and recover from epidemiological setbacks. Whereas Europe was able to weather and eventually overcome the long demographic stagnation imposed by the Black Death from 1348 until at least 1450, Native Americans by contrast were at a severe cultural disadvantage for doing so, quite aside from the sheer number, severity, and timing of the epidemics themselves. For example, it has been asserted that both European and Native American societies responded to major disease outbreaks with terror, fear, and despair; I have argued elsewhere, however, that such a characterization has been grossly exaggerated when describing the European response to the Black Death in the late Middle Ages. An assortment of humanists, doctors, artists, mystics, and even clergymen began formulating alternatives to the obsessively morbid "guilt culture" that supposedly imbued late medieval Europe in the aftermath of the Black Death.[23]

On the other hand, such fatalistic attitudes are more believable in the New World in the context of the intersection between the Black Legend and disease. Contemporary reports, mostly from European observers, do testify to natives who succumbed to suicide, self-inflicted abortions, reluctance to reproduce, and other symptoms of a demoralized and defeated mentality. The mood seems captured by the Yucatan *Book of Chilam Balam of Chumayel*, which bemoans, "Great was the stench of the dead. After our fathers and grandfathers succumbed, half of the people fled to the fields. The dogs and vultures devoured the bodies. The mortality was terrible. . . . So it was that we became orphans, oh my sons! So we became when we were young. All of us were thus. We were born to die!"[24] Smallpox was very conducive to this depressed outlook among survivors because of the disfigurement it produced, to which some Native American cultures that apparently prized the beauty of their complexions were particularly sensitive. Studies of the impact of "virgin soil" epidemics in the Hawaiian islands during the eighteenth and nineteenth centuries, where smallpox was perhaps the most feared of all diseases that also included measles, mumps, whooping cough, chickenpox, influenza, and tuberculosis, nonetheless conclude that declining birth and fertility rates and high male-to-female ratios were primarily responsible for the drastic population declines in the region. Sterility caused by venereal diseases such as syphilis and gonorrhea are largely held to blame, but a collective cultural suicidal impulse brought on by racial oppression from white *haole* colonists and missionaries—expressed in the form of abortions and suicides induced either deliberately or through simple neglect or "anomie"—are also believed to have played a role, particularly in skewing the relative proportions of the sexes. Venereal diseases may likewise have been facilitated by cultural attitudes such as the reputed open sexual mores of the Hawaiians.[25]

Even when Native American responses to disease are similar to those in other cultures, the fact that these responses were not allowed to express themselves in isolation but were impinged upon by the responses of a completely different culture changes the dynamics of the outcome. A good example of this is the typical explanation of disease as the product of the displeasure of the gods, an outlook that natives in the New World shared with the new arrivals from the Old World. As if the wrath of one's own gods was not bad enough, Native Americans were also told that the rival Christian God likewise caused disease, so that they were then caught in an epidemiological catch-22, being subject to some kind of epidemic punishment no matter whom they worshipped. I think it also possible that the differential mortality and morbidity with which a disease like smallpox afflicted Native Americans as compared with Europeans (for whom, at least during the Middle Ages, smallpox seems to have behaved like a relatively mild childhood disease) encouraged New World societies to view their gods as defeated by the one God of the Christians,[26] especially since they already viewed their own gods as sometimes battling each other, such as the Aztec legend of the defeat and banishment of Quetzalcoatl by Tezcatlipoca.

Another parallel set of responses that actually turns out to be dissimilar is the tendency to flee any occurrence of a disease, even when it occurs among one's own family, which we have seen was widely reported in Europe during the Black Death and was likewise observed among Native Americans during smallpox epidemics. (Only in the Muslim Middle East does there seem to have been a cultural antipathy *against* flight.) Yet, here again, the experience was not the same. Not only did flight threaten to disrupt the traditional communal bonds holding together a society, as Giovanni Boccaccio complained it did in Florence during the Black Death, but also to this was added in the New World the humiliating spectacle of some Europeans, such as the Jesuit missionaries, being more charitable toward the natives than the natives themselves as they stayed behind to nurse the sick. It is quite likely that European medicine at this stage was no more effective in treating smallpox than native healing methods. Although some have blamed the traditional indigenous practice of resorting to sweat lodges alternating with cold baths or immersions in lakes for fatally exacerbating the illness, European observers tended to view any kind of bathing with suspicion on both moral and humoral grounds, while some European doctors, such as a Master Bernard of Frankfurt and Theobaldus Loneti of Besançon, advocated their own sweating regimens as a cure for plague.[27] But because European healers in the New World such as the Jesuits had the great advantage of being seemingly immune to a disease like smallpox, they were able to fill a void left by native shamans and *hechicheros* who had failed to cure illnesses with their own brand of magic and so were able to persuade many natives to abandon their own belief systems, as one study of the impact of disease upon native culture in northwestern New Spain has found. In addition, agents of colonialism such as the Jesuits already had an ideological framework in place with which they could readily explain and rationalize epidemics of smallpox.[28]

Even as the symbiotic relationship between disease and cultural imperialism was playing itself out in the New World, smallpox was once again gaining in virulence in the Old World, perhaps as a result of the reimportation of a new *Variola major* strain from the Americas back to Europe. From the second half of the sixteenth century, smallpox epidemics started to recur more frequently, until by the close of the seventeenth century smallpox had become the predominant disease in Europe, apparently bypassing plague, leprosy, and syphilis as the leading killer throughout the Continent. Much of this was aided by the fact that urban populations were rising and warfare was incessant, both of which facilitated the spread and prevalence of a disease like smallpox.[29] During the eighteenth century, however, Europeans finally acquired the tools to combat the rising tide of smallpox: the century was bracketed by the introduction of the technique of inoculation at its beginning and the discovery of vaccination by its end.

Inoculation, also known as variolation, is the deliberate introduction of a weakened form of smallpox into the patient in order to induce a mild case of the disease and so create immunity to it and was widely practiced in Istanbul toward the end of the seventeenth century, after the Turks learned of it from the Chinese or the Persians. By the dawn of the next century, several European observers in Istanbul began communicating their newfound awareness of the practice, the most famous being Lady Mary Wortley Montague, wife of the British ambassador to Turkey, who eventually introduced it to England in 1721. Around this same time, inoculation also found its way to the American colonies, when the Reverend Cotton Mather of Boston learned of the practice from his West African slave, Onesimus, and from other slaves in Boston who reported that it was long and widely practiced in western Africa. Later, inoculation was to play a role in the American Revolution, when General George Washington had his soldiers inoculated in order to forestall germ warfare from the British, who were generally more immune to the disease.[30]

Then, on May 14, 1796, Dr. Edward Jenner performed his famous vaccination of a patient, an eight-year-old boy named James Phipps, with cowpox lymph taken from a sore on the hand of a milkmaid, Sara Nelmes. This was by no means the first recorded vaccination, but it was the most influential in that Jenner demonstrated that it could induce immunity to smallpox without the side effects of inoculation. Indeed, it is even claimed that vaccination can be traced all the way back to ancient Ayurvedic medicine in India. During the nineteenth century, vaccination became compulsory in many European countries, even though there was opposition mainly on the grounds of safety in terms of other diseases that might be communicated with the vaccine, and on the grounds of efficacy in that the immune response generated by vaccination was not lifelong, as in the case of inoculation. Ironically, the drastic decline of smallpox in Europe only facilitated antivaccinators' objections due to the waning urgency of vaccination itself.[31] These objections were largely overcome through the development of better vaccines and revaccination programs. It should also be pointed out that, despite the advent of vaccination, smallpox continued to devastate "virgin soil" populations throughout the nineteenth century in the Americas, the Pacific Islands, and among the Aboriginal peoples in Australia, while a more virulent strain of the disease wreaked havoc in West Africa even though it had been endemic there for centuries.

Resistance to nineteenth-century vaccination programs was encountered by European governments not only at home but also in its colonies abroad. A prime example of this is the British experience in India, where expectations were high that vaccination would be gratefully and joyfully received by natives as a benevolent marvel of Western medicine and so help cement imperial political rule in the country. But as with its later measures against the Third Pandemic of plague, the British disastrously underestimated the extent of native resistance to vaccination. These included some Hindu religious objections that were unique to India, such as that arm-to-arm transmission of the cowpox lymph might violate caste taboos and reverence for the sacred inviolability of the cow, but they also shared some of the same concerns that motivated protests in Europe, such as the unreliability of the vaccine. India also had a strong and ancient local tradition of variation and of religious rituals centered on the smallpox goddess, Sitala. Even though British medical authorities regarded native inoculators, known as *tikadars*, to be their rivals in terms of implementing their own vaccination programs, eventually they were forced by fears of widespread political unrest to adopt a more low-key, collaborative policy whereby they recruited *tikadars* as vaccinators. It was not until the end of the century that vaccination because more available and widespread in India.[32]

Another "vaccination revolt" in a former European colony famously occurred in Rio de Janeiro in Brazil in November 1904. Here the European-influenced government of Rodrigues Alves, advised by a young bacteriologist named Oswaldo Cruz, regarded vaccination as a humanitarian blessing of the new, modern, scientific approach to disease, just as the British did in India. However, the city's Afro-Brazilian population preferred its native practice of variation inherited from Africa, while socialists and other political opponents of Brazil's oligarchic regime protested the "sanitary despotism" of such public health measures being imposed by the government.[33] Antivaccination sentiments have not gone away even in this day and age; during the writing of this book, I saw a bumper sticker that said, "Say No to Forced Vaccinations." Today, the issue primarily concerns vaccines developed for influenza, of which more will be said in chapter 5.

The final chapter of the history of smallpox is the successful eradication of the disease during the twentieth century. By the time the Smallpox Eradication Program was announced by the World Health Organization (WHO) in 1966, with a goal of global eradication in ten years' time, smallpox was still endemic in South America, sub-Saharan Africa, and the Indian subcontinent and archipelagos of Southeast Asia. Almost miraculously, the program completed its eradication campaign on schedule, with the last case of *Variola major* reported in Bangladesh in 1975 and of *Variola minor* in Somalia in 1977. Complete, certifiable eradication was finally announced by WHO in 1979, which was achieved largely by a "surveillance-containment" strategy that focused only on vaccinating those who were in contact with known cases of smallpox.[34]

Today, the only controversy that still exists with respect to smallpox is whether or not to destroy the last known remaining stocks of the virus at the U.S. Centers for Disease Control in Atlanta and at the Russian State Research Center of Virology and Biotechnology in Novosibirsk. Originally, WHO had scheduled the final execution of the virus to take place on June 30, 1999, but a stay of execution was granted indefinitely at the behest of the administration of former U.S. president George W. Bush in 2001 in the immediate aftermath of the September 11 terrorist attacks. On the one hand, execution makes sense if only to avoid tragic mishaps with the virus, such as happened in Birmingham, England, in 1978, when the virus escaped from a research laboratory there, killing one person and driving another, the man in charge of the laboratory, to suicide. There is also the fear that some of the remaining supplies could somehow end up in the wrong hands and become an agent of bioterrorism, in which the virus would act almost like a virgin soil epidemic, since it has been three decades now since anyone got the disease or has been vaccinated. The dangers of even waste material from the laboratory was illustrated in 2000, when eight children at Vladivostok in Russia were diagnosed with a mild case of smallpox after playing with glass ampoules containing expired smallpox vaccines at the city's garbage dump. On the other hand, others, including Donald Hopkins, perhaps the greatest authority on smallpox, who has authored a history of the disease and participated in the Smallpox Eradication Program, argue for keeping stocks of the virus alive for research purposes and as insurance in case somehow another epidemic should break out that would require developing more or better vaccines. In 2004, for example, WHO approved genetic manipulation of the smallpox virus in order to develop drugs for treating the disease, once again in response to renewed fears of possible bioterrorism attack.[35] (To date, no cure is available for smallpox, only a vaccine.) All this shows that, once again, smallpox plays a differential role in history, even at the very putative end of its existence, when its fate is in the hands of only two countries that still have stocks of the virus. We can only hope that, regardless of the outcome of this debate, smallpox as a disease will remain consigned to the pages of history.

CHAPTER 3

Tuberculosis

Tuberculosis (TB) is an ancient disease that probably emerged in humans with the domestication of animals some ten thousand years ago at the start of the Neolithic period. Tuberculosis, like smallpox, is a crowd-dependent disease, needing a critical mass of victims in order to become endemic in a population; this would have been achieved in both animals and humans only when herds and cities would have created the prerequisite densities and contacts required. It seems that the crossover from animals to humans in tuberculosis occurred with our domestication of goats rather than cows, since the goat strain of *Mycobacterium bovis* that causes the disease in animals is more closely related to the human bacterial agent *Mycobacterium tuberculosis* than is the strain in cows.[1] However, it is entirely possible that tuberculosis occasionally afflicted Paleolithic man, since *Mycobacterium tuberculosis* has been discovered in the remains of a seventeen-thousand-year-old bison.[2] As with smallpox, the physical evidence of tuberculosis has been found in ancient Egyptian mummies and other Neolithic burial remains, particularly in the bone decay produced in their spines, giving them a humpbacked appearance. The ancient Greeks called the disease *phthisis*, which Hippocrates in his *Aphorisms* described as a wasting illness characterized by such symptoms as the coughing up of bloody sputum, loss of hair, and diarrhea. In the Middle Ages, tuberculosis was commonly referred to as scrofula or the "king's evil," in which the swelling of the neck caused by inflamed lymph nodes was believed to be curable with the miraculous touch of the royal hand, as was claimed by both the kings of France and England.

But it was not until the modern era that tuberculosis apparently reached epidemic proportions in Europe. At the end of the Middle Ages, in the late fifteenth century, tuberculosis was already the leading cause of death among the monks of Christ Church Priory in Canterbury, England, accounting for almost a third of all cases of disease diagnosed in the community.[3] By the seventeenth century, hospital and other records indicate that "consumption," as the disease became known at this time, caused a fifth of all deaths in Britain, and perhaps as much as a quarter of Europe's population was infected by the disease.[4] It should be no wonder, then, that the English author John Bunyan should famously call consumption the "captain of all these men of death" in his fictional biography *The Life and Death of Mr. Badman* published in 1680. By the next century, consumption was thought to be causing fully a third of all deaths in Europe, and mortality and morbidity from the disease probably peaked at the end of the eighteenth and during the first half of the nineteenth centuries, before beginning a long, slow decline from the 1860s on the Continent and from the 1870s in Britain.[5]

The bacillus responsible for tuberculosis was not discovered until 1882 by the German physician Robert Koch (who in the next year also uncovered the *Vibrio* bacterium that causes cholera). Koch's claim to have found a cure for tuberculosis, a solution containing killed bacteria that he called "tuberculin" and which he unveiled in 1890, proved to be premature, but it did form the basis for a skin test of the disease that is used to this day for diagnostic purposes.[6] (Only those who have been infected will develop an allergic reaction to tuberculin.) A true cure for TB had to wait until 1943, when the first of the antibiotic drugs effective against the disease, streptomycin, was discovered by a Rutgers University biochemistry professor, Selman Waksman, and his laboratory assistants, Albert Schatz and Elizabeth Bugie.[7] This was later followed by other drugs that are now frequently used in conjunction with streptomycin to treat tuberculosis, including para-aminosalicylic acid (PAS), isoniazid, and rifampin. In the meantime, a vaccine for tuberculosis was developed by two Frenchmen who headed up the Pasteur Institute at Lille, Albert Calmette and Camille Guérin, who first tested their formula containing an attenuated form of the tuberculosis bacillus, known as *bacille* Calmette-Guérin (BCG), in 1921. Even now, however, after nearly a century of trials, there is considerable debate among medical experts as to whether BCG does, in fact, provide any effective immunity; some contend it actually does more harm than good by making it difficult to diagnose whether a patient has active or latent TB.[8] It did not help that, early in BCG's history, a batch contaminated with live tuberculosis bacteria was mistakenly given to 249 babies in Lübeck, Germany, in 1930, with disastrous consequences. Tragic accidents like this one continue to be the bane of modern vaccination programs down into quite recent times, such as the association of a 1976 swine flu vaccine in the United States with a rare paralytic disease, Guillain-Barré syndrome (see chapter 5).

Yet, the steady decline of TB for almost a century prior to 1943 does pose something of a mystery. How could this happen in the absence of antibiotics? Before 1882, doctors did not even have a clear understanding of the real causes behind tuberculosis. Contagion was accepted by some, just as it had been with respect to plague since the Middle Ages, but this had to compete with other explanations, including heredity; social/moral behaviors that could predispose a person to the disease, such as alcoholism or promiscuous sexual intercourse (resulting in syphilis); and a host of environmental factors, including poor hygiene, stress, overcrowding, and poverty.[9] Even after Koch's earth-shattering discovery of *Mycobacterium tuberculosis*, debate continued as to just how the microorganism was communicated person to person; we in fact know that environmental factors such as overcrowding do make one more susceptible to tuberculosis, as the disease is rampant today in prison populations, particularly in Russia, where prisoners must sleep in shifts since there are as many as three inmates for each bed in a cell.[10] Belle Époque Frenchmen were quite right to campaign against spitting as a hygienic measure against tuberculosis, as we now know that the bacterium, in its dried form, can more easily penetrate to alveolar sacs deep inside the lungs carried on dust particles stirred up in the air rather than in larger liquid droplets emitted by contacts, and poverty naturally makes such conditions more likely.[11] We also know from recent experience that TB can behave like an opportunistic infection glomming on to other diseases, particularly AIDS, that are largely based in social and moral behaviors.[12] Finally, since it is as yet imperfectly understood why only one in ten people who are infected with the bacterium actually develop full-blown TB, while in the rest of the population the invading organisms are "walled off" in the lung in caseous or fibrous nodes known as "tubercules," there still seems to be a role to play by individual predispositions, such as heredity.[13]

Even by the standards of what was known at the time, preantibiotic treatment of TB was woefully ineffective. Bleeding was a standard medical response right up until the mid-nineteenth century; it is sometimes claimed that a phlebotomy could alleviate the symptom of haemoptysis, or the coughing up of blood from the lungs, which was taken as a sure sign of tuberculosis (made famous by the self-diagnosis of the English poet John Keats, who called the blood on his pillow "my death warrant"). However, I know from my own personal experience with this symptom (the result of chronic bronchiectasis, not tuberculosis) that only antibiotics can truly alleviate it, as the seeping of blood into the lungs will persist so long as bacterial infection remains and inhibits the healing of any scarring into the blood vessels surrounding the alveolar sacs. But starting in the second half of the nineteenth century, the sanatorium movement began to take over as the preferred method of treating the tubercular, first in Germany and then in Switzerland, where the resort at Davos became the most famous, visited by international luminaries, and that served as the setting for the novel by Thomas Mann, *The Magic Mountain*. By the end of the century, these were joined by the "cottage system" of Saranac Lake in the Adirondacks in upstate New York, founded by a physician who was himself suffering from the disease, Edward Livingston Trudeau.

The early sanitoria operated on the principle that a supervised regimen of rest and mild exercise in the bracing mountain air, supplemented by a nourishing, if not gluttonous, diet of at least three full meals a day would give the body an opportunity to exert its own natural healing powers and effect a cure of tuberculosis. The principle was not a new one, as it could be found going back to at least ancient times, and the idea of retreating to a special climate for tuberculosis was the fashion among consumptives in the earlier part of the century who favored the warmer climes of Italy, southern France, or Spain. Trudeau's famous experiment with rabbits notwithstanding, it is not clear that the sanitoria did much beyond confirm the natural progression of the disease in the patient; not even the much vaunted benefit of isolating patients from the general population is as clear cut as it might seem. Patients were usually released after a six-month period, when they were still very much infectious, and only a small minority ever had the privilege of visiting the sanatoria in the first place, as these were usually limited to early, "curable" cases of the disease or to those who could afford to pay, although some charitable institutions were set up in Britain and the United States, which survived on donations or the free labor of their inmates.[14]

The last phase of tuberculosis treatment before the advent of antibiotics was perhaps the most brutal and was not any more demonstratively effective: this was the "collapse therapy" of performing an artificial pneumothorax on the patient by inserting a hollow needle into the pleural cavity of the chest and introducing a measured amount of air in order to collapse the lung. (Sometimes injections of paraffin wax or oil were substituted for air to try to make the collapse more permanent.) Although the procedure was first introduced during the nineteenth century, it reached the height of its popularity during the 1920s and 1930s and was based on the same theoretical principles as the sanatoria (where most pneumothorax operations took place): that the lung would benefit from a resting period when it would allow itself to heal. Although a collapsed lung would, in theory, deprive the bacteria of oxygen needed for growth, this was a dangerous procedure prone to complications, such as a gas embolism in the circulatory system when the needle was not inserted correctly, which could result in death. It was also not painless, especially after the effects of local anesthetic wore off, when patients commonly described the feeling of having a "mule kick" or a "knifelike pain" delivered to their chest, and it was a procedure that had to be repeated with "refills" of air injection on a regular basis if the lung was to remain collapsed for long periods. In frequent cases where the lung adhered to the pleura due to the normal fibrous scarring of tuberculosis, open chest surgery had to be performed, with even greater risks of fatal side effects. At its most extreme, this surgery entailed removing part of the rib cage entirely, a procedure known as thoracoplasty, and cutting or removing the phrenic nerve, which paralyzed the diaphragm, in order to achieve permanent collapse, but patients ran a high risk of severe blood loss and shock. Overall, what follow-up studies were done of pneumothorax and thoracoplasty surgery showed that 50 percent or less of patients were still alive a few years later to justify such radical intervention; in a large minority of cases, it was estimated that it was completely unnecessary to the patients' chances of recovery.[15]

Given these dismal results, it still remains to be explained why incidences of tuberculosis continued to decline even before proven antibiotic treatments took effect. The most likely explanation is the general improvement in living standards of populations in the West during the second half of the nineteenth and first half of the twentieth centuries, including better housing, diet, work conditions, and so forth.[16] This makes sense if one considers that the height of the tuberculosis epidemic during the hundred years or more just prior to its protracted decline coincided with the rise and advance of industrialization in Western countries, with its attendant environmental degradation, dramatic shifts of population from rural to urban settings, and untrammeled exploitation of workers, especially children.[17] This is further indicated by setbacks to the disease that occurred when living standards temporarily fell in times of crisis or national emergency, such as during the First World War. The bare fact of this decline, more than almost any other aspect, demonstrates that tuberculosis was, and remains today, a "social disease" that depends on more than mere biology for its behavior in a given population.

Yet another efflorescence of tuberculosis's dependency on societal factors is the romantic reinvention of "consumption" during the early nineteenth century, when it was in very great danger of being nearly perceived as not a disease at all. One could in fact say that consumption at this time became almost fashionable, when it was imagined that one could simply waste painlessly away into a version of Keats's "easeful death" (the reality, as patients drowned in their own blood or gasped frantically from air hunger, was obviously quite different), and apparently some even wished to get sick in order to acquire the delicately pale looks so admired in consumptives and that even today seem to be strived for by bulimic fashion models.[18] By the end of the nineteenth century, consumption had lost most of its romantic associations, signified by the mere fact that the more prosaic term of "tuberculosis" was coming into greater usage, which was probably a function of the increasingly scientific approach to the disease following Koch's explication of its bacterial cause and of the fact that poverty was being seen more and more as the natural environmental context of tuberculosis. But until then, consumption touched the lives of many of Europe's leading artists of the romantic period, including Keats, Percy Shelley, Frédéric Chopin, Robert Schumann, the Brontë sisters, Robert Louis Stevenson (who was a patient at both Davos and Saranac Lake), and, in the United States, Edgar Allen Poe, Ralph Waldo Emerson, and Henry David Thoreau.[19] Even though many an artist's life span was prematurely cut short by the disease, it was widely believed at the time that their genius actually benefited from feverish bouts of activity induced by consumption, and indeed it is entirely possible that the tragically doomed creators' awareness of their impending demise lent a sense of urgency to their work. Tuberculosis also has a starring role in much of nineteenth-century literature, afflicting the characters of Charles Dickens, Victor Hugo, Anton Chekov, and Fyodor Dostoyevsky. Aside from Mann's *Magic Mountain*, perhaps the most well-known example is Alexandre Dumas fils's *The Lady of the Camillias*, in which tuberculosis claims its self-sacrificing heroine, Marguerite Gautier (based on Dumas' acquaintance with an actual courtesan who died of consumption at age twenty-three, Marie Duplessis). Dumas' novel and subsequent play became the inspiration of Giuseppe Verdi's opera *La Traviata* and in more modern times of the films *Camille* (1936), starring Greta Garbo as Marguerite, and *Moulin Rouge!* (2001), starring Nicole Kidman as Satine, a character clearly based on Marguerite.

An interesting footnote to this cultural aspect of tuberculosis is the disease's contribution to the vampire legend, particularly in New England. Sometimes, the decomposition of the body after death, which in the case of a disease like tuberculosis is most pronounced in the lungs, can apparently result in blood seeping from the lips, giving the impression that the corpse is still alive and achieves this feat by feasting on victims.[20] Added to this would be the suspicious circumstance, especially in an age that imperfectly understood disease contagion, of several members of a family succumbing to consumption within a relatively brief period of time. The allegedly voracious sexual appetite of tuberculosis victims may have also contributed something to the infamously sensual aspect to the legend. From the late eighteenth through to the end of the nineteenth centuries, in Rhode Island, eastern Connecticut, and my home state of Vermont, the graves of both men and women were disinterred in order that a ghastly ritual might be enacted upon the occupants, which was believed to have the power to end their supernatural scourge: this consisted of none other than cutting out the heart (often described as full of blood) of the exhumed victim and burning it to ashes nearby. It seems that nearly all of such "corpse killer" incidents were initiated by consumption running rampant through a family, giving rise to the belief that one of the deceased was now preying on the remaining members who were sickly but still alive. Part of this ritual apparently included a healing rite in which the ashes of the suspected vampire were fed to the ailing family member in the hopes that this might yet save his or her life. In at least one instance, that of Mercy Brown of Exeter, Rhode Island, whose months-old body was violated in March 1892 in an attempt to save her brother, Edwin, who likewise was to succumb to tuberculosis, this ritual occurred almost exactly ten years to the day from when Koch had announced his discovery of the bacterium that was truly sucking the life force from consumption victims.[21] On my own farm in Vermont, one can still see the traces of such desperate attempts to escape tuberculosis when walking in the woods, only to suddenly stumble upon abandoned stone walls and cellar holes that stand like ghostly sentinels to their former inhabitants' retreat halfway up the mountain in search of healthier air.

The romantic disposition of tuberculosis stands in evident contrast to that of plague and smallpox, and also of cholera. The reason for this is not hard to find: I believe it can be traced back to the physical symptoms of each disease. We have already seen how bubonic plague and smallpox can cause horribly painful and disfiguring eruptions on the body; both diseases can also be terrifyingly swift and sudden in their assault on the body's defenses. We will also see that cholera is devastatingly rapid in its progression and produced symptoms that were particularly repulsive to nineteenth-century Western sensibilities. By comparison, tuberculosis could lie hidden and dormant, scarcely noticed by the victim, for years, and, when and if it did finally emerge from its latent phase into a virulent one, it typically caused the "pale, wan, frail look" (hence the name by which tuberculosis was commonly known, the "white plague" or the "white death") that actually was admired and aspired to by fashionable beauties for at least the first half of the nineteenth century. Even the most visible symptom, the coughing up of blood, could apparently be discreetly hidden, until perhaps the very end, by a strategically placed handkerchief. Thus, tuberculosis was, for much of its romantic history it seems, the perfectly acceptable disease from which to die. The interconnectedness of the clinical and societal aspects of tuberculosis illustrates the fine line to be drawn between positivist and relativist interpretations of disease.

The latest chapter in the history of tuberculosis, which is still being written, is the emergence within the last few decades of epidemics of a multi-drug-resistant strain of the disease (known by its acronym as MDR-TB), and now an even extensively drug-resistant variety (XDR-TB). This is when TB bacteria, which are hard to kill because of their waxy coating, develop resistance to one or more antibiotic drugs by means of genetic mutations. (Keep in mind that hundreds of millions of these bacteria are usually present in a victim.) Such a scenario arises only when treatment regimens for TB fail to eliminate all bacteria that have been exposed to the drugs being used (which is said to be usually the fault of the doctor rather than the patient). Any number of circumstances may be responsible: the patient does not complete the full course of treatment (the usual "short course" of a combination of TB drugs lasts six to nine months); the doctor prescribes the wrong or insufficient dosage of drugs to correctly treat the patient's TB; the drugs have been manufactured badly (such as in a form that cannot easily be absorbed by the patient or with not enough active ingredient); or treatment centers, particularly in Russia and the third world, do not have enough drugs to allow patients to complete their recommended course. In essence, the patients now become an incubator for a far more deadly form of the disease than before they started treatment, and they can now pass this form on to other victims. It is perhaps no coincidence that, at the very same time that MDR-TB was arriving on the scene during the 1980s, a frightening, new disease called AIDS started taking its toll, which, as we will explore in more detail in chapter 6, destroys the body's immune system; AIDS makes it easier for the patient to not only contract TB but also become an incubator of MDR-TB. (Currently, tuberculosis is the most common "opportunistic infection" that actually kills off patients with AIDS.) As the first decade of the twenty-first century comes to a close, the World Health Organization (WHO) reports that a third of the world's population is currently infected with TB, with one new person becoming infected every second, and that 5 to 10 percent of those infected will go on to develop an actively virulent form of the disease. As of 2005, southeast Asia had the highest number of cases, nearly three million, or 34 percent of the world's total, followed by Africa with two and a half million, or 29 percent of all cases globally; it is no accident that these places also have some of the highest incidences of AIDS. TB strains resistant to at least one antibiotic drug have been documented in every country surveyed by WHO, and strains that are resistant to *all* major antibiotic drugs have by now emerged. More usually, MDR-TB is defined by WHO as strains resistant to the antibiotics isoniazid and rifampin; it is most prevalent apparently in the former Soviet Union.[22]

The case that is usually cited in the literature to illustrate the current MDR-TB crisis is an epidemic of both regular and MDR tuberculosis that occurred in New York City from approximately the mid-1980s to the mid-1990s.[23] At the height of the epidemic in 1992, New York had nearly four thousand TB cases, comprising 14 percent of all cases in the United States, a third of which were MDR-TB, comprising 61 percent of those in the country at large. Moreover, 23 percent of patients contracted MDR-TB without ever having been treated before, proving that the drug-resistant strain was spreading independently of its "home-grown" origins, and over 40 percent of New York's TB patients were also infected with AIDS. Whereas TB infection rates had previously been falling or holding steady, the number of cases tripled in that one year. Yet, most see the origins of the crisis as going back to the 1970s, when the U.S. Congress stopped setting aside money solely for fighting TB and allowed states to spend it at their discretion. In most places, including New York, other priorities took precedence out of a sense of complacency that epidemic TB was a thing of the past, a victory celebration that proved premature.

Eventually, New York City's TB epidemic was brought under control, largely through a policy known as directly observed therapy (DOT), in which patients complete their drug course under supervision, and which has now been adopted by WHO as its preferred method for treating TB. For MDR-TB, this strategy must be tailored to the patient by first testing to determine which drugs the bacteria are immune to and then prescribing specific second-line drugs against them, a regimen known as DOTS-plus (the acronym stands for directly observed therapy short course). Using the DOTS technique, New York City's health department was able to reverse the poor compliance rates for completing treatment, which had stood at less than half of all patients at the height of the epidemic and in some places, such as Harlem, was as low as 11 percent. By the mid-1990s, compliance rates were now at 90 percent and cases of MDR-TB saw a correspondingly dramatic decline, down 91 percent.[24]

But this remarkable achievement came at a price, and not just in monetary terms of the one billion dollar price tag for the program; although most patients completed treatment voluntarily, after signing a contract agreeing to do so that was sweetened with incentives such as free medications and food and transportation coupons, a tiny minority—forty-seven patients in all—had to be coerced into completing treatment by being detained in special wards at hospitals, such as the twenty-five-bed facility at Goldwater Memorial Hospital on Roosevelt Island. New York City's health code was amended in 1993 to allow for such detention in cases of active tuberculosis where it was deemed there was a "substantial likelihood" that the patient might transmit his or her TB to others and would not complete treatment, based on "past or present behavior." Some argue this was nonetheless a "sensitive solution" since patients had the right of appeal and were even provided free legal counsel; moreover, the mere threat of detention was perhaps a persuasive tool for voluntary compliance, thus obviating the need for enforcement in many cases, although no hard evidence has been produced to this effect.[25] However, others insist this was an unprecedented infringement of liberties, since it was based on the principle of noncompliance rather than an immediate and quantifiable threat to the public health, as was the previous standard with all mental illnesses and other contagious diseases, and since less restrictive alternatives were not tried beforehand.[26]

Historical parallels have been drawn with comparable dilemmas in the past, such as the infamous "Typhoid Mary" case, in which the New York City health department forcibly detained an Irishwoman, Mary Mallon, in quarantine at a hospital on North Brother Island for the last twenty-three years of her life between 1915 and 1938 because she was a healthy but highly infectious carrier of typhoid fever. Although some might consider Mary's fate to have been cruel, she did infect a total of fifty-three people (three of whom died) during her career as a cook. (Typhoid, like cholera, is spread through contaminated feces, which Mary would have had on her hands since hand washing was not widely practiced at the time.) After her first period of incarceration from 1907 to 1910, Mary was granted her freedom despite a court ruling that upheld her detention in the face of a habeas corpus legal challenge filed by a lawyer on her behalf; her release was on condition that she sign an affidavit promising to cease employment as a cook, a condition she subsequently violated under an assumed name (at a hospital, no less). Yet, there is more to Mary's case than simply the biological issue of protecting the public from deadly germs, for it does not explain why hundreds of other healthy carriers besides Mary were allowed to go free, including a "Typhoid John" in the Adirondacks who infected thirty-eight victims, two of whom also died. An indefinite, involuntary detention of a healthy person as a public health threat was in fact unprecedented. It seems that the New York board of health was determined to make Mary an example of how someone who was in perfect health could nonetheless be a walking carrier of disease; Mary's misfortune was simply to be the first such healthy carrier to be so identified. Moreover, as a single, female, sexually active, working-class Irish immigrant with a physically imposing presence who refused to cooperate with authorities or even admit she was a carrier, Mary also posed a social threat to contemporary preconceptions of acceptable feminine behavior; she certainly did not get along with George Soper, the sanitation engineer who first tracked down Mary and who came from a middle-class, Protestant, educated background, almost the exact opposite of hers.[27]

If we go just a little further back in history, we have already seen that Britain's attempts to take extraordinary measures to combat plague in its empire in India at the turn of the twentieth century encountered widespread opposition among the native population there, to the point that they were rendered almost counterproductive (chapter 1). This was partly the result of a lack of conviction that these efforts were truly effective and partly because they ran counter to traditional cultural values and domestic sensibilities. It could be argued that, in this day and age, transmission of a disease like tuberculosis is far better understood and that modern Western culture is far more accepting of the authority and encroachments of medical science into our daily lives. The courts, press, and the public at large all, with few exceptions, seemed to endorse NYC health department's drastic actions taken ex officio to combat MDR-TB, the threat of which seemed to far outweigh any constitutional objections that might appeal to tender consciences. But we must remember that only a few people on the margins of society were directly affected; what would happen if large numbers from mainstream society had to be coerced, and if close family members had to be separated in the process? Although such scenarios might be the fodder for simulation exercises and Hollywood films, they have yet to be tested in the real world.

Despite New York City's success story, the way forward in the campaign to eradicate TB is far from clear. Not everyone, for example, is enamored of the DOT approach; in Russia, which has the third largest number of MDR-TB cases in the world, largely owing to its severely crowded prison system that serves as an incubator for the disease, there was much cultural resistance to DOT until relatively recently. This was because many in the Russian Ministry of Health were convinced of the necessity to go back to the old, Soviet method of treating TB, which operated on a ponderous, case-by-case basis that relied primarily on X-ray diagnosis and surgery.[28] Perhaps for reasons of sheer national pride, Russia's reluctance to adopt DOT was not overcome until 1995, and even then universal, countrywide application of DOT was not to be achieved until 2007. Not coincidentally, it was not until the last decade that the growth rate in number of new TB cases has finally slowed in Russia. Yet, problems remain, including ineffective detection and notification of new cases, poor compliance and success in DOT administration, spectacularly high TB rates in prisons (where overcrowding and poor air quality conditions remain despite attempts at reform), and considerable coinfection with HIV (human immunodeficiency virus).[29]

Others suggest that DOT demands an allegedly too "paternalistic" and "authoritarian" approach to compliance for some cultures and that alternative treatment methods should therefore be considered, such as voluntary administration of "fixed-dose drug combinations" (which presumably would encourage completion of treatment through the ease of taking just one pill).[30] Developing and getting new drugs to market that may be effective against TB is often a challenge when drug companies see "a high investment with little commercial return," since "the vast majority of people with TB are young and poor and live in developing countries."[31] (This is the subject of the 2005 film *The Constant Gardener*.) Recent sequencing of the TB genome holds some promise for targeting "hibernating" bacteria that can lie dormant in the body and thus resist antibiotics, only to be reactivated at a later time, but the full fruits of this research are probably years away. More promising in the near term is perhaps efforts under way to develop a more effective BCG vaccine, which would allow for targeted eradication on the model of the successful campaign against smallpox.[32]

Then there are underlying causes of TB, such as poverty, which are far more intractable problems to solve, especially since TB and poverty are closely linked in a mutually reinforcing cycle: TB is said to flourish in the overcrowded, malnourished, unhygienic environments that poor people are most susceptible to, while at the same time the disease hits poor families the hardest in terms of lost wage income and increased expenses for medical treatment, often as the result of delayed and incorrect diagnosis.[33] Yet, with the many possibilities of global spread of TB (such as on airline flights), the current crises in poorer nations simply cannot be ignored by richer neighbors. Since TB can be spread so rapidly and easily, with one contact potentially infecting dozens of others in short order, time is of the essence in the fight against the disease. Much of this challenge is of humankind's own making, particularly in the case of MDR-TB, where ironically the cure is also our curse. But the consensus seems to be that society can conquer TB, if only it can muster the will, money, and ingenuity to do so.

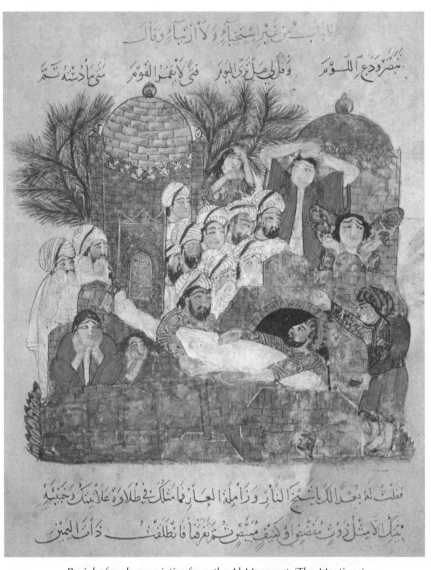

Burial of a plague victim from the Al Maqamat *(The Meetings)*
by Al-Hariri, Persian school, fourteenth century. Getty Images

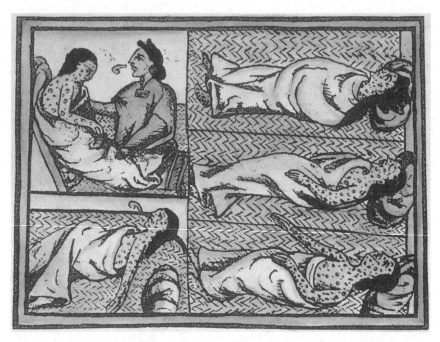

Smallpox epidemic in Mexico. Aztec natives with smallpox contracted from Spaniards are ministered to by a medicine man. Illustration from Father Bernardino de Sahagun's sixteenth-century treatise, A General History of the Things of New Spain. *The Granger Collection, New York*

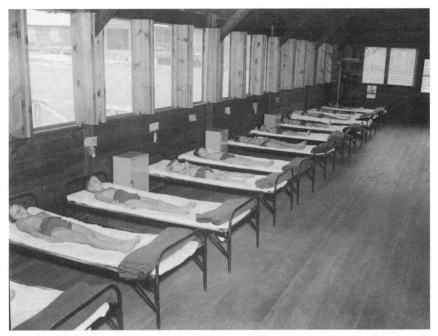

Tubercular children taking enforced rest for fifteen hours each day at a tuberculosis camp in Washington, DC, in 1938. Note the many wide-open windows designed to let in fresh air. © Bettmann/CORBIS

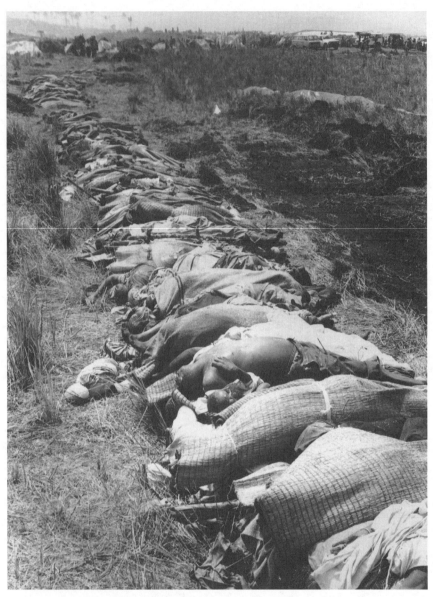

Bodies of Rwandan refugees, who died in a cholera epidemic that spread through refugee camps at Goma in July 1994, await burial in a mass grave near Kibumba camp, Zaire. © Howard Davies/CORBIS

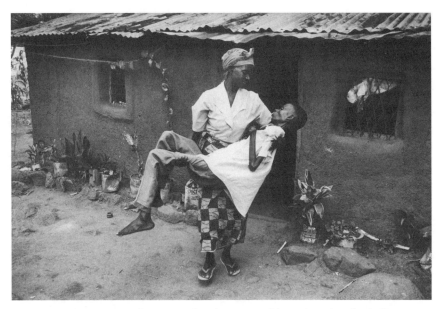

A Tanzanian mother carries her thirty-year-old son, Joseph, who is ill with AIDS, outside to sit in the shade, c. 2000. © Gideon Mendel/CORBIS

CHAPTER 4

Cholera

Like tuberculosis, cholera is a disease often associated with the nineteenth century and is likewise caused by a bacterium, in this case, the comma-shaped *Vibrio cholerae* that was identified by Robert Koch in 1883 after conducting autopsies on victims in Alexandria, Egypt, and Calcutta, India.[1] Cholera, whose name comes from *choler* or yellow bile, the humor often associated with digestive illnesses, made its impact not so much through its mortality as through its especially dramatic symptoms. In Europe, Russia, and the United States, death rates from cholera probably never exceeded 2 to 3 percent, although they were considerably higher in other parts of the world, particularly India and Southeast Asia, North Africa, the Caribbean, and South America, where they could reach 10 to 15 percent.[2] Nonetheless, cholera was feared even in Europe as almost a second Black Death, largely due to the terribly sudden onset of some truly horrific symptoms, which include uncontrollable defecation and vomiting, painful muscle spasms, and an alarming bluish tinge to the skin (hence the name "blue death") and gaunt appearance to the face. All this is the result of rapid dehydration caused by a toxin released by the bacteria that reverses the osmosis process through the lining of the small intestines, creating the salty fluid on which the bacteria thrive. Although *Vibrio cholerae* is normally destroyed by acids and enzymes in the stomach and even in saliva, making the disease hard to contract, some of the bacteria if ingested in sufficient numbers will reach the intestines, where their assault starts peeling away the lining, resulting in "rice-water" stools. The disease is then passed on to other victims typically when sewage containing contaminated feces seeps into a population's untreated drinking water, although the bacteria can also be transmitted and live for days or even weeks in contaminated food. Complete prostration due to a sudden drop in blood pressure and shock can occur within hours, so that it was said a man healthy in the morning could be dead by evening, or a person could simply collapse in the street lying in his own excrement. (Roughly half of all victims afflicted by the disease died.)[3] Cholera was therefore a particularly humiliating, not to say agonizing and terrifying, disease to die from by the standards of nineteenth-century sensibilities, which presented quite a contrast to the romantic associations with the "easeful death" of tuberculosis. Only bubonic plague and smallpox could probably equal or surpass it in terms of the terror the spectacle of its symptoms could inspire.

Cholera has been a worldwide phenomenon but is said to have its endemic home in India, more specifically the Bengal region, where nearly every pandemic seems to have originated. (This is why the disease is sometimes known as *Asiatic* cholera.) Historians count seven separate pandemics of cholera to have occurred throughout history, the first beginning in 1817 in Bengal, India; earlier occurrences of the disease no doubt existed, although it is hard to distinguish these in the record from other gastrointestinal diseases, such as dysentery or diarrhea. Lasting until 1824, the first pandemic was largely confined to India, Southeast Asia, China, Japan, the Middle East, and southern Russia. It was not until the second cholera pandemic of 1827 to 1835 that the disease directly impinged itself upon the consciousness of Europe and the United States, particularly in the crucial year of 1832. The third pandemic from 1839 to 1856 brought the disease for the first time to South America, especially Brazil, and to much of North Africa as far west as Tunis. During the fourth pandemic of 1863 to 1875, much of sub-Saharan Africa was ensnared in cholera's worldwide net. By the time of the fifth and sixth pandemics of 1881–1896 and 1899–1923, greater understanding of the disease largely confined its worst mortalities to the east, including Egypt and the Arabian peninsula, Persia, India, and the Philippines, although some notable epidemics did occur in Europe and Russia, including an outbreak in Hamburg, Germany, in 1892 and in Naples, Italy, in 1910–1911. The seventh, and last, cholera pandemic first began in 1961 in Southeast Asia with the appearance of an alternative strain of the disease, named El Tor (after the quarantine camp in Egypt where it was first identified in 1905), and persists to the present day.[4] As of 2007–2008, cholera has been reported in India, Iraq, Vietnam, and throughout much of sub-Saharan Africa. Recent epidemics of cholera, however, are characterized by much lower infection and mortality rates than in the past, but the disease is persistent and endemic in some parts of the third world largely because of poor sanitation and poor access to safe drinking water supplies.[5]

Cholera, like tuberculosis, lends itself particularly well to a social interpretation of disease. What exactly that interpretation should be, however, has been much debated by historians. Traditionally, cholera has been seen as dividing nineteenth-century European society into two camps, those who preferred to explain it as the product of person-to-person contagion and those who saw it as caused primarily by environmental factors, such as miasma, poverty, filth, and so on. Each explanation in turn produced its respective champions in terms of how best to combat cholera. Contagionism, typically associated with conservative members of the ruling class, advocated quarantine, while anticontagionism, also referred to as localism or infectionism, which was taken up by bourgeois captains of commerce and political liberals and free traders, recommended sanitation measures and better hygiene. Both had their antecedents in Europe's medieval and Early Modern past during the fight against plague. In reality, as more recent historians have argued, etiologic approaches to cholera did not always fall so neatly along these lines; often, in fact, the two might blur together within the same explanatory system, which perhaps best reflects the true epidemiology of cholera, and became known as "contingent contagionism."[6]

Nineteenth-century cholera also presents historians with an opportunity to study the possible connections between disease and social conflict. The epidemic in Europe during the 1830s in particular coincided with social upheavals, such as the aftermath of the 1830 July Revolution in Paris that overthrew the Bourbon monarchy of Charles X in favor of the Duke of Orleans, Louis Philippe. Antagonisms between the social classes opened up by the revolution, which can be traced back even further to the French Revolution of the previous century, are believed to have been exacerbated by the sudden and unexpected arrival of cholera in the Paris capital in June 1832. Workers and populist elements tended to deny the existence of the disease or attribute it to a poisoning conspiracy on behalf of the government and ruling class; accusations of poisoning to explain disease of course go back to the medieval Black Death, but in the case of cholera it was particularly apropos since the observed gastrointestinal symptoms seemed to make it medically likely, and the recent economic theories of Thomas Malthus, which took a complacent attitude toward disease as a necessary check on population, seemed to supply a motive. This time, doctors became the main target of the mob's scapegoating ire as potential agents of the government's campaign to supposedly improve the "public health," and rioters tended to congregate outside cholera hospitals. Meanwhile, bourgeois and upper-class elements might see the disease as an excuse for greater state intervention and control of their social inferiors, not only on the grounds that cholera could incite rioting and other threats to public order, but also because the very conditions of poverty and filth associated with the lower classes were viewed as an integral cause and essence of the disease and thus opposed to Enlightenment progress and civilization. This became of particular concern as cholera began spreading from the poor slums where it began to more genteel enclaves. But by the time of the third cholera pandemic in 1849, despite coming hard on the heels of the socialist revolutions that swept across Europe in 1848, these connections between cholera and social tensions are seen to have been severed, largely due to greater empathy and rapprochement on the part of the bourgeoisie toward the poor, higher confidence among the ruling class that saw itself as less threatened by the Catholic Church and other potential enemies, and a shift in focus toward socialism as the main threat to the existing order, rather than disease. Poison accusations and hostility toward the medical profession also considerably abated, at least in France.[7]

However, poison hysteria and riots did break out in 1832 in other countries, such as Russia, where the scapegoat was mainly foreigners, but there such upheavals did not lead to any long-term social changes or reform, except perhaps in a blossoming of Enlightenment medicine along Western lines.[8] In Britain, popular fears and suspicions in connection with cholera were directed, as in France, against hospitals and physicians, but for different reasons. Instead of accusations of poisoning, there was concern that cholera victims were not receiving proper burial but instead were being diverted to anatomy schools for dissection, which was normally reserved only for criminals and those denied Christian burial. The disease just happened to coincide with a rash of "resurrectionists" or body-snatchers, gangs of criminal elements who robbed graves or even worse in order to supply subjects for anatomy students; the most notorious incident occurred in Edinburgh in 1827–1828, when two men, William Burke and William Hare, murdered a total of seventeen victims and delivered them to Dr. Robert Knox of the Edinburgh medical school. (Burke, the man who was hanged for these crimes on Hare's testimony, subsequently lent his name to "burking" and "burkers," as body-snatching and its practitioners became popularly known from then on.) During the cholera epidemic itself, the body of a four-year-old boy who had died at the Swan Street cholera hospital in Manchester was discovered in his coffin with a brick in place of his head, which had been removed for dissection purposes by the resident surgeon, Robert Oldham. Ironically, the boy's grandfather, who led an avenging crowd of three thousand that rioted in front of and inside the hospital, was another Irishman also named Hare.[9]

Once again, it is hard to argue for long-term trends in later cholera outbreaks, for popular discontent in Britain rapidly subsided after the passing of the Anatomy Act by parliament in 1832, the same year that the Reform Bill greatly expanded the electorate and eliminated "rotten boroughs." One study of a severe cholera outbreak in Hamburg, Germany, in 1892, which claimed over eight thousand lives (mostly among the working-class poor), has argued that the lack of any civil disturbances in the city, despite the panicked flight of some forty thousand middle-class citizens and a prior history of rioting during previous cholera epidemics, proves that by this time European populations had become "medicalized," or resigned to authoritarian efforts to contain disease as necessary sacrifices of individual liberty and local customs on behalf of the general welfare.[10] But the argument from silence here may be deceptive. An epidemic in Naples in 1884 provoked a poisoning "phobia" directed mainly against Gypsies, while another in 1910–1911, the last outbreak in Europe that claimed an estimated eighteen thousand lives in Italy, sparked a widespread popular resistance movement known as the *locandieri* to the government's heavy-handed health measures throughout the central part of the country. In Naples itself, the local populace and the press apparently collaborated in city authorities' efforts to deny the disease's existence entirely, a cover-up so successful that Naples' early twentieth-century bout with cholera went undocumented by historians until relatively recently. But if this is an example of a population's "medicalization," then it is a rather perverse one.[11]

Yet another reason for historians to study cholera during the nineteenth century is that it is an irresistible case study of how disease can become a "tool of empire" or, in other words, the role that disease can play in the imperialist policies of European powers in their colonies in the Americas, Africa, and Asia. This is particularly true of the British empire in India, the endemic home of cholera, where medical authorities (who adopted an anticontagionist line) mainly took a sanitary approach to combating the disease, as they were to do later during the Third Pandemic of plague beginning in 1896. However, even more so than in the case of plague, the British were hampered in their medical intervention in India and never seem to have seriously attempted to carry out what were considered the necessary measures, such as restricting pilgrim traffic at Hindu shrines like the temple of Jagannath at Puri, due to the costs involved, fears of offending native sensibilities (particularly after the Sepoy Mutiny of 1857), and remaining uncertainties about the etiology of cholera. This was in spite of the fact that an international sanitary conference held at Constantinople in 1866 had declared pilgrimages to be "the most powerful of all causes" of cholera, an assertion seemingly backed up by the severe cholera outbreak that occurred in Mecca, one of the most popular pilgrimage sites in the world, in 1865, when fifteen thousand pilgrims died of the disease.[12]

An important difference between cholera and plague in terms of British policies in India is that, when cholera first broke out in the Bengal region in 1817, native Ayurvedic and Western medical approaches were quite similar, both being based on humoral and miasmatic theories of disease; British doctors, despite maintaining the superiority of their medicine, were quite willing to borrow from local Indian practices. With later cholera outbreaks, however, the attitude of India's imperialist masters began to change, as the disease was identified to be of

Asian origin and became associated with lower standards of Asian hygiene (emblematic, in Western eyes, of an inferior "civilization") and greater Asian propensities toward superstition. By 1831, a Frenchman, Alexandre Moreau de Jonnès, connected Indian Hindu pilgrimages with the spread of cholera and greatly exaggerated cholera deaths there (to as much as eighteen million), while a British sanitary commissioner remarked in 1868 that the Jagannath temple car at Puri presented a "tawdry and contemptible" spectacle.[13] Yet, we have seen how European populations, especially in 1831–1832, could likewise give in to irrational beliefs, such as that their own doctors were poisoning them, and resist, sometimes violently, their own government's attempts to "medicalize" them.

By the mid-nineteenth century, however, Britain and Europe, through the efforts of medical pioneers such as John Snow, were making great strides in understanding the true causes of cholera, although differences of opinion still remained, so that it is hard to argue that "gentlemanly capitalist" interests behind the British Raj were solely responsible for keeping these advances from saving millions of lives in India.[14] Rather, the very history of British policies toward cholera in India stood in the way of a drastic remolding of native medicine in line with the model provided by the colonial mother country, as was tried in response to plague at the end of the century. Britain therefore never had to learn the hard lesson that there were limits to what its superior medicine could do against the cholera in India, because it never really tested those limits where cholera was concerned. In turn, from the very beginning of cholera epidemics, native opinion in India tended to blame British violations of local Hindu customs and native acquiescence in colonial rule for its own susceptibility to the disease.[15]

By contrast, the United States did learn this hard lesson with cholera when, after the Spanish-American War in 1898, it took over the Spanish colony of the Philippines, where a terrible epidemic of the disease—killing an excess of one hundred thousand people—occurred in 1902, hard on the heels of a three-year-long war of independence or insurrection against U.S. rule. As with the British experience with plague in India, the United States discovered that its heavy-handed attempts to control cholera, such as isolating victims and their contacts in segregation camps and destroying or disinfecting their houses and possessions, were only counterproductive, inspiring Filipinos to flee or conceal victims of the disease, thus prolonging and even spreading the epidemic, and American authorities were forced to back down and make concessions to native sensibilities.[16] The case of Tunisia in North Africa, however, demonstrates that native resistance to Western medicine against cholera did not always fall so neatly along colonial lines but perhaps more in the way of traditionalist objections to the forces of modernism. Since the eighteenth century, the local *beys* ruling Tunisia had championed Western medicine and science as superior to local Muslim custom. Quarantine, for example, which was administered by a Sanitary Council dominated by Europeans, was held to be responsible for Tunisia being largely spared the cholera pandemic of the 1830s. But in 1848–1850, quarantine proved incapable of preventing the disease from spreading to Tunisia from Egypt and Arabia, and it was resisted by both European anticontagionists and local Muslims who, as in Europe, spread rumors of poisoning by foreign doctors. The fact that religious invocations by forty *sharifs* named Muhammad—who all claimed descent from the Prophet—seemed to halt the epidemic in the summer of 1850, where medical efforts had failed, only served to reinforce local Muslim prejudices that assimilated or privileged older, traditional concepts of disease, such as that the *jinn*, or demons, could pierce victims with their arrows and thus give them cholera. By the time of the next cholera outbreak in 1856, the new ruler, Muhammad Bey, expressly forbade quarantine or indeed any of the other measures recommended by the Sanitary Council that had been taken during the last epidemic; yet, in the long run this did not dislodge the continued influence and acceptance of European-style medical reforms in Tunisia.[17]

Finally, cholera demonstrates, like plague, that worldwide pandemics of disease are greatly facilitated by modern methods of transport, such as the railways and steamship travel that were coming into their own during the nineteenth century. But to my mind, one of the most important lessons of cholera, and it is a very heartening one, is how solutions were found for cholera—solutions that haven't been bettered even to the present day—even when society was decades away from the germ theory and the modern technology of antibiotic treatment. In 1854, for example, a Yorkshire surgeon practicing in London, John Snow, was able to map out a cholera epidemic in the city that proved conclusively that the disease was spread by "animaculae"-infected drinking water. (Snow was inclined to reject the dominant miasmatic theory through his work as an anesthesiologist.) Two companies that supplied water to the same districts from the River Thames, one site contaminated with sewage and the other not, resulted in dramatically different infection rates regardless of class or other factors. Most famously, Snow mapped out cholera infections that radiated out from the Broad Street pump in the Soho area where he himself had formerly lived, a pump that had been contaminated by a dead child's soiled nappies washed into a cesspool that leaked into the well. Those nearby who didn't use the well, such as the denizens of a workhouse and the employees of a brewery, remained free of the disease even though their moral or social status might make them ideal potential victims, while Susannah Eley, who lived four miles away from the city in Hampstead, nonetheless got infected and died because she had a nostalgic taste for the water from the pump just outside her late husband's percussion cap factory in Broad Street. When Snow persuaded the parish's Board of Guardians to remove the handle of the Broad Street pump, the epidemic disappeared.[18] Snow's demonstration that cholera could be fought and conquered simply by altering the environment in which the disease was transmitted finds its parallel in twentieth-century efforts to eliminate yellow fever and malaria by targeting their mosquito insect vectors, such as was achieved in 1905–1906 by William Gorgas, chief sanitation officer during the completion of the Panama Canal by the United States.[19] (Malaria's recent resurgence, which is particularly acute in sub-Saharan Africa, is partly due to the fact that pesticides used to keep down mosquito populations, such as DDT, have unintended harmful side effects that complicate their use.)

Yet, it has been observed that Snow's evidence published in his *On the Mode of Communication of Cholera* reads more convincingly to us than it did to his contemporaries—nor was cholera invariably the spur to public works projects, such as were taken up by local boards of health in England and New York City, that eventually eliminated the disease.[20] Authorities in London did not act upon Snow's water-borne theory until 1866, after his death, and sewage renovation in the city was as much inspired by the "great stink" that occurred in 1858, when private toilets overflowed the existing system.[21] Not even Koch's discovery of *Vibrio cholerae* in 1883 proved decisive in all cases: during the cholera epidemic in Hamburg in 1892, Koch's personal presence in the city nonetheless did not ensure that all his recommended measures were effectively carried out, and the National Epidemics Law that he championed was not to be passed until plague threatened Germany in 1900.[22] Naples's cover-up of its cholera outbreak in 1910–1911, motivated largely by its desire to maintain its lucrative emigration traffic, undoubtedly hindered its low-key efforts to contain the disease and finds modern parallels in Bangladesh and the Philippines, which stopped reporting cholera cases in the 1980s over fears of trade embargoes and declines in tourism, and in China's initial silence about SARS (severe acute respiratory syndrome) when an epidemic broke out in the Guangdong province in 2002.[23]

In the same way, the most effective therapy for cholera, direct injection of saline solution into the veins of the victim, was devised and successfully tested as early as 1832 by an obscure physician from Leith, England, Thomas Latta.[24] To this day, fluid replacement therapy is the most widely used treatment for cholera, especially as the bacteria develop resistance to antibiotic drugs, such as tetracycline.[25] Yet, because Latta's chemically based therapy did not fit easily into any existing medical tradition, such as the humoral theory, it was not widely adopted during his own lifetime. Meanwhile, some spectacularly unsuccessful, and indeed quite harmful, treatments were being employed, such as bleeding (still practiced as late as the Hamburg epidemic in 1892) and administration of laxatives and other purgatives, which, while perhaps endorsed by long tradition going back to ancient times, had exactly the opposite desired impact in a disease that was already draining the body's available fluids. Other "remedies" were simply bizarre, such as bunging up the anus with beeswax in a futile attempt to stem the involuntary gastrointestinal flow.[26] All this demonstrates that, while the means of prevention and cure of a disease may be prematurely available to human society, it does not always have the wisdom, foresight, or perhaps the mere psychological readiness to avail itself of them.

CHAPTER 5

Influenza

Influenza is a viral disease, like smallpox, but the viruses that cause influenza are far more unstable genetically than *Variola major* and *minor*, and consequently there are far more, ever-shifting varieties of the microbe that make it a much more challenging disease to combat by means of vaccination. Like a "moving target," influenza viruses are constantly mutating in the process of replicating copies of their RNA (ribonucleic acid) that they can only achieve by invading a host cell in order to harness its biological machinery; it is estimated that within a single cell an influenza virus can manufacture and then release up to a hundred copies of itself within five or six hours. It is because of this high rate of reproduction (without any ability to "proofread" or correct copies of its genes as in the case of deoxyribonucleic acid, or DNA) that influenza viruses remain so elusive, since the protein molecules or antigens comprising the viruses' outer coat or capsid, which are recognized and engaged by the antibodies of our immune defense system, are constantly evolving in both minor and major ways, known respectively as antigenic *drift* and antigenic *shift*. For this reason, we will probably never "conquer," or entirely eliminate, influenza as was achieved against smallpox in the 1970s, and in this respect, influenza is more akin to the human immunodeficiency virus (HIV) that causes AIDS (acquired immune deficiency syndrome) and that will be the focus of the next chapter. Interestingly enough, it has also been recently discovered that the influenza virus can target and suppress the body's immune system, much as HIV does in AIDS, in order to give the virus time to replicate within the lungs.

Due to their complexity, influenza viruses have earned an elaborate classification system whereby they are divided into three main "types," known as A, B, and

C (based on the nucleoprotein antigen), of which the type A viruses are the only ones known to cause large-scale pandemics in humans. Within type A, influenza viruses are further classified on the basis of their outer protein coats that allow them to enter and exit a host cell: these are the hemagglutinin (H) and neuraminidase (N) glycoproteins, of which fifteen varieties are known of the former and nine of the latter. This is how various influenza viruses get their names in the news and other literature that talk about the agents responsible for particular pandemics; for example, the H1N1 virus is believed to have caused both the 1918–1919 pandemic and the recent one that made the rounds in 2009. What is not so clear is if influenza viruses only drift and shift in a cyclical manner, within the relatively limited number of antigenic combinations identified thus far, or if we are doomed to encounter ever new proteins as these constantly evolve.[1]

Influenza is perhaps the most contagious of any infectious disease we know of; it is more transmissible than smallpox because influenza viruses, like the rhinoviruses that cause the common cold, specifically target cells in the upper and lower respiratory tract, although they can subsequently be distributed to other parts of the body, such as the brain and central nervous system, where they cause other symptoms typically associated with the disease. Influenza is therefore particularly well suited to person-to-person communication by means of sneezing, coughing, or simple breathing. And since a virus is five hundred times smaller than a bacterium, many more infectious agents are emitted by a victim of influenza with each cough or sneeze than one afflicted with a bacterial respiratory disease such as pneumonic plague or tuberculosis; this makes it far more likely not only that a person nearby will contract influenza but also that it will penetrate deeper into the lungs where it cannot easily be ejected by the cough reflex. (This is why gauze facemasks recommended by Dr. Wu Liande that protected his medical staff during the pneumonic plague outbreak in Manchuria in 1910–1911 proved not so effective against the influenza pandemic in 1918–1919.) In addition, the influenza virus can remain infectious for up to forty-eight hours outside the host, so that one can also contract influenza by breathing in contaminated dust particles or by touching contaminated objects such as doorknobs and utensils and then ingesting the microbial agents on one's hands. Recent experience with avian flu has likewise demonstrated that influenza can be spread, at least from animals to humans, via the gastrointestinal tract as a result of eating infected poultry products or drinking contaminated water.[2]

As soon as one or two days from infection, the typical flu symptoms will manifest themselves, which include high fever, chills, headache and other bodily aches and pains, prostration, lethargy, and sometimes vomiting or diarrhea. In the worst-case scenario, bacterial or viral pneumonia will later emerge, due to the fact that a certain amount of synergy exists between flu and pneumonia: flu can prepare the way for pneumonic infection and vice versa.[3] It is important to note that the victim is infectious even before these symptoms appear, and some people can be infected by flu without showing hardly any signs at all, becoming in effect asymptomatic carriers of the disease.[4] But flu symptoms are so general that it is quite difficult to make a positive diagnosis of historical epidemics on that basis alone; usually a pattern of high morbidity accompanied by low mortality that is typical of influenza will confirm its presence in most scholars' minds.[5] Influenza usually runs its course through the human body in three days, after which the patient can generally be expected to make a full recovery. Death from flu is rare, occurring on average in only one-tenth of 1 percent of all victims during most outbreaks; these unfortunates also tend to be either the very young or the very old, people already at high risk in premodern times. The exception, of course, was the 1918–1919 pandemic, when average mortality rates jumped to 2.5 to 5 percent or higher in some places, and many more victims came from among those in the prime of life, roughly between twenty and forty years of age. Morbidity rates for this pandemic were likewise unprecedented for normal influenza, comprising anywhere from 25 to 50 percent of populations, although such statistics are notoriously hard to pin down since cases of sickness were less rigorously reported than actual deaths.[6]

A seasonality of incidence is also associated with influenza, which strikes typically during the winter months in the northern and southern hemispheres and during the rainy or monsoon seasons in tropical zones. At times, however, influenza can come on in waves, as it did in 1918–1919. In this particular outbreak, historians have noted three successive waves of the disease, a first and mild one occurring in the spring to midsummer of 1918, the second and most severe wave starting almost immediately thereafter in the late summer and autumn, and finally a third and again mild wave during the early months of 1919.[7] The flu pandemic that ran its course in the United States during the latter half of 2009 peaked in September and October, rather than during the usual bad months for flu of December and January. A combination of social and environmental factors are thought responsible for flu's seasonal behavior. Certainly, overcrowding of populations that tend to occur with the onset of bad weather will greatly facilitate spread of influenza, but the virus also does best in conditions of low humidity and sunlight such as we find in winter. Human immune systems are also more likely to be compromised as the body fights off the effects of cold or rain. Yet, a certain amount of mystery remains in this regard: laboratory experiments with mice have found flu behaving seasonally even when conditions of temperature and humidity are equal.[8]

Such are the bare epidemiological facts about influenza that distinguish it from other infectious diseases we have discussed thus far. Compared to those of plague, smallpox, or cholera, its symptoms are not especially memorable, dramatic, or enduring. In most cases, an entire epidemic or even pandemic comes and goes quickly, in a matter of months, leaving behind relatively few to mourn and those at the life-expectant margins of society. This has made it easy for both past and present cultures to overlook influenza, seeing it, perhaps, as no worse than a severe cold. And yet the 1918–1919 pandemic overturned all these expectations about this otherwise seemingly benign disease, for in that one outbreak influenza swept across as many categories of society as the "danse macabre" of plague; in some unforgettable cases, it brought on the heliotrope or blue-black cyanosis of the face so typical of cholera, and it marked its survivors with a trauma as tangible, even if not as visible, as the pockmarks of smallpox. Remarkably, influenza in this particular instance behaved both like the worst of infectious diseases in the minority of cases it did kill, striking with a virulence that invited comparisons with the Black Death, *and* like any other flu outbreak in terms of the usual pattern of low mortality and high morbidity: horrifying as the deaths from flu were, the vast majority of people still recovered from or did not get the disease. In a sense, here was influenza on the grand scale, with a much higher incidence of the disease than normal and across a broader spectrum of the population, accompanied by a higher mortality rate within that subgroup, in a particularly far-reaching pandemic that left practically no part of the world, even in its remotest spaces, untouched. In other words, influenza was still influenza, only this time morphed into a monstrous version of itself that, of necessity, impinged upon the consciousness of all. Although the historian Alfred Crosby has dubbed it the "forgotten pandemic" among its own contemporary generation, the outbreak of 1918–1919 has since cast a long shadow over almost every subsequent pandemic threat of influenza.[9] It is quite simply the deadliest single outbreak of disease in history, surpassing even the Black Death in terms of sheer numbers of people directly killed by its onslaught, with the most recent estimates ranging anywhere from fifty to one hundred million dead worldwide. Why and how this happened are mysteries that are still in the process of being answered.

Before we get to the infamous 1918–1919 pandemic, however, it is advisable to trace the prior history of this disease. Influenza viruses have been around for millions of years, where their natural host reservoir has been and continues to be ducks and other aquatic wildfowl, which are generally immune to the disease and instead act as carriers, continually shedding viruses in their feces. When humans began domesticating ducks around four thousand years ago, the influenza virus was then able to make this species leap, even though the current human strains of influenza had already emerged toward the start of the Neolithic age another four thousand years earlier. As humans domesticated other animals, particularly pigs and chickens, influenza was able to make its endemic home in human populations across much of the ancient world. (In addition to the above species, influenza epidemics are also known to afflict horses, dogs, and cats.) However, the source of most new outbreaks of human influenza, both then and now, is thought to be China and Southeast Asia, due to its ancient practice of rice grow-ing and fish farming, where live ducks living in the water were used for weeding and their feces as fertilizer and fish food. When pigs were added to this microbial stew, passage of the influenza virus from animals to humans became much easier, since pigs, having an anatomy much closer to humans than do birds, were able to be infected by both human and avian strains of influenza and thus became a kind of "mixing bowl" for emerging flu pandemics.[10] Yet, the influenza virus can and does pass directly from birds to humans, and indeed this is what is now thought to have occurred during the influenza pandemic of 1918–1919, as well as in the current outbreaks of avian flu that have menaced the world for at least the past decade.

The ancient Greek physician Hippocrates provides perhaps our first written description of influenza in his *Epidemics* composed sometime during the fourth century B.C.E., and down through to the Middle Ages flu outbreaks may have been subsumed under references to "fevers," "rheums," and "catarrhs." The term "influenza" itself was apparently first introduced from the Italian in 1504 to describe any general disease epidemic that afflicted large numbers of people due to the "influence" of the stars; the modern sense of the word does not seem to emerge, however, until the eighteenth century, when the "grippe" also came into usage to refer to the disease. Some convincing descriptions of influenza epidem-ics in Britain and Europe can be produced for the sixteenth and seventeenth centuries, but it is quite likely that any such outbreaks were sporadic and not very widespread.[11] There may be any number of reasons for this. One explana-tion that has not been considered thus far is that, at this time, health manuals, plague treatises, and dietary regimens all advised that people steer clear of water-fowl, such as ducks and geese, not only on the grounds that their "watery" meat would produce watery, easily corruptible blood but also because they fed on unclean, noxious things in often foul, stagnant waters.[12] While of course igno-rant of the fact that waterfowl were the natural hosts of the influenza virus, such medical prescience may nonetheless have limited the opportunities for the virus to become endemic in human populations, at least in Europe, where this advice was proffered. Moreover, human traffic to the Far East, presumably the ancient home of influenza, would have taken too long and would not have been of high enough volume to really sustain too many pandemics.

Influenza did not really come into its own as a pandemic disease until the eighteenth century, when the more rapid transport of peoples and the worldwide scope of wars began to make global outbreaks more likely. Unlike bubonic plague, a rat- and flea-based disease that could follow the movements of grain and merchandise shipments, influenza had to wait until modern technology made human-to-human transmission across long distances possible. Also, cities now began to greatly increase in size and density, especially in the latter half of the century with the advent of the industrial and agricultural revolutions. Pandemics are thought to have occurred in 1729–1730, 1732–1733, 1761–1762, 1781–1782, and 1788–1789, with the one in 1781–1782 particularly severe. The pandemic of 1761–1762 also coincided with the Seven Years' War of 1756–1763, the first truly global conflict that pitted the European powers and their colonies in the Americas and India against each other. These pandemics were characterized by the high morbidity and low mortality typical of influenza, although firm figures are hard to come by. A months-long, east-to-west spread of flu across Europe, with an origin typically in Russia, was noted in this century, albeit an Asian source of the disease began to be suspected by the 1780s; flu also came to the Americas from Europe in the course of these pandemics but after a delay of as much as a year. And while this century saw more detailed and accurate diagnoses of influenza outbreaks and a more enlightened approach to the medical profession, the old ideas of the miasmatic spread of disease and of contagion still applied, and bleeding and cupping were still the norm in terms of treatment. However, because influenza was a relatively mild disease, at least compared to plague or smallpox, that killed few people, invasive purgative remedies may not have been as intensive, and doctors seem to have recommended above all that their patients rest and consume nourishing foods, advice that still holds true to this day.[13]

The nineteenth century saw all these trends noted in the previous century continue and indeed accelerate: Travel across oceans and continents grew far swifter with the advent of steamship and railroad technologies; European colonialism and imperialism established far-flung empires in every corner of the globe; and cities and populations expanded exponentially as the industrial revolution moved into full swing. All these developments, of course, greatly favored the outbreak and spread of influenza. At the same time, exciting and unprecedented new approaches to the medical explanation and treatment of infectious diseases emerged, such as smallpox vaccination programs and the awareness and identification of various disease-causing bacteria. And yet, such advances did not really apply to influenza and may, in fact, have given doctors a false sense of superiority over the disease. In the earlier part of the century, the miasmatic rather than the germ theory and even bleeding treatments still held sway. But greater sophistication and reliability of statistics, at least in terms of excess mortality from influenza in Europe and the United States, now became available. A major influenza pandemic occurred in 1831, at the same time as cholera swept across Europe, with a second and third wave striking in 1833 and 1837, the last causing much higher mortality than in the previous outbreaks. Finally, another influenza pandemic striking in three successive waves occurred in 1889–1891, with a last gasp of a related strain possibly following in 1899–1901. Russia was once again blamed for this pandemic's origins (hence its popular name as the "Russian flu") although scholars now believe it came from southern China. Best estimates are that a million people or more died in Europe and the United States. People exposed to this pandemic may have gained some immunity to the horrific outbreak of 1918, which tended to target people in the prime of life (who would have been young children in 1889), and some scholars believe that the H2N2 flu strain that circulated in the 1957 pandemic may also have been active at the end of the nineteenth century.[14]

We now come to the greatest influenza pandemic of them all, the one that engulfed the entire world in three waves in 1918–1919, with remarkably high morbidity *and* mortality. It has become the pandemic against which all succeeding ones are measured, especially in recent times with fears of avian flu (H5N1) and the latest pandemic of the H1N1 strain in 2009. It is certainly the "forgotten pandemic" no longer, with a plethora of narrative histories appearing on the publishing scene in the wake of Crosby's groundbreaking study of 1976.[15] But in addition to the usual anecdotes that are typically set in the United States or Europe, a lot more information is now available about the pathogenic and social impact of flu elsewhere around the globe.

For example, the one part of the world that seems to have suffered the most from the pandemic was India, where recent estimates place its death toll at close to twenty million, which is nearly double the number of deaths India suffered during the Third Pandemic of plague. If we accept a figure of fifty million for flu deaths around the world, then India's share alone would account for 40 percent of that total. The Indian experience with influenza illustrates a strong connection between the disease and poverty, since lower castes of Indian Hindu society suffered disproportionately compared to the higher castes, which was probably due to their poorer nutrition and lack of good nursing care that could have helped the body resist opportunistic bacterial infections. In addition, India shows how a place far removed from the front of World War I and not mobilizing on a grand scale for war could nonetheless suffer tragically during the pandemic. In India's case, influenza's spread seems to have been greatly facilitated by the railroad network installed by the British and by overcrowded conditions in the cities, while its high mortality rate (for flu) of 6 to 10 percent was perhaps owing to the failure of the monsoon rains during the summer of 1918 that made famine, instead of war, the synergistic partner of disease.[16] All three factors—disease, war, and famine—were in bed together in Tanzania, a German colony in Africa that was taken over by Britain during the war and where troop and refugee movements both spread the flu and pillaged agricultural lands, which then could not be re-planted as farmers succumbed to the disease, resulting in mortalities comprising 10 percent of the population.[17] War likely impacted the response to influenza in India in a more indirect way, by distracting the British government from taking more effective measures against the disease, for which it was criticized by the native press. Instead, the British relied on cooperation with voluntary, nongovernmental organizations (NGOs) to provide what medical and hospitalization services were available during the epidemic, which was perhaps a lesson it learned from the outbreak of plague in Bombay in 1896. In addition, since Western medicine proved woefully ineffective in explaining or treating the disease despite being newly armed with the germ theory, native traditions of Ayurvedic and Unani medicine were favored by voluntary hospitals and other groups offering medical care, which nonetheless still faced suppression from the government under the delusion "that it had all the answers."[18]

Other places in the third world, such as the Belgian Congo, Ghana, and the Dutch East Indies (present-day Indonesia), suffered mortality rates comparable to India's. But influenza reached even isolated regions of the globe, such as the hinterlands of Alaska and the Canadian subarctic as well as islands in the South Pacific, such as Western Samoa and Tonga, where influenza acted like a "virgin soil" epidemic much as smallpox did in the New World in the sixteenth century, wiping out 50 or even 100 percent of local populations. This was not all due to native lack of prior exposure to the disease, however. A study of the influenza pandemic in the Canadian subarctic, for example, found that families stricken by the flu also suffered from lack of food and wood fuel, as they were dependent on distant supply lines to the Hudson Bay Company stores, which had collapsed with the onset of the disease; the hunger and cold that resulted certainly amplified susceptibility to the flu. In other, distant parts of the world, such as Australia, the American Samoan islands, and the city of Fairbanks, Alaska, quarantine was successful in preventing or containing outbreaks of influenza.[19]

Among the more sensational developments to take place in research into the influenza pandemic of 1918–1919 is the genetic re-creation of the virus responsible from autopsy samples preserved at the Armed Forces Institute of Pathology in Rockville, Maryland, and in the Alaskan permafrost. The samples in question were taken from two young soldiers who died at their army bases in the United States in September 1918 and from an Inuit woman who succumbed to the pandemic in November 1918 in a village bordering the Bering Strait where all but eight of the inhabitants died. Between 1996 and 2005, a research team at the institute was able to complete the eight-gene sequence of the virus from the samples and then use it to resurrect a live 1918 virus that was then tested on laboratory mice.[20] Not everyone was so enamored of this Frankenstein-like experiment on so lethal a viral monster,[21] yet it did provide some valuable historical information. It was found that the 1918 H1N1 strain was uniquely virulent, in that it was able to rapidly reproduce inside the lungs—as much as several thousand times faster than a normal influenza virus—which in turn provoked a correspondingly uncontrolled immune response, known in modern medical parlance as a "cytokine storm." (Cytokines are molecular substances that trigger our white blood immune cells or leukocytes to hurry to wherever the infection is located in the body, and a circular process then ensues as the immune cells produce yet more cytokines.) This only made matters worse, as the lungs began to fill up with a combination of immune cells as well as blood and fluid leaking into the alveolar sacs where tissue had been damaged. The resulting suffocation of the victim is currently called acute respiratory distress syndrome (ARDS). This is precisely what was observed in numerous autopsies conducted in 1918–1919, when lungs and sometimes the entire body cavity were found to be full of a bloody, frothy liquid, which had produced some of the most dramatic and alarming symptoms of the disease, such as a blue-black cyanosis of the face and skin (the result of a failure of oxygen to reach the blood) and blood pouring from the nose and ears.[22] Just such cytokine responses are nowadays produced in newly emerging viral diseases that are likewise highly fatal, such as Ebola and other hemorrhagic fevers, hantavirus pulmonary syndrome (HPS), and severe acute respiratory syndrome (SARS).[23] As if this wasn't bad enough, the 1918 virus also laid the groundwork especially well for bacterial pneumonia, which is always a danger due to its synergistic relationship with influenza.

What is still left unresolved, however, is from where exactly this atypical influenza virus originated. Researchers at the Armed Forces Institute came to the conclusion that the 1918 virus arose suddenly from a direct adaptation of avian flu to humans, rather than through an intermediary swine influenza strain, as was previously thought.[24] This would increase the likelihood that the source of the 1918–1919 pandemic was China or Southeast Asia, the ancestral home of human avian flu strains since it is where the most contact between waterfowl and humans has traditionally occurred. As early as December 1917 and January 1918, a pneumonia-like disease was reported in the Shanxi province of China along the Mongolian border; it is argued that this was pneumonic plague rather than influenza, since it was diagnosed as such by Dr. Wu Liande, the man who had headed up the response to the 1910–1911 outbreak of pneumonic plague in Manchuria. However, Wu's diagnosis of plague was contested at the time. He made it in some chaotic circumstances, since his unauthorized autopsies sparked rioting among the local population, and although bacteria were found in sputum and spleen samples, they were allegedly not *Yersinia pestis*. We have already noted that bacterial pneumonia is an opportunistic disease of influenza, and in any case, the exceptional virulence of the 1918 flu pandemic would seem to mimic that of pneumonic plague. Another possibility includes Haskell County, Kansas, a small, isolated, rural community where influenza broke out suddenly in January and February 1918, well before the first soldiers came down with the flu three hundred miles away at Camp Funston in Fort Riley, Kansas, on March 4, 1918. A third alternative is that the virus originated in Etaples, France, where British soldiers stationed at a camp there came down with what was described at the time as "purulent bronchitis," accompanied by a "heliotrope cyanosis" that was later noted in flu victims, during the winter of 1916–1917; when influenza subsequently swept over Europe during its second, deadly wave in the autumn of 1918, doctors who had performed autopsies on the earlier "bronchitis" victims became convinced they had died of the same disease that was now killing in a vast pandemic. What is more, the base camp at Etaples was supplied by food markets that included ducks, geese, chickens, and pigs, and utilized gas weaponry that had mutagenic properties (i.e., the ability to mutate genes). However, no autopsy samples from Etaples currently survive in order to confirm the presence of the influenza virus, and some British doctors stationed there at the time were not convinced that the bronchitis was contagious, since it did not spread.[25] Of course, it is always possible that the 1918–1919 pandemic of influenza had several points of origin at once.

While the latest microbiological detective work into influenza is all very impressive, there is still a role to be played by the historical context of the 1918–1919 outbreak. The most obvious component of that context is the First World War, which came to a close in November 1918 just as the terrible second wave of flu was in full swing. The fifteen million or more military and civilian deaths directly caused by the war were of course dwarfed by the worldwide totals for influenza, although if we restrict ourselves to Europe, where most of the action during the war took place, then flu mortalities would be just a fraction of the war's impact. Certainly, influenza and World War I seemed to exist in a mutual, symbiotic relationship. After flu broke out in its first wave during the spring of 1918 among American soldiers mustering in camps across the country, it then spread to Europe as the doughboys disembarked at Brest in France. By late spring and summer, flu was playing its role in the war as the German offensive stalled at the Marne thirty-seven miles from Paris; according to the memoirs of General Eric von Ludendorff published later in 1919, the "blitzkatarrh" was to blame for the failure of German muster and morale at this turning point in the war. As the Allies began their counteroffensive in late summer and autumn, the second wave of the flu began sweeping through both sides. U.S. president Woodrow Wilson has been criticized by historians for refusing to delay troop movements in October 1918 as was urged by medical advisers; a delay could have saved many lives by denying to flu its tinder of mass numbers of men in cramped quarters. But given the enormous pressure and demand for American troops to seal an Allied victory, at a time when Britain and France were exhausted and spent, there was perhaps little choice left for the president to make. However, America did learn the hard lesson that it needed to provide better medical support services to its troops and not build hospitals at its bases last.[26]

Even countries in the very thick of the fighting, such as France, found it was the logistics of war, rather than the war itself, that most contributed to influenza, as troops were transported to and from the front and civilian populations were starved of supplies that were sent instead to the soldiers, thus facilitating both the spread of the disease and host susceptibility to it. And yet Spain, a neutral country in the war, apparently suffered equally from influenza, to the point that the epidemic in Europe began to be called the "Spanish Flu" or the "Spanish Lady," an unfair designation as Spain was simply one of the few countries publishing its statistics on the disease. Counterintuitively, war could even be a benefit to a country struck suddenly and unexpectedly by influenza, as was found to be the case in New Zealand where a heightened state of preparedness during wartime helped mobilize emergency relief efforts in response to the disease. The connection between flu and other factors, such as overcrowding and socioeconomic disparities, could likewise be called into question on the basis of figures from Britain, which show flu mortalities being distributed fairly equally.[27] But how else to explain the fact that India's death rate from the flu was twelve times higher than that of the United States or Europe, unless a completely different strain of the virus prevailed in Asia, which seems unlikely?[28] This conundrum of flu needs to be solved if we are to draw the right lessons from 1918, to wit, if the flu's mortality was largely biological, as was the case with plague in Europe during the Middle Ages or smallpox in the New World during the sixteenth century, when human populations had little immunity to these diseases, then experts think it quite likely, indeed almost inevitable, that another such devastating pandemic will occur. If, however, flu deaths were primarily the product of the unique historical context of 1918–1919, including the First World War and its aftermath, bad weather and widespread crop failures, inadequate medical knowledge of and preparedness for the disease, and so forth, then there is hope the disaster will not be repeated.[29] I think the odds are that it was a combination of both: the emergence of an unusually virulent strain of influenza in 1918 and circumstances that greatly facilitated its spread and mortality, especially from opportunistic diseases like pneumonia. If this is the case, then at the very least we can expect to mitigate (or else amplify) any future flu's impact, even one as deadly as that in 1918. Then there is also the possibility that, in our current climate, the two sides of the equation are inextricable: that some of our more destructive social behaviors, such as environmental degradation or factory farm-ing and food production, are in fact creating the very conditions in which new biological strains of influenza, and of other exotic viral diseases, can occur.

Historians have noted that the 1918–1919 flu pandemic broke all the rules. In some ways, it acted like any other influenza outbreak, striking most places with high morbidity and relatively lower mortality, but in other respects it fla-grantly bucked the trend of the way flu was expected to behave. One of the more shocking things that was happening at the time was that people in the prime of life, between twenty and forty years of age, were the ones being most struck down, which wasn't normally supposed to happen in a typical flu outbreak; as already explained, this was due to the unique cytokine response that the 1918 virus induced, which would be most expressive in robust, healthy adults. This was an anomaly noted all over the world, but it should be remembered that virtually all age groups, including the very young and the very old that were typically targeted by flu, were experiencing above-average mortality at this time. Flu was behaving like the Black Death of the Middle Ages in this respect. Life expectancies were set back by ten years or more even in advanced industrialized countries not directly invaded by the war, such as the United States, and gener-ally women (particularly those who were pregnant) seem to have lost their lon-gevity advantages over men.[30] When influenza's effects are combined with losses from the war, which also targeted the most productive (in this case male) mem-bers of society, it is easy to see why this became the "lost generation" of its time. The spectacle of corpses stacked like "cordwood" in hospital corridors and bod-ies lying unburied due to lack of space or a shortage of gravediggers naturally evoked memories of plague, as did reports of panicked flight and scapegoating early in the pandemic, which quickly subsided once it was realized that no one was exempt and there was nowhere to run. Like the Black Death, the influenza pandemic of 1918–1919 was both an urban and a rural phenomenon. Doctors once again found themselves utterly impotent for all their recent advances in bacteriology. Discovery of a potential cause of the disease in "Pfeiffer's Bacillus," a bacterium allegedly found in flu patients by the German physician Richard Pfeiffer, proved premature and discouragingly anticlimactic; the first flu virus was not to be isolated from human subjects until 1933. On the other hand, fe-male nurses found themselves empowered due to the fact that simple bed rest and nursing care proved the most effective remedy, or at least provided some comfort to suffering victims in their last hours, especially in an age that preceded antibiotics as a "miracle cure" for pneumonic infections.[31]

Campaigns to improve sanitation and hygiene, such as local laws that for-bade coughing and spitting, were reminiscent of what was tried during cholera epidemics in Europe in the previous century. In an even earlier throwback to

the time of plague, authorities also proscribed communal spaces—now to include schools and movie theaters in addition to churches (but not bars, since
alcohol and tobacco were believed to be prophylactic against the flu!). And
predictions of the apocalypse, or end of the world, once again came into fashion, as they had been in the Middle Ages. Influenza even inspired its own
nursery rhyme, comparable to the "ring around the rosy" ditty composed during the London plague of 1665, which was sung in 1918 by my grandmother-
in-law and which proved remarkably prescient, given what we now know about
the probable avian origins of the virus:

> I had a little bird
> And its name was Enza
> I opened up the window
> And in-flu-enza!

Some aspects of the 1918–1919 pandemic also foreshadowed future concerns
about disease: for example, some American cities mandated the wearing of gauze
masks, but when these proved ineffectual, civil liberty suits were brought because
they were uncomfortable or embarrassing for some. The millions of dollars in
business losses, such as were sustained by the life insurance industry, as death rates
soared in 1918 added an economic dimension on a scale that was to become a
familiar one in the calculations of the impact of all subsequent pandemics.[32]

Above all, the influenza outbreak of 1918–1919 is unique in terms of how
contemporaries chose to historicize this disease. In contrast to the plague, for
example, it became the "forgotten pandemic" and not just in the United States
or Europe but also in other countries around the globe, such as Senegal. Why
this is so has been variously explained. For much of the Western world, the unprecedented violence and brutality of the previous four years of war perhaps in-
ured it to the "just another millions" more deaths from influenza, which did not
produce the political and diplomatic legacy of Versailles, or maybe the quiet
deaths from disease were not heroic or dramatic enough even for a generation
that had lost its romantic love affair with war. The nature of influenza itself also
encouraged collective amnesia about it. As Crosby notes, it came and went relatively quickly, and compared to a more deadly disease per incidence like plague,
it did not inspire the same degree of terror when most people who contracted it
could still expect to survive, even in 1918. In the end, people may simply have
wished to forget its horrors, after everything else they had been through, and
remember it just like any other influenza.[33] Yet, this is now no longer the case.
Since 1976, the recovered memory of what happened in 1918–1919 has cast a
long shadow, as dark and ominous as the Black Death, over every real and potential pandemic of the flu.

After 1919, influenza pandemics seemed to subside for the next three decades: During that time, viruses were successfully scanned by the new technology of electron microscopes, antibiotics were discovered and first tested on humans, and the World Health Organization (WHO) was formed in 1948, with a World Influenza Center established the following year, in order to coordinate world-wide responses to disease and share information from laboratories in forty-five countries around the globe. Thereafter, an influenza pandemic looked set to be occurring once a decade with the advent of airline travel and an ever-shrinking world: pandemics occurred in 1946–1949—in the aftermath of World War II; in 1957; and in 1968—the so-called Hong Kong Flu. All these pandemics were considerably milder than the one in 1918–1919, conforming once again to flu's typical pattern of targeting the very young and the very old, and WHO demonstrated that vaccination programs could be coordinated on a global scale, experience it was to use to good effect in its smallpox eradication campaign of the 1970s. But the disturbing thing about these pandemics was that they demonstrated the rapidly mutating capability of the flu virus. The one of the 1940s was a H1N1 strain to which many must have had some immunity from the 1918 pandemic; those of 1957 and 1968, however, were caused by entirely new strains (antigenic shift) of H2N2 and H3N2 respectively, which successively crowded out earlier ones. These pandemics are also believed to have come from the Far East, specifically China, and to have come on in waves, like in 1918, with the second wave seemingly more virulent (both in terms of morbidity and mortality) than the first, showcasing an evolutionary process whereby the virus was evidently adapting itself more successfully to humans. Yet, as in 1918, those who caught the flu in the first, milder wave seem to have acquired some immunity to later incidences of the disease, and it is thought that the strains of 1957 and 1968 may have circulated in the late nineteenth century, conferring some protection to the older generation who were most susceptible. This time the viruses responsible are thought to have arose through "reassortment" of human and avian strains in a third host, such as pigs, rather than making a direct leap from birds to humans as in 1918, which means that these later pandemics would act less like "virgin soil" diseases in human populations and were less likely to provoke in them uncontrolled immune responses, such as a cytokine storm. Yet, all was not smooth sailing, as Communist China under Chairman Mao Zedong maintained a closed-door policy with respect to reporting flu cases, a pattern that has continued recently with avian flu; to this day, we still do not know how many Chinese died in 1957, with some scholars believing that a good proportion of the thirty million who died during the "Great Leap Forward" collectivization program between 1958 and 1961 may be attributed to flu. Even in Western democratic developed countries, such as Britain, authorities were slow to follow

WHO recommendations and close schools, which has been proven to halt epidemics, and hospital facilities and staff were at times overwhelmed.[34]

The postwar experience of a flu pandemic occurring once every decade looked set to continue when in January 1976 more than two hundred army recruits at Fort Dix in New Jersey came down with an H1N1 "swine flu" strain, although several dozen victims were also infected with the H3N2 virus that had last circulated in 1968. Of great concern at the time was that the swine flu virus was demonstrated to be transmissible from person to person and that it seemed to be related to the exceptionally virulent strain of 1918, since serum obtained from individuals over fifty years of age, who were likely to have been exposed to the earlier virus, contained antibodies to the present one. This also meant that much of the population, particularly the younger generation, would have no immunity to this virus since they had been born after the strain of 1918 had ceased circulating, which raised the specter of another "virgin soil"–type pandemic. As it turns out, we have already seen that recent biomolecular archaeology on autopsy samples from victims of the 1918 flu indicate that it was an avian strain, not a swine one, yet this information was simply not available in 1976; in fact, this "epidemic that wasn't" was the first to demonstrate that a major antigenic shift can occur in an influenza virus without producing a widespread outbreak. This was probably because the virus passed directly from pigs to humans without recombination or reassortment in swine with a human viral strain, which would have made it far more transmissible person to person.[35]

However, while doing nothing was simply not an option, some at the time did counsel caution: Albert Sabin, who helped develop the polio vaccine in the 1950s, recommended to the Centers for Disease Control (CDC) and in testimony before Congress that only high-risk groups be initially targeted for vaccination and that in the meantime extra doses be stockpiled, while WHO failed to report any further outbreaks of flu cases around the world. Yet, dissenting voices were deliberately excluded from the blue-ribbon panel advising U.S. president Gerald Ford. As a consequence, an ambitious, $135 million program to mass vaccinate the entire U.S. population of roughly two hundred million people was quickly signed into law by Ford in April, and implementation began with the first shots administered in October. A number of factors went into this decision to vaccinate on such an unprecedented scale. Chief among these seem to have been fears of a repeat of 1918, with its huge potential losses in lives and treasure, this time ranging in the millions of deaths and billions of dollars. Historical writing about the flu also played its part. It was said that the secretary of the Department of Health, Education, and Welfare, David Mathews, read Crosby's new book about the 1918 pandemic, *Epidemic and Peace*, and warned his colleague, James Lynn, director of the Office of Management and Budget, that "we will see a return of the 1918 flu virus." In addition, the 1957 and 1968 pandemics had demonstrated the costs in thousands of lives lost when vaccine was delivered too late or in too few doses. But this was also an election year (as well as America's bicentennial), and Ford faced strong challenges first during the Republican primary from California governor Ronald Reagan and then in the general election from his Democratic opponent, Jimmy Carter. Editorials in the *New York Times* indeed accused the vaccination program of being primarily motivated by politics. In the event, the ensuing "fiasco" or "debacle," as it was called, probably cost Ford more in political capital than he gained. When an epidemic failed to materialize in the fall, this only reinforced his popular image as an incompetent bungler.[36] I still remember watching a satiric spoof of the U.S. presidential debates by the *Saturday Night Live* comedy program, in which comedian Chevy Chase appeared as Ford with a vaccine shot still stuck in his arm! (A picture of Ford receiving his flu shot was published on the wire, perhaps to increase confidence in the vaccine.)

By mid-December the vaccination program was canceled, largely due to fears of side effects when several hundred vaccinated individuals came down with a rare and sometimes fatal neurological disease called Guillain-Barré syndrome. Although subsequent studies claim that those receiving a vaccine had a five times higher (yet still pretty remote) chance of contracting Guillian-Barré than those who did not, a more than circumstantial connection has still to be proven with this particular vaccine, since such complications can occur with any foreign substance introduced into the body.[37] Despite this setback, some would argue that the 1976 vaccination was a success, in that it demonstrated how a large number of vaccine doses—over forty-three million, representing 50 percent of the high-risk group (double what is normally covered in most vaccine programs) or nearly a quarter of the general population—could be mobilized in a short amount of time. Edwin Kilbourne, who served as medical adviser and advocate of the program, summed up his justification, and that of the CDC, thus: "Better a vaccine without an epidemic than an epidemic without a vaccine."[38] Two National Immunization Conferences were also held in the immediate aftermath of 1976 under the succeeding Carter administration, which resulted in proposals for a permanent flu vaccination program supervised by the federal government as well as increased awareness of the necessity for better immunization against other infectious diseases, such as polio, measles, and diphtheria.[39]

But aside from the monetary cost, these benefits did not come without a price. Hostility to government vaccination programs was given free rein during the presidency of Reagan in the 1980s, which helped scuttle funding for immunization against the flu as well as against other preventable diseases like measles, while the initiative for developing future vaccines was hereafter surrendered to private industry.[40] The experience of 1976, however, proved this to be a mistake, for pharmaceutical companies found they could not get insurance on their own to cover their liabilities from potential lawsuits (to date over six hundred million dollars in filed claims), which instead had to be covered by a special appropriation from Congress, and difficulties ensued with the distribution and administration of the vaccine, which was left up to local state control and was therefore very uneven. A more general fallout, but no less tangible for that, was a loss of public confidence in vaccinations, which was due to not only medical complications but also faulty manufacturing, in which one set of trial lots of the vaccine was made up with the wrong virus. All these misunderstandings could probably have been avoided or at least mitigated with better sharing of information amongst the media and the public, especially in the context of the widespread disillusionment with the federal government engendered by the recent Watergate scandal.[41] It is a failure that still haunts vaccination efforts against flu to this day.

In recent years, fears have been raised about a possible pandemic of avian flu, caused by the H5N1 virus. The virus first came to the world's attention in 1997 with an outbreak in Hong Kong, where an epidemic was averted by the culling of about one and a half million market poultry, a policy that Hong Kong has adopted ever since in response to any reported outbreak of avian flu. As of the end of 2009, WHO reported a total of 467 human cases of avian flu around the world, resulting in 282 deaths, representing a mortality rate of just over 60 percent.[42] Some would argue, however, that this vastly overstates the virulence of avian flu, since many more cases where flu symptoms are quite mild simply go unreported. Over half of the known cases occurred in Indonesia and Vietnam, with the next most numerous cases occurring in Egypt, China, Thailand, Turkey, Cambodia, and Azerbaijan, in that order. Again, this may reflect honesty of reporting just as much as actual cases. Typically, those who have come down with avian flu contracted it directly from domestic birds, who are likewise highly susceptible to the virus (to date millions upon millions have died); in most cases, the virus was transmitted either by eating infected poultry products (such as raw duck blood, considered a delicacy in Vietnam) or by breathing in dust particles contaminated with bird feces, within which the virus is shed in huge numbers. However, clusters of cases of human-to-human transmission have also occurred, although these are usually confined to family members where close contact with infection sources likewise seems to be a prerequisite and where the virus seems to have weakened in virulence with each subsequent transmission. Some flu victims exhibited symptoms of a cytokine storm, or immune overreaction to the virus, much like what happened during the 1918 pandemic, but in other cases symptoms were delayed or much less severe; such variations seem to be due to different genetic responses to the virus in respective hosts.[43]

There is much debate about whether an avian flu pandemic is likely to occur outside what so far have been very localized outbreaks. Some say it is inevitable that the H5N1 virus will undergo a genetic shift and thereby evolve an ability to pass directly from human to human in a far more efficient manner than hitherto, since this has always been the past history of influenza. Others counter that the "not if but when" fears of an avian flu pandemic is all a hoax perpetrated largely by the media establishment and the pharmaceutical industry, who stand to benefit substantially from manufacturing an avian flu vaccine or antiviral drugs.[44] In this scenario, avian flu will simply be a dead-end disease in its animal hosts, never breaking out widely in humans because its unique genetic and protein makeup is incompatible with that of human cells, as seems to have been the case with the overblown "swine flu" of 1976. In the case of avian flu, it is thought that the surface proteins of the virus are unable to bind to the sugar molecules in the cells of our nose and throat but can do so once the virus is deep in the lungs in the alveoli; this is why it is hard to contract yet is deadly once it happens. A sanguine view of avian flu also depends on the notion that a genetic hybrid or mixing (reassortment) of bird and human strains in a third host, such as a pig, is naturally impossible, which hasn't stopped recent efforts to artificially create one in the lab in the hopes of heading off its occurrence in nature, another Frankenstein's monster experiment that, as with the resurrection of the 1918 virus, is controversial.[45]

A further focus of debate concerns the source pools of infection for avian flu. In most literature this has been identified as the poor, rural areas of southern China, such as the Guangdong province, where human populations mingle with huge flocks of domestic ducks, geese, chickens, and turkeys that roam freely or are transported across vast areas of land with ample opportunities for contact with wild birds harboring the H5N1 virus; from there, the virus is then alleged to spread out to Hong Kong, Korea, Japan, and Southeast Asia. However, as was noted toward the start of this chapter, China's poultry farming practices go back to time immemorial, and so far, it does not seem that the virus has migrated with wild bird flocks outside its endemic areas, perhaps because most carriers die before they can get very far, as happened to wild geese and other waterfowl in some of China's nature reserves in 2005. Although other H5 and some H7 bird flu strains have appeared in the West, including the United States, Canada, Italy, Ireland, and, most recently in 2003, the Netherlands, these have been confined to animals or have not been very deadly to humans.[46]

An alternative hypothesis places the blame squarely on the industrialized production of food and factory farms, or Concentrated Animal Feeding Operations (CAFOs), the so-called bird jails where enormous numbers of poultry are kept confined at close quarters in cages and often in contact with other animal populations, such as pigs. This "livestock revolution" has been a relatively recent phenomenon, cresting, it has been noted, in the 1990s at the same time that avian flu first made its appearance. It is associated with Asian conglomerates such as Charoen Pokphand (CP) based in Bangkok, Thailand, and with American versions such as Tyson Foods and Perdue. These food monopolies produce mass quantities of chicken manure, which are sometimes used as fertilizer or otherwise present run-off hazards for the environment; appropriate or drive out smaller, free-range family farms; use antibiotics or genetically engineered embryos to maintain product quality (while increasing the risk of drug-resistant viral strains); adopt risky feeding practices such as the chopped-up remains of other animals (which is how bovine spongiform encephalopathy, or "mad cow disease," emerged); and can best absorb the costs of governmental oversight aimed at preventing or halting disease migration from animals to humans, such as the culling of at-risk herds or monitoring programs such as the National Animal Identification System (NAIS) proposed by the U.S. Department of Agriculture. Although claims are made that such confinement operations are healthier because they keep their animals separate from wild reservoirs of disease, it is just as likely it is the other way around, that wild birds have picked up exotic viruses from chance encounters with artificial environments that receive little ventilation or sunlight and whose denizens are forced to defecate on each other and otherwise live in incredibly unhygienic, not to say inhumane, conditions.[47]

What is the solution, or rather denouement, to the avian flu dilemma? Even if we don't have to worry about a pandemic of avian flu, we probably would be wise to keep searching for better ways to medically prevent and treat the disease. Some antiviral drugs, like oseltamivir and zanamivir that inhibit the N protein responsible for new viral copies budding out from the host cell, may have some effect against avian flu, but the most they do is alleviate symptoms—they are not a cure. The drugs' main use, if stockpiled and administered shortly after flu symptoms appear, is to buy some time for vaccine development and distribution. Current vaccines for H5N1 are only 50 percent effective and must be administered in doses twelve times higher than that for regular vaccines, which increases the likelihood of side effects and makes them almost impractical for inoculating large numbers of people quickly in response to an emerging pandemic. Avian flu vaccines are notoriously hard to produce because they naturally kill off the fertilized chicken egg cultures in which the formulas are usually grown; genetically engineered vaccines may get around this problem and would also be far easier to manufacture at short notice. Another possibility is to use the antibodies of those who have survived or who happen to be immune to avian flu; this possibility parallels similar work being done with AIDS. Still a third alternative in the vaccine arsenal uses the harmless adenovirus to carry the H surface protein of avian flu, which seems to be effective against multiple strains caused by antigenic drift since it stimulates both antibodies and immune cell activity in the host. This would make for a vaccine that could be effective year to year, until a major genetic shift occurs. The holy grail of this kind of vaccine would be one that focuses on a protein common to all flu strains, meaning that one shot would confer immunity to flu for all time.[48] This would then set up an eradication campaign for flu equivalent to what was done for smallpox in the 1970s.

Until and if that happens, however, the socioeconomic and cultural dimension of avian flu cannot be ignored. This means that, for the time being, perhaps flu can best be fought with lifestyle and behavioral changes that limit the opportunities for flu to make the leap from animals to humans. Within the endemic foci of avian flu in Asia, this would entail changing farming practices in order to better respect the boundaries between wild and domestic fowl, increasing hygiene at live poultry markets and farms, scrupulously reporting cases of sick birds or humans, and changing the ways in which poultry products are handled, cooked, or consumed. These policies have already been proven to be successful in Thailand, for example, after avian flu returned to Southeast Asia in 2004. But we must also recognize that currently there are major disincentives for doing almost all these things, such as the loss of families' livelihood and food source should their flocks be culled, or the potential damage to developing countries' economies in terms of tourism and exports should flu outbreaks be made public. Probably the only way to counter these negatives is with financial compensation forthcoming from the richer nations of the world, and perhaps the only way to persuade others to render such aid is by casting avian flu as a health problem that affects us all as part of a global network of disease, in the same way that attempts have been made to mobilize a global response to the environmental disaster of global warming. This also means that the inhabitants of the wealthier West will not be exempt from making similar social, economic, and cultural choices, such as shifting consumer patterns away from mass-produced foods and toward locally sustainable sources.[49] (This is indeed the subject of the 2009 documentary *Food, Inc.*)

The many issues surrounding flu were recently brought back into focus with the occurrence of an H1N1 pandemic in 2009, the first flu pandemic to occur in over forty years, if one does not count the 1976 scare. The first wave in the spring was first reported in Mexico, where flu may have been present as early as January, with a second wave occurring in the autumn. (A third wave expected for the winter–spring of 2010 never materialized.) By June of 2009, the flu was officially declared a pandemic by WHO and the CDC. In the United States alone, it is estimated that to date forty-seven million people have come down with "swine flu," representing about 15 percent of the total population, and that over two hundred thousand victims have been hospitalized and almost ten thousand people have died.[50] While this is by far the largest number of flu mortalities reported in any country in the world, anecdotal evidence suggests that the flu was a lot more severe and deadly in developing countries, where access to vaccines and quality health care is quite a bit lower than in the United States.[51] Moreover, the designation of "swine flu" by the media to this pandemic is an unfortunate misnomer, since the genetic makeup of the virus has been revealed to contain elements from swine, avian, and human influenza strains. Although the virus has been found in pigs in some countries, it is only transmitted person to person and has not been communicated from pigs to humans, nor by eating pork products. Nonetheless, this has not stopped some countries, such as Azerbaijan and Indonesia, from banning imports of pork, and Egypt decided to slaughter all pigs in the country (numbering over three hundred thousand) in April, despite reporting no flu cases.

In terms of socioeconomic and cultural responses, the flu of 2009 produced an interesting mix of reactions, some familiar and some new. The fact that most flu deaths have occurred among healthy, vigorous adults aged between eighteen and sixty-four and among pregnant women raised fears of another pandemic like the one of 1918, even though mortalities, at least in the United States, have actually been below what is to be expected in an average flu year. In some cases, victims indeed succumbed rapidly to a cytokine storm as their robust immune systems overreacted to the new strain. Yet, the superior, modern health care now available—at least in developed countries mostly in the West that have better diagnostic techniques and treatment therapies, such as antiviral drugs like Tamiflu and antibiotics to ward off bacterial pneumonia—and the fact that this time most people's nutritional health and immune systems are not being compromised by a world war, seems to have kept such deaths to a minimum compared to 1918. Some countries, such as China, Japan, Australia, Egypt, Russia, and Taiwan, have adopted or announced quarantine measures against travelers suspected of harboring the virus, isolating them in their hotels or on cruise ships, and new technologies, such as thermal imaging systems that can detect feverish conditions in the body, have been employed at airports to keep pace with worldwide airline travel. Wearing of masks once again came into fashion, particularly in countries like Japan, where they are culturally accepted and often used to ward off pollution. Some countries have also felt a severe economic fallout from the pandemic. In Mexico, for example, the local tourism industry, such as to Cancún and other popular destination resorts, simply collapsed during the summer in the wake of its spring scare, and the country has received millions of dollars in loans from the World Bank to cope with the crisis, partly it seems as a reward for its brave, early reporting of the outbreak. In spite of fears to the contrary, the pandemic did not dim proceedings at the 2010 Winter Olympic games in Vancouver, Canada, which is currently ranked ninth in the world in terms of flu incidences and deaths. And yet, this flu has also defied expectations and posed some continuing challenges: it is still not known whether the flu will come back as a cyclical, seasonal virus or if it was just a one-off occurrence; in a high proportion of cases there were no telltale symptoms of fever and cough even though the victims were still highly infectious and remained so for up to three weeks after recovery; and, as already noted, there was a great discrepancy around the world in severity of the pandemic based on the availability of vaccines and medical care.[52]

Here in the United States, responses have been mostly organized at the local school and state level, some of whom had already in years past been making similar preparations in expectation of a pandemic of avian flu. At the college where I teach in Vermont, for example, regular e-mail updates on the pandemic and information fact sheets were posted campuswide, and student health services geared up for a 30 percent infection rate. Advisories included commonsense precautions, such as the washing of hands and face, coughing or sneezing away from others, self-isolation at home—if infected—for at least twenty-four hours after symptoms fade (even though this particular outbreak of flu can be contagious for far longer than that), seeking medical help if symptoms persist beyond three days or are extreme, and so on. This also meant I had to suspend my normal absentee and assignment deadline policies, which I'm sure my students appreciated! A massive vaccination program, one not seen since the polio vaccine of the 1950s, was geared up by WHO and the U.S. government in response to the pandemic, although here in the States delivery of the vaccines came late, in November, when the second wave of the flu had already struck in early autumn. This was attributed to difficulties in culturing the vaccine in fertilized chicken embryos; the virus was claimed to be exceptionally slow to replicate. It is also possible that delays came from elaborate testing protocols and safeguards for the vaccine, given the experience of 1976. An underground drumbeat against vaccination surfaced on September 26, 2009, when political commentator and cable TV talk show host Bill Maher published a brief broadside on Twitter: "If u get a swine flu shot ur an idiot." In the second week of January 2010, U.S. president Barack Obama declared it by proclamation to be "National Influenza Vaccination Week," and the U.S. Department of Health and Human Services editorialized in local newspapers to encourage people to get vaccinated for swine flu, indicating that we are still haunted by the ghosts of 1976. But just like back then, the state delivery system of the vaccines has also been very uneven. In my home state of Vermont, H1N1 flu clinics were mobbed, and the state ran out of vaccine early due to higher than normal demand. I remember standing outside in the cold for two and a half hours to get my own shot. But in New York City, the *New York Times* reported that flu clinics were deserted, which again echoes 1976, when New York had only a 10 percent vaccination rate. There has also been some debate about who should get the vaccines and who should administer them. In Vermont, vaccines were, at least initially, restricted to certain "priority" or high-risk groups, which included pregnant women, health care workers, those aged between six months and twenty-four years, and those with preexisting health conditions that made them more susceptible to flu (of which I was one). But if fulminant cases of flu are also striking down healthy, prime-age adults in other categories due to their vigorous immune systems, shouldn't vaccines also be made available to them (perhaps on a first-come, first-served basis), especially since they would be the ones, through their active lifestyles in the workplace, who would be most likely to spread the flu? At the Vermont college where I teach, for example, I attempted to get an H1N1 vaccine offered at health services, but I was told that shots were restricted to students. This makes sense if students are spreading flu in their dorms, but professors are also at the "flashpoint" of this pandemic and their sick leaves, it could be argued, will have a greater impact on the continued viability of campus life, particularly in terms of instruction. In the event, hundreds of elementary and secondary schools throughout the country did temporarily close in response to the pandemic, in spite of CDC recommendations against this. I also question the delivery method of special public clinics for the vaccines, since the holding area where my wife and I along with dozens of other families were milling around filling out paperwork seemed a perfect environment for spreading the flu. Instead, perhaps flu shots and live vaccine nasal sprays would have been better administered at general practices, where staggered appointments could be made. Despite these difficulties, however, my overall impression as of 2010 is that the pandemic was successfully contained. The disaster that some of us anticipated did not happen, and 1918 was not repeated. Indeed, the fact that a pandemic has taken so long to reemerge, whereas previously a pandemic was to be expected every decade, is a very hopeful sign. We can all congratulate ourselves for that. But there are still some lessons to be learned with regard to the next flu pandemic, when and if this should occur.

CHAPTER 6

AIDS

Of all the deadly infectious diseases that are discussed in this book, acquired immune deficiency syndrome (AIDS) is perhaps the most culturally constructed one, whose ever-shifting "metaphors" relative to each society's attitudes and behaviors are intimately connected with the clinical and biological manifestations of the disease. There is no better illustration of this than the tale of "two AIDS" that can be told in the three decades since its discovery at the dawn of the 1980s. One tale takes place in the countries of the West, primarily the United States and Western Europe (what are sometimes called Pattern I countries by those tracking the global spread of AIDS), while the other is set mainly in sub-Saharan Africa and the Caribbean (Pattern II). What will happen in those countries where AIDS is still emerging, such as Eastern Europe, Asia, and the Middle East (Pattern III) remains to be written. Indeed, the differences between these tales is so striking that some "AIDS dissenters" go so far as to say they are about two different diseases entirely, which of course is not true. But let us look at each of these tales in turn.

First, we should briefly recount what we know thus far about the unique biology and origins of this complex disease. AIDS is caused by the human immunodeficiency virus (HIV), which, like the viruses that cause influenza, mutates rather prolifically, about once in every replication cycle, making the disease difficult to counteract with a vaccine or a cure. However, HIV is different from smallpox or influenza viruses in that, with the aid of an enzyme called reverse transcriptase, its RNA is able to make DNA copies of itself, which it then incorporates into the nuclear chromosomes of the host cell so that it manufactures more viral RNA and hence more viruses. Microbes with this ability are called retroviruses, because they actually reverse the normal order of cell biology, which is to transcribe DNA into RNA. The advantage for the retrovirus is that the cell can keep functioning and remain alive to serve the replicating needs of its viral guest, rather like a body taken over by some alien avatar or possessing spirit, whereas other viruses would kill off their host once the lysis or release of new copies from the cell membrane is complete. (Retroviruses instead "bud out" from the cell in immature form without apparently compromising the membrane's integrity.) Retroviral DNA can also lie hidden or dormant within their cellular crypt, doing nothing for years until suddenly and mysteriously called back from the dead to compel the cell to do its replicating bidding once more.

Within this devious family of retroviruses, HIV has the further dastardly capacity of specifically targeting cells that are crucial for marshaling our immune defense system. These are namely the helper T-lymphocytes, or T-4 cells, which signal other cells to start producing antibodies in our blood and which also mobilize a cellular immune response to the virus; yet, T-4 cells are particularly prone to invasion by HIV because they contain CD4 protein molecules on their surfaces with which HIV happens to bind. Another type of immune cell called macrophages, which are phagocytes or white blood cells that devour other, viral-infected cells, also contain the CD4 receptor and thus can be infected by HIV. Unlike other retroviruses, however, HIV usually kills off the T-4 cells after it has used them to replicate, although in some of these cells and in macrophages it becomes latent, only to be reactivated later. So far as we know, HIV and related viruses in animals—including monkeys, cats, sheep, goats, and horses—are unique in terms of this immune-suppressing quality, forming their own genus or subclass of retroviruses known as lentiviruses (meaning slow to cause disease). HIV is therefore a particularly insidious kind of disease organism in that it seeks out and destroys or else incapacitates the very cells upon which our bodies rely in order to fight off an infection. And unlike any other microbes that simply compete with the body's immune defense system for control of our nutritional resources, HIV actually harnesses that system to manufacture more of the virus it is supposed to be defending against, thus turning our body's would-be saviors into its own worst enemy.[1]

But because HIV is a latent and slow-acting virus, usually patients will go for long periods, often years, without any noticeable symptoms (and are therefore called asymptomatic), during which time they might be blissfully unaware that they have the disease even as they are still infectious in terms of the virus passing through their blood, semen or vaginal secretions, and breast milk, although it should also be pointed out that HIV's presence in these fluids is often low or variable. However, some do show symptoms immediately upon infection with

HIV, which can include a flulike illness and swollen lymph glands, or what is called acute infection syndrome, which is nonetheless practically indistinguishable from many another disease. Later, some more characteristic symptoms might manifest themselves, including low T-4 cell counts, night sweats, persistent low-grade fever, diarrhea and loss of appetite (often brought on by thrush) accompanied by a dramatic drop in weight, and general nausea and fatigue; these symptoms were originally referred to collectively as AIDS-related complex (ARC), but this term is now no longer used in the field because it tends to confuse people as to whether or not patients actually have AIDS. Instead, experts prefer to see ARC as part of a continuum eventually leading to full-blown AIDS, especially given that the same symptoms can reappear at that time.

Eventually, full-blown AIDS emerges because the body, left helpless without a properly functioning immune defense system, is prone to opportunistic or secondary infections—far more deadly and aggressive than normal—which is what the AIDS patient usually dies from, rather than from HIV itself. Absent the intervention of some kind of antiretroviral therapy (ART), such cases of full-blown AIDS will typically appear within ten to twelve years from infection with HIV, although considerable variation within that time frame is possible. Some patients can develop AIDS fairly quickly, within two years from infection due to contributing lifestyle factors (such as drug use) or coinfection with other blood-related illnesses such as hepatitis; but in 5 percent of cases certain "nonprogressors" can go for a dozen years or more without manifesting AIDS, perhaps because their immune system is especially good at fighting HIV or because they are infected with a less reproductive form of the virus. Once a patient does come down with a case definition of full-blown AIDS, he or she has anywhere from six months (usually in Pattern II countries) to two years to live without treatment. Some of the more typical opportunistic infections in a case definition of AIDS include the following: protozoan illnesses such as toxoplasmosis (which attacks and inflames brain tissue) and cryptosporidiosis (infecting the intestines, causing severe and prolonged diarrhea); fungal diseases such as *Pneumocystis carinii* pneumonia (PCP), cryptococcosis (a form of meningitis), and candidiasis (or thrush); and bacterial diseases, particularly tuberculosis. Many of these organisms are already present in the body but are usually kept under control by a normally functioning immune system. AIDS patients are also susceptible to cancers often caused by coinfection by a member of the herpes virus family, such as: Kaposi's sarcoma, an otherwise rare skin cancer that produces purplish lesions or tumors on the body, similar to the disseminated intravascular coagulation (DIC) of septicemic plague; lymphomas or cancers that originate in the immune system that are caused by the Epstein-Barr virus (which also causes mononucleosis in young adults); and cytomegalovirus infection, which

commonly leads to blindness. Female patients also often contract cervical cancer. Most of these infections can be treated independently of HIV with antibiotics and chemotherapy; they are also specifically associated with simultaneous
HIV infection, since they show up again and again in AIDS patients out of all
the diseases to which a compromised immune system is potentially vulnerable.
Furthermore, HIV causes on its own some potentially life-threatening illnesses
without help from other microbes. One is called AIDS-dementia complex, in
which the patient suffers memory loss, headaches, disorientation, depression,
personality changes, and other neurological symptoms due to the fact that HIV
hidden in macrophages can invade the cells of our brain. Finally, the patient will
lapse into a coma and die; damage to the spinal cord and peripheral nerves can
also cause paralysis and burning, tingling sensations or numbness in the extremities. A couple of other HIV-related conditions include HIV wasting syndrome (also known as "slim disease"), in which the patient suffers dramatic
weight loss of 10 percent or more of total body mass, often accompanied by
persistent diarrhea, high fever, night sweats, and loss of appetite; and lymphade-
nopathy syndrome, whereby the patient suffers prolonged swellings of the
lymph glands in the neck, armpit, or groin, akin to the symptoms of bubonic
plague but apparently not as painful.[2]

Transmission of HIV from person to person is now well understood and
documented. Fortunately for us, HIV is a fragile virus that cannot long survive
outside the host; therefore, it must be passed directly in certain bodily fluids
from one contact to another. Since HIV is mostly present in blood, semen,
vaginal secretions, and breast milk (while only present in tears and saliva in trace
amounts), this means it can be spread through limited routes of entry into the
body that can mostly be regulated by a conscious choice of social behaviors. The
most efficient mode of transmission is transfusion of HIV-tainted blood, with a
90 percent infection rate, but since 1985 all blood products in the United States
have been screened for presence of the virus (as detected by an antibody test), so
this is currently a rare mode of transmission, at least in Pattern I countries. However, blood transfusions may still play a significant role in new HIV infections
where screening is not affordable or practical, such as sub-Saharan Africa, and it
has undoubtedly contributed to the historic spread of the virus prior to our scientific awareness of it. Some patterns of injected drug use can also mimic the
transfusion method of transmission, such as when addicts share syringes with
which they have pulled back the plunger to mix their blood with the drug (in
order to make sure they have found a vein or that all of the drug is being injected). Reusing of injection equipment in poorer countries with limited supplies
is also highly dangerous for the same reason, in that some amount of blood will
remain in the syringe after each use. Worldwide, injecting drug users (IDUs)

account for less than 5 percent of all HIV infections, indicating that this is a problem easily solved by disinfecting needles, where these have to be reused, but until quite recently it has remained the primary mode of transmission in Asia and Eastern Europe. On the other hand, accidental needlestick injury represents a rather low risk of infection, at 0.3 percent (or three out of one thousand incidences), perhaps because actual injection of syringe contents into the victim usually does not take place. Mother-to-child transmission (MTCT) either during pregnancy and birth or afterward by means of breast-feeding is likewise a highly contagious mode of HIV infection: it is estimated that a child has anywhere from a 25 to 50 percent chance of contracting HIV from its infected mother by such means, provided that neither is treated by antiretrovirals. Finally, there is unprotected sexual intercourse as a mode of transmission of HIV; compared to most other methods discussed above, it has a relatively low rate of infection, yet this can be highly variable depending primarily on the way the act is performed and with whom. Vaginal intercourse has the lowest rate of infection, at 0.33 to 1 per 1,000 exposures for men and 1 to 2 per 1,000 exposures for women, but if there are genital lesions due to accompanying venereal infections such as syphilis or gonorrhea, the rate can be much higher. Also, if one has multiple or even daily concurrent sex partners (as in the case of commercial sex workers or prostitutes), the risk of infection will greatly increase. These factors, of course, also hold true with anal intercourse (whether homosexual or heterosexual), which on its own has a much greater rate of infection, at 5 to 30 per 1,000 exposures, than vaginal intercourse, mainly due to the greater risk of trauma to the protective epithelial barrier against the virus (which can not only receive infection but also give it, since HIV-tainted macrophages can be present in mucosal linings). And yet, other sexually transmitted diseases (STDs), such as syphilis and gonorrhea, have an even greater risk of transmission during unprotected vaginal sex than anally passed HIV, at 20 to 40 percent per exposure.[3] As we will see, MTCT and heterosexual transmission seem to be the norm in sub-Saharan Africa, while homosexual and IDU modes have historically been the most prevalent in Pattern I and III countries.

The usual strategy of combating an infectious virus like HIV is to develop vaccines, as has been done with smallpox and influenza. However, HIV presents an unusually challenging microorganism to vaccinate against, for both biological and some socioeconomic reasons. As we have already seen, HIV integrates its genome into the DNA of the host cell, where it can lie dormant or hidden for years safe from any antibodies generated by a vaccine. Once activated or triggered, HIV then replicates rapidly within the cell and thus mutates quite easily, making it a moving target for vaccination, much like influenza. There is also concern about whether inactivated HIV used in a vaccine could become active again, as does indeed happen in people naturally infected by the virus. Another possibility is that an AIDS vaccine could harm the immune system just as much as priming it against HIV, since antibodies would have to mimic the same CD4 proteins that HIV binds to on T-4 cells and macrophages. Given these difficulties, some have argued for developing a "therapeutic" vaccine rather than a "preventative" one, which would stimulate the immune system to fight and eliminate the virus once it is established inside the body, thus preventing progression to the full-blown disease of AIDS rather than warding off HIV infection itself. This would also have the advantage of reducing the risk of person-to-person infection, including MTCT. But other difficulties besides biological ones have intervened to forestall HIV vaccine development: difficulty in finding animal models and human volunteers to undergo vaccine trials, length of time involved in demonstrating the efficacy of the vaccine, ethical questions with regard to control groups and conducting trials in poorer countries, and economic disincentives such as liability issues and threat of lawsuits, high costs of development, low rates of return in developing countries—where most of the vaccine market is currently located rather than in the more affluent West—and, after years of trying to find a vaccine, simple disillusionment and discouragement in the wake of failure.[4] Nonetheless, a six-year trial that concluded in 2009 found that a combined vaccine that stimulated both a cellular T-4 immune response as well as an antibody response had a 26 to 31 percent effectiveness rate in preventing HIV infection, rekindling hopes that eventually a viable vaccine will be found.

Of more proven effectiveness to date have been ARTs that reduce the viral load in the blood. These include reverse transcriptase inhibitors (which interfere with the production of viral DNA), such as azidothymidine (AZT), also known as zidovudine or retrovir; protease inhibitors (which interfere with the assembly of the protein coat in new viruses); fusion inhibitors (which prevent HIV from fusing with a host T-4 cell); entry inhibitors (designed to prevent HIV from entering a host cell); and cytokine-based drugs such as interleukin-2 that help stimulate the production of more T-4 cells in the body's race against viral replication. Usually, a "cocktail" combination of such drugs is prescribed to AIDS patients who can afford it (at a cost of fifteen to thirty thousand dollars in the West) in order to circumvent the potential emergence of HIV resistance. As we will see, this highly active antiretroviral therapy, known by the acronym of HAART, has greatly prolonged the lives of AIDS sufferers in Pattern I countries and transformed the disease into something that is still chronic but manageable, instead of one that has invariably spelled impending death. ART has also demonstrated its ability to prevent MTCT. And yet, it must be emphasized that ART is not a cure for AIDS, because HIV will eventually and inevitably acquire resistance to any drug cocktail due to its mutating ability. It is for this reason that new drug therapies must constantly be devised for HIV—for example, at least ten nucleoside and nonnucleoside reverse transcriptase inhibitors, such as nevirapine, are currently being marketed in addition to AZT—and why ART is now started only after an HIV-infected patient has become symptomatic, rather than administering it to one whose viral count is already low. Nonetheless, antiretrovirals have made hefty profits for the pharmaceutical industry precisely because they must be administered over long periods of time in ever-changing varieties, as opposed to vaccines that theoretically confer lifetime immunity after just one dose. Now that all nine genes of the HIV genome have been mapped and identified, gene therapy may provide a promising alternative to drugs or vaccines in the future.[5]

Last but not least, we should consider the geographical origins of AIDS. This is a controversial topic owing to the stigma attached to any part of the world held responsible for giving birth to so dreaded a disease. We have already seen how, in the nineteenth century, India was blamed as the "home of cholera," which naturally associated the perceived filthy living conditions of the natives with its fulminant diarrheal symptoms that were so disgusting, at least to Western sensibilities. But there is also a biological and historical basis for making such identifications, which can help advance our knowledge of the disease and ultimately our ability to combat it. We have to remember that AIDS is still a very new disease in humans, especially compared to other ills such as plague or tuberculosis that have been around for centuries. With time, the stigma attached to the endemic origin of AIDS in western and central Africa, which currently is still a topic that must be tiptoed around with caution at AIDS conferences, will fade. No one now thinks any less of Central Asia for being the probable origin of the Black Death; it is simply a historical question to be explored and elucidated. We are still coming to terms with living in a world marked by the presence of AIDS.

The scientific evidence for AIDS originating in sub-Saharan Africa is strong. Much research has been done on the simian immunodeficiency virus (SIV) found in monkeys native to Africa. Three of the SIV strains isolated from chimpanzees have been found to be genetically very close to the three groups of the HIV-1 virus that cause almost all cases of AIDS in humans. (The M group alone is responsible for 99 percent of cases, while the O and N groups have been found in patients in Gabon and Cameroon in West Africa, exactly corresponding to the natural range of chimpanzees harboring the SIV strains.) It is therefore believed that HIV first crossed over into humans from chimpanzees, much like smallpox or influenza have historically crossed from cows, birds, and pigs. Africa also holds the most genetic diversity of HIV anywhere in the world. It is the only region to contain all ten subgroups of the M version of HIV-1 as well as the most recombinant strains of these subgroups, and an HIV-2 strain confined to West Africa is practically identical in its genetic makeup to that of an SIV strain found in local sooty mangabey monkeys. (The relative prevalence of all these strains of HIV may partly explain why AIDS behaves differently in various parts of the world.) Since chimpanzees in the wild do not normally develop AIDS, despite having a genome that is over 98 percent identical to that of humans, it seems clear that chimps have evolved a mutual adaptation with the virus, just as waterfowl have with influenza, and that their resistance mechanism can perhaps be of future benefit to us. This is also, of course, an argument for respecting and preserving the natural boundaries of these animals, as likewise holds true for wild birds as the endemic source of influenza. The oldest HIV-positive blood result has been obtained from a native of Kinshasa on the eastern border of the Democratic Republic of Congo (formerly known as Zaire) who died in 1959. Genetic mapping of progressive changes in the HIV genome indicates that the first infection of humans from chimpanzees probably took place during the 1930s, which coincided with massive conscription of natives for railroad construction in the French colonies of west-central Africa, where famine forced workers to consume wild animals, including monkeys. From its "ground zero" point of contact, HIV then spread rapidly in human populations throughout Africa and around the world through the new, interconnected global networks of the second half of the twentieth century. The most likely means by which HIV was able to cross over from chimps to humans was through a sore or wound on a hunter handling the bloody remains of "bush meat" used to supplement the diet of those living in rural areas of Africa. Transmission of SIV (not AIDS) to hunters was found to be still taking place in Cameroon in the early twenty-first century. The theory that AIDS was cultured by Western labs in the Congo that used the kidney cells of chimpanzees to develop and test a polio vaccine during the 1950s has an attractive air of ironic drama to it—modern medicine in the very act of trying to use its technology to save lives gives birth to a new plague!—along with overtones of political correctness in terms of chronicling the ongoing negative impacts of Western imperialism in the third world.[6] But it has now been proven that there is no connection between AIDS and the Congo polio vaccine. Independent laboratory analyses of frozen samples of the original vaccine found no traces of either HIV or chimpanzee cells—the vaccine was actually cultured in Asian macaque monkeys; moreover, the chimpanzees from the region of the Congo where the scientists originally worked do not harbor the ancestral SIV of AIDS. Historically speaking, it now seems quite likely that the crossover occurred before the polio trials of the 1950s. Contaminated needles used for medicinal or vaccination purposes may still have played a role, however, in rapidly cycling SIV through African populations, allowing it to be converted into HIV.[7]

A word here should be said about "dissident" scientists, such as Peter Duesberg, who cast doubt on whether HIV causes AIDS or that the disease originated in Africa. Setting aside the more far-out conspiracy theories such as that AIDS came from outer space or that it was intentionally developed by Western laboratories as a biological or racial weapon, Duesberg's dissidence has to be taken seriously because he is a respected research scientist at the University of California at Berkeley who specializes in cancer-causing viruses, although he is also known within the scientific community for his contrarian views. Duesberg does not deny the existence of HIV but rather contends that it is a harmless passenger in the bodies of infected victims and that the disease of AIDS is instead brought on by lifestyle "stressors" such as poor diet and nutrition, recreational drug use, or even by the very antiretroviral therapies currently used to control and manage the disease. This is not simply the harmless hypothesis of a marginalized crank, because although opposed by the "mainstream" scientific community, Duesberg's theory has been taken up by a handful of other "dissident" scientists, including his cancer research colleague David Rasnick; the Columbian physician and specialist in tropical infectious diseases Roberto Giraldo; the Belgian professor of pathology at the University of Toronto Etienne de Harven; the mathematical biologist Rebecca Culshaw; and the Nobel prize–winning chemist Kary Mullis, some of whom have formed their own advocacy group called "Rethinking AIDS." In addition, AIDS dissidence has been championed by some "investigative" journalists, such as John Lauritsen, Henry Bauer, and Janine Roberts, and most prominently outside the United States by the former president of South Africa Thabo Mbeki, who provided a forum for Duesberg at the 2000 AIDS conference in Durban and who opposed ART implementation in his country largely on the strength of Duesberg's objections, despite drastic price concessions from pharmaceutical companies supplying AIDS drugs. Therefore, it could be argued that this is no mere academic debate but rather one with the lives of millions of men, women, and children at stake. In popular culture, Duesberg's ideas also receive a hearing in the news media, science journals, and through Duesberg's own publications, such as his 1996 book *Inventing the AIDS Virus* and his own personal website (augmented by the publications and websites of other dissidents). Complicating this controversy is that the lifestyle cofactors favored by Duesberg do seem to play a role in the onset of full-blown AIDS after HIV infection, and that viral loads in asymptomatic AIDS patients can be so low as to be virtually undetectable, even though a diagnostic test for HIV infection can still be devised by measuring antibodies. AIDS denial also perhaps plays into a wish fulfillment to blot out the horrors of this world, akin to the motives of some deniers of the Nazi Holocaust.

One of Duesberg's most cogent criticisms is that HIV does not fulfill scientific protocols for identifying a disease agent, such as the "postulates" drawn up the bacteriologist Robert Koch in 1890. It should be pointed out that even Koch could not fulfill all of his postulates when identifying the bacterial causes of cholera and leprosy, and that to a certain degree we have to accept practical limits on how well the correlation between a given microbe and a disease needs to be proven before it can be accepted and put to use. Moreover, HIV is an extraordinarily complex microbe unlike any that Koch had to face. Its fragility outside the host cell, for example, makes it extremely difficult to grow the virus pure in culture, as one of the postulates insists. Even so, some would argue that in fact all of Koch's postulates have by now been fulfilled with respect to AIDS, including the one in which the disease must be reproduced by artificial introduction into a human host. While a deliberate experiment in this regard is ethically untenable in the case of a deadly, incurable disease like AIDS, three laboratory workers who tragically exposed themselves by accident to HIV did indeed go on to develop AIDS. A large amount of circumstantial evidence also supports linking HIV with AIDS, such as that HIV can be tested in all patients with full-blown AIDS while almost no one who is HIV negative has gone on to develop the case definition of the disease; likewise, in no country around the world has AIDS appeared without HIV infection manifesting itself first. We also have to recognize that AIDS is a unique illness, in that it comes about through a latent suppression of the body's immune system and by means of coinfection with an opportunistic disease or cancer. There is therefore no direct, immediate cause and effect from a single microbial invasion, as in the case of most other infectious diseases.[8] Despite the dispiriting counterblast with which Duesberg opens his 1996 book—"By any measure, the war on AIDS has been a colossal failure"—in fact, the lives of countless AIDS patients around the world have been almost returned to normal by the very antiretroviral therapies he condemns. HIV may well be an ancient microorganism centuries or even millennia old,[9] as Duesberg contends, but this still doesn't explain how the virus established itself in the human community, and the recent emergence of the current AIDS pandemic argues for a strong connection with recent historical trends that are particularly apropos to sub-Saharan Africa, such as encroachment on wild animal habitat, widespread migrations of human populations and disruptions of their settlement patterns, and the relaxing or changing of traditional sexual mores. A crossover from monkeys as the natural reservoirs of the virus to humans in Africa remains so far the most plausible explanation of the origin of AIDS.

The focus of most historical narratives on AIDS has been the United States and sub-Saharan Africa. It was in the United States that public awareness of the emerging AIDS pandemic began, even though the crisis in sub-Saharan Africa has by now completely eclipsed the epidemic in Pattern I countries. The first notice taken of the new disease seems to have occurred in June 1981, when the Centers for Disease Control (CDC) published an article in its *Morbidity and Mortality Weekly Report* that detailed the strange case of five young gay men from Los Angeles who all had come down with a rare lung disease, PCP, as a result of a "profoundly depressed" immune system. This was shortly followed up in July with two dozen more cases of PCP in conjunction with an equally rare skin cancer, Kaposi's sarcoma, occurring once again in gay men with dysfunctional immune systems, most of them from New York City. By the following year, 1982, hundreds of cases of the new disease were being reported to the CDC, representing a doubling in the size of the epidemic every six months, and of these cases 40 percent or more were dying. We now know that these cases had probably been incubating for a decade or more since the late 1960s and 1970s. A teenager who died in St. Louis, Missouri, in 1969 of symptoms that suggest PCP and Kaposi's sarcoma was confirmed as perhaps the first American victim of AIDS when his frozen blood and tissue samples tested positive for the virus in 1986. It was also becoming evident by 1982 that the disease was now affecting populations aside from gay men. The CDC came out with its so-called 4H high-risk groups of heroin addicts or IDUs, hemophiliacs, and Haitian immigrants, in addition to homosexuals. In this same year, the CDC officially adopted AIDS as its preferred name for the disease over other alternatives such as gay-related immune deficiency (GRID). By 1983 and 1984, it was becoming clear that AIDS could be spread by heterosexual intercourse and MTCT, which meant that theoretically almost no part of the general population could assume itself to be safe from the disease; meanwhile, the gay community, particularly in San Francisco and New York, began modifying their "risk" behaviors, such as by reducing the number of sexual partners and increasing their use of condoms, so that by 1985 the number of new cases among gays began leveling off. At the same time, greater medical understanding of AIDS was quickly emerging, especially with the announcement of the discovery of HIV, which was jointly attributed to Luc Montagnier of the Pasteur Institute in Paris and Robert Gallo at the National Cancer Institute in the United States, although it is now conceded that most of the credit should go to the French. The shelved cancer drug AZT was also found to be the first effective antiretroviral treatment for AIDS, which was administered to human subjects in 1985. The death of movie star Rock Hudson in October of that year raised awareness of and seemed to give a public face to the disease.[10]

The rest of the 1980s decade saw many of the social issues associated with AIDS play themselves out on the American stage. Some of the leading actors in this drama were the Gay Men's Health Crisis (GMHC) in New York and the AIDS Coalition to Unleash Power (ACT UP), both founded by the activist Larry Kramer. While GMHC pursued what could be called a low-key role as an AIDS service organization (ASO) or informational and resources clearinghouse for AIDS victims, ACT UP took a much more confrontational approach toward its political agenda, such as by performing "zaps" against perceived obstructionist targets, which famously included the seat of the Catholic archdiocese of New York at St. Patrick's Cathedral, where a communion mass was disrupted in 1989. A central focus of AIDS advocacy at this point was to preserve civil liberties, particularly confidentiality and privacy concerns, in the face of public health imperatives to contain an epidemic through such measures as testing, contact tracing, and occasionally quarantine. Remarkably, AIDS activists were able to reverse a long precedent, going back in the United States to almost a century with respect to infectious diseases like syphilis, influenza, and tuberculosis, whereby individual rights had been superseded in the interests of preserving the public health. Instead, AIDS testing and notification, using the enzyme-linked immunosorbent assay (ELISA) and the "Western Blot" tests, first developed in 1985, were to be strictly voluntary with certain exceptions, such as recruits to the U.S. military or applicants to the diplomatic corps. Even by 1997, only half the states in the union required reporting by name of individuals who tested positive for HIV. A number of circumstances were responsible for this AIDS "exceptionalism," including concerns about false positives (although when used together the two tests were nearly foolproof), the self-defeating specter of AIDS patients being driven underground for fear of discrimination, the unproven efficacy of past public health efforts, and the recent example provided by civil rights agitation in the 1960s and 1970s (including the gay liberation movement beginning with the Stonewall uprising in 1969). A recurring refrain at this time was that anyone could get AIDS and thus any oppressive measures would potentially encompass everyone, but this claim was rather specious given that already by the late 1980s evidence pointed to the epidemic, at least in the United States, becoming entrenched among certain sectors of the population who engaged in "high-risk" behaviors, namely, unprotected anal intercourse, multiple sexual encounters (i.e., prostitution), and IV drug use. By the early 1990s, it was clear that AIDS was not going to break out into the general population and become the universal scourge that everyone so feared, especially when it was estimated that the vast majority of Americans had five lifetime serial sex partners or fewer. Yet, the interests of continued AIDS funding dictated that the threat-to-all orthodoxy be maintained even by medical authorities who knew better, and it was debunked only by a vilified few, such as Michael Fumento, author of *The Myth of Heterosexual AIDS*.[11] One myth that was worth debunking, however, was that AIDS was supposedly spread by casual contact, such as coughing, sneezing, touching, kissing, sharing of surfaces or public spaces, mosquito bites, and so forth. On the contrary, the difficulty with which AIDS is spread—as well as the fact that its contagion is largely determined by premeditated and voluntary social behaviors—made it much less of a compelling health threat than, say, a disease like tuberculosis that is communicated involuntarily by airborne droplets. Yet,

AIDS paranoia did not stop the installation of "touchless" hand dryers, soap dispensers, faucets, and toilets in public restrooms, which were to become ubiquitous, and, in the end, completely unnecessary. It also did not help the public health cause that some made extreme recommendations, such as perennial presidential candidate Lyndon Larouche, whose ballot initiative in California to quarantine all AIDS victims (presumably for life) went down to resounding defeat, or the conservative commentators William F. Buckley and Ann Coulter, who proposed tattooing HIV-positives on the buttocks or genitals. On the other hand, it is also undoubtedly true that, due to civil rights agitation, some opportunities to contain the scope of the epidemic were tragically missed. The notorious San Francisco bathhouses, for example, which served as almost perfect breeding grounds for AIDS with their abundant opportunities for anonymous, promiscuous sex, were finally closed down by the city's Public Health director, Mervyn Silverman, in 1985 with little fanfare or protest, but by then it was largely a moot gesture as most of their clients had already made the conscious choice to change their "high-risk" behaviors.

There were plenty of other social conundrums with respect to AIDS. Housing and job discrimination against AIDS patients, which had received the tacit blessing of the attorney general, Ed Meese, was overturned by the Supreme Court on the grounds that their condition qualified them for handicapped or disabled status, and yet misinformed bigotry continued to occur nonetheless, such as doctors and ambulance personnel refusing to treat people known to be HIV infected, police officers wearing gloves and other protective gear when forced to interact with people with AIDS, insurers denying coverage on the basis of membership in one of the "high-risk groups," and immigrants denied entry on the basis of AIDS screening, which played havoc with attempts to host international conferences in the United States on AIDS. (This last policy has only now been reversed by the administration of U.S. president Barack Obama.) Particularly heartbreaking were the so-called innocent victims of AIDS, namely, hemophiliac children (who relied on blood products combined from many different donors) denied access to schools after they tested HIV-positive, owing to false fears that they could spread the disease in certain (highly unlikely) scenarios, such as bloody sports contact. Such was the case of Ryan White of Indiana, or the Ray brothers from Arcadia, Florida, whose family quit town after their house was burnt down.

Aside from civil rights, another major agenda of ACT UP at this time was to improve access to experimental treatments for AIDS patients, whose mortal outlook obviated the usual bureaucratic protocols surrounding new drugs and who often lacked the financial wherewithal to pay for them. Thus, "die-ins" were staged at regional offices of the Food and Drug Administration (FDA), and a group of protestors chained themselves to the VIP balcony at the New York

Stock Exchange. It could be said that the impact of these protests produced the desired result, for the FDA subsequently approved AZT relatively quickly, in a matter of months rather than the usual years, and Burroughs Wellcome, the manufacturer of AZT (with considerable help from the National Cancer Institute), nearly halved the original ten-thousand-dollar-per-year price tag of its drug. Anthony Fauci, director of the National Institute of Allergies and Infectious Diseases (NIAID), earned praise for his championing of an unprecedented "parallel track" approach designed to get investigational new drugs (INDs) into the hands of AIDS patients excluded from clinical trials or "compassionate use" programs from drug manufacturers. At the same time, however, Fauci was heavily criticized for failing to produce any new effective treatments from his AIDS Clinical Trials Group (ACTG), and sometimes the side effects of the new drugs were so severe that patients preferred to die rather than continue treatment.[12]

In terms of presidential policy, the Republican administration of President Ronald Reagan betrayed considerable insensitivity to the plight of AIDS victims, since the disease itself was not publicly acknowledged by the president until 1987, undoubtedly due to its strong associations with the gay community. And yet, for a fiscally conservative administration, the federal AIDS budget grew astronomically during the Reagan years, from $5.5 million in 1982 to over $900 million by the end of the presidency in 1988. Meanwhile, Reagan's outwardly staid surgeon general, C. Everett Koop (known for his signature bow ties), surprised everyone with his AIDS report in 1986 that recommended comprehensive and "value-neutral" sex education in all primary and secondary schools as part of an effort to combat AIDS spread, which nonetheless proved unpalatable to the majority of U.S. households, especially in the conservative heartland. The subsequent administration of a more moderate Republican, President George H. W. Bush, signaled a greater willingness from the president to empathize with AIDS patients and champion antidiscrimination laws, even as he was criticized for failing to provide substantial leadership in the fight against AIDS. Appointing the HIV-positive basketball star Earvin "Magic" Johnson to the National AIDS Commission might be called an empty gesture, but the administration did put its money where its mouth was, increasing federal funding for AIDS-related research to over two billion dollars by 1992 and passing the Ryan White Care Act in 1990, which helped funnel special AIDS funds to the neediest cities. Indeed, AIDS funding could be said to be enormously disproportionate when compared to that for other diseases. The amount spent per AIDS death was four to five times higher than that for the next most expensive diseases, despite the fact that AIDS afflicted a relatively small number of patients, at 120,000 in the United States in 1992, a small fraction of the fifty million estimated Americans suffering from the leading ills of heart disease, stroke, and cancer. The succeeding Democratic administration of President Bill Clinton naturally continued or amplified these trends, yet even Clinton found there were limits to what he could do in terms of AIDS policy. He backed away from federal funding of needle exchange programs, despite the fact that they were proven to be effective in limiting the spread of HIV among drug users and that such programs were already in place in several dozen cities, often in defiance of state laws.[13] He also failed to secure passage of universal health care legislation, which was needed to help poorer patients gain access to ever more expensive treatment regimens for AIDS and to relieve the financial burden on Medicaid (where each patient on triple combination therapy cost the program thirty thousand dollars per year). Although universal health care reform was finally passed under President Obama, it remains to be seen how it will be implemented on a local level in each of the fifty states, some of which are pursuing legal challenges to the new law.

The Clinton era of the 1990s represented a seismic shift in the medical treatment of and overall culture surrounding AIDS. In 1996, a new treatment regimen was announced, called "combination therapy," in which a drug "cocktail" of two different reverse transcriptase inhibitors, such as AZT, nevirapine, or dideoxyinosine (ddI), was combined with one of the newly developed protease inhibitors, such as Crixivan, in order to deliver a triple knockout blow that was found to reduce viral loads to undetectable levels for over a year, in effect eliminating all traces of the virus. Its drawbacks were an extraordinarily complicated pill-taking regimen, which increased chances of noncompliance and hence potential drug resistance in HIV; increased possibilities of side effects; and an exponentially greater expense, which posed a problem for the increasing proportion of AIDS patients too poor to afford the drugs. Nonetheless, combination therapy held out the promise of a return to an almost normal lifestyle, with potentially decades added on to an AIDS victim's life expectancy. This in turn necessitated a reconfiguration of support services for AIDS patients, from end-of-life issues to now more mundane concerns of continued housing, employment, financial planning, and so on. Indeed, so successful was combination therapy in turning AIDS into a chronic and manageable disease that a sense of complacency now crept in among both infected victims and "at-risk" groups. In the gay community, AIDS was transformed from the "gay plague" into the "gay diabetes," and there was a noticeable "backsliding" in safe sex practices and precautions that had been championed earlier, perhaps under the mistaken belief that undetectable viral loads in the blood meant that the disease could not be transmitted. As a consequence, new infections among the gay community began to rise once again during the 1990s.[14] Thus, combination therapy achieved some dramatic benefits in the years immediately following its introduction, but in the long term it seems to have brought us to no more than an impasse or deadlock in relation to the disease. By the end of the 1990s, for example, the number of new HIV infections and AIDS deaths in the United States as reported to the CDC had fallen to forty thousand and less than twenty thousand, respectively, down from highs in the first half of the decade at eighty thousand and fifty thousand. Since then, however, these numbers have scarcely changed: As of 2007, new AIDS diagnoses stand at just over 37,000 while annual deaths from the disease are at roughly 14,500 or maybe higher. Currently, over half a million people have died of AIDS in the United States, and more than a million are estimated to be living with the disease.[15]

There were other ways in which the late 1990s foreshadowed trends that were to emerge in the third decade of AIDS in the United States, or in other words the first decade of the third millennium. If there was a certain complacency toward AIDS among the gay community as a result of its being perceived now as a successfully treatable disease, this was even more noticeable among the general population at large. AIDS can now be said to have earned the title of "forgotten epidemic" that was formerly reserved for influenza. Partly, I think this has been the result of an inevitable backlash against the overhyped threat of AIDS in its early days, as the general public intuited data that suggest that the disease had yet to make much headway among the majority heterosexual population. AIDS was also bound to fade from the public consciousness as its morbidity and mortality rates declined and then leveled off and as it was no longer perceived as a death sentence due to new and improved antiretroviral therapies. This growing obliviousness toward AIDS was reflected in popular culture. Attention garnered by AIDS perhaps peaked in the late 1980s and early 1990s, as the AIDS quilt was unveiled several times at the national mall in Washington, D.C., and made regional tours throughout the United States, while the mainstream Hollywood film *Philadelphia*, released by TriStar Pictures in 1993, earned an academy award for best actor for Tom Hanks, who portrayed a gay lawyer suing his firm for unlawful dismissal after coming down with AIDS, and who was represented by an initially homophobic black colleague, played by Denzel Washington. But by 1998, AIDS was given absolutely no mention in the comedic film *The Wedding Singer*, which was steeped in 1980s nostalgia, and the 2009 "mockumentary" *Brüno*, about a fictional gay Austrian fashion journalist who interacts with real people primarily on homoerotic themes, mentions chlamydia, but not AIDS. (When asked on the online interview program Digg Dialog to name "the hottest illness around now," Brüno cited "bulimia," the joke being that this is really a noninfectious eating disorder rather than a disease proper.) And yet AIDS historian Susan Hunter warns in a 2006 book, *AIDS in America*, that there is the potential for AIDS to flare up again in the United States with even greater force than in the early 1980s and to spread far more deeply than ever before into the mainstream white heterosexual population. Hunter's claims rest on a number of contentions that are mainly supported by anecdotal evidence, such as that large numbers of heterosexuals secretly practice homosexual intercourse on the "down low," that teens engage in promiscuous anal and oral sex as a way of technically fulfilling abstinence-only pledges, and that AIDS statistics reported by the CDC vastly underestimate the true scope of the epidemic. It is undeniable, however, that young people and women are making up greater proportions of new HIV infections; that unprotected intercourse, prostitution, and drug use continue to grow as contributing factors of infection; and that AIDS has established a disproportionate presence in America's growing prison population.[16]

An additional factor in the marginalization of AIDS is the continued marginalization of its "high-risk" groups. Even as AIDS was making a resurgence in the gay community in the late 1990s, it was also migrating toward racial minority groups, namely, blacks and Hispanics, a trend that had commenced since the late 1980s. At the end of the 1990s, blacks' overrepresentation in HIV infections was becoming quite dramatic, at 45 percent of all new cases, even though blacks made up only 12 percent of the general population. This disparity was also evident in the subpopulation of HIV-positive black women, who outnumbered their white female counterparts by a ratio of fifteen to one in 1995. These trends have hardly changed in recent times. As of 2007, blacks made up 44 percent of all people living with AIDS, while whites constituted the next largest group at just over 35 percent; and Hispanics, at 19 percent. Male-to-male homosexual contact was allegedly behind 47 percent of these existing AIDS cases in the United States, while high-risk heterosexual contact and injection drug use are roughly equivalent at 24 and 22 percent respectively.[17] Even though it has been speculated that blacks have a genetic predisposition to AIDS, it is in fact far more likely that certain environmental cofactors are responsible for the higher rates of HIV infection among blacks through IV drug use and homosexual and heterosexual intercourse, such as higher rates of needle sharing and greater prevalence of STDs, including syphilis, chancroid, genital warts, and herpes. (On the other hand, researchers have found that a significant minority of the Caucasian population do have defective genes encoding the CCR5 coreceptor for HIV, which gives them partial or almost complete immunity to the disease. The theory that this was inherited from European ancestors immune to the Black Death is, however, almost pure speculation.[18]) Some argue that to lower AIDS incidence among blacks, efforts should be focused on improving their socioeconomic status and tailoring educational materials to their specific culture. It is likewise claimed that black churches and communities have historically been reluctant to face up to issues of sexual promiscuity, drug use, and homophobia, which have only contributed further to the furtive advance of AIDS. In addition, substantial percentages of surveyed minorities profess themselves disposed to believe in erroneous conspiracy theories about AIDS, such as that the disease was manufactured in government laboratories as an instrument in racial or biological warfare, perhaps because their faith in institutional medicine has been compromised by such real scandals as the Tuskegee syphilis experiment.[19] Meanwhile, research on heterosexual transmission, such as that conducted by Nancy Padian in San Francisco, suggests that women are up to twenty times more susceptible to HIV transmission than men due to a combination of factors: greater presence of the virus in semen as opposed to vaginal secretions, prolonged exposure of the vagina to semen ejaculations, and higher incidences of the vaginal wall being compromised through STDs (which are more likely to remain undetected in women as opposed to men) and through violent or prolonged penetrative intercourse as occurs during sexual assaults and recreational drug use.[20] Even when drug use is not of the intravenous variety that can directly transmit HIV, it can act as a cofactor of sexual transmission of AIDS by impairing the cognitive ability to select safe sex behaviors—and also, in the case of certain drugs such as cocaine, methamphetamine ("crystal meth"), and ecstasy, by enhancing sexual performance and thus the likelihood of epithelial trauma during "dry sex."[21] Many of the issues identified in AIDS transmission among black and female populations in the United States serve as a microcosm for the larger tragedy unfolding in sub-Saharan Africa.

The gay community, which originally bore the brunt of the AIDS epidemic in the United States and continues to do so to this day, is faced with an ongoing ambivalent legacy from its close association with the disease. On the one hand, the AIDS epidemic threatened to set back by at least a decade greater public acceptance of and civil rights for gays. Early in the epidemic, for example, some despicable comments were made by conservative commentator Patrick Buchanan and Moral Majority leader Jerry Falwell that suggested AIDS was a just punishment for the gay lifestyle, all of which were very much in the mode of medieval pronouncements about plague as divine retribution for humanity's sinful behavior. (Indeed, a popular acronym used by the political right at this time for the disease was wrath of God syndrome, or WOGS.) Even though most church congregations tried to balance their moral and humanitarian impulses in their responses to AIDS patients, violent assaults on gays were on the rise, and the political climate seemed ripe for discrimination, if not outright oppression, under the guise of preserving the public health. Yet, we would be less than honest if we failed to point out that at least some of the harm was self-inflicted. There is a certain amount of nihilistic disregard for one's own bodily health in indulging in hundreds of anonymous sexual partners every year, as the patrons of bathhouses were allegedly doing (just as there is in injecting drugs into one's veins), and even before the advent of AIDS, an astonishingly high incidence of STDs in the gay community was already laying the groundwork for the emergence of a more fearsome disease. But the moral opprobrium expressed by the Christian right never saved any lives, and it had long before proved its impotence against syphilis, when the target had been prostitutes. One also has to understand that, for the gay community, promiscuity was a sign of its liberation and "coming out" in the face of an adversarial society during the 1970s. And yet AIDS could equally well be said to have opened the door of opportunity to gays in the United States in terms of galvanizing them for civil rights advocacy in a way that still eludes that other major victim group of the disease, drug users. Perhaps as a result of the necessity of changing risk behaviors in response to AIDS and caring for sick loved ones, the gay community seems to have shifted its agenda in recent years to agitating for recognition of partner benefits and same-sex unions and marriages. While some, even in the gay community, may deplore this domestic agenda as depriving gays of their distinctive identity, it does seem to be facilitating greater acceptance of gays in mainstream society, even as the old political fault lines still seem to apply. My home state of Vermont was the first to recognize civil unions that extended full partner benefits and rights to same-sex couples (although a more watered-down version of "reciprocal beneficiary registration" had been available since 1997 in Hawaii), and Vermont is now one of five states that allow same-sex marriage, in spite of the federal Defense of Marriage Act that restricts marriage to members of the opposite sex. These achievements, it could be argued, might not have come about if not for AIDS.

A final aspect to consider in the so-called third phase of AIDS policy in the United States is the greater emphasis upon surveillance and coercion toward HIV-positive individuals since at least 1997. This coincided with the year of the Nushawn Williams case in New York, where an HIV-positive man was reported to have infected thirteen women, most of them teenage girls, out of some fifty to seventy-five sexual contacts over a two-year period, despite allegedly knowing of his own seropositive status. This led to the adoption in New York and in least twenty-six other states of laws requiring names reporting, contact tracing, or even criminalization of sexually active people who test HIV-positive. Further impelling this change of policy was the stated motive of improving access to new and improved treatments and more accurate monitoring of new AIDS cases. Yet, accepting public assistance now meant that AIDS patients had to submit to far greater surveillance and control. From 2003, the CDC announced that HIV testing of at-risk populations would from now on be the focus of its prevention efforts, and it pressured community-based organizations receiving its funding to "elicit number of partners and contact information" when providing counseling and referral services. It should come as no surprise that the George W. Bush administration's assault upon civil liberties during its so-called war on terror should extend to people with AIDS, but AIDS advocacy groups also seemed to surrender the initiative and abandon the stance on AIDS exceptionalism. The push for an abstinence-only approach to sex education and a continued ban on needle exchange programs were also criticized for being counterproductive and against all the evidence on HIV/AIDS prevention.[22]

AIDS also has a very personal resonance with me, for its social history in the United States that I have just outlined above happens to almost exactly coincide with my own most socially and sexually active years and experience. I remember that when I graduated from college and first entered the workforce as a journalist in 1985, AIDS was simultaneously cresting in public awareness and paranoia in the United States. Fears about this new disease were almost palpable, largely due to the big unknowns still surrounding AIDS and the fact that medical authorities at this point made only qualified statements with regard to its transmission and spread. What was especially terrifying was that here was an invariably fatal disease but one that liked to linger, drawing out its death sentence into a long, exquisite torture. (Unlike our medieval ancestors, we seem to prefer the mercifully quick kill.) Particularly tragic and heartrending were victims who had to tell their families for the first time that they were gay and then immediately inform them that they had AIDS, exposing themselves to a double indemnity of prejudice. As I helped prepare a monograph on *AIDS: The Workplace Issues,* I heard stories of people refusing to touch coffee cups or sweaty keyboards used by an office mate rumored to be infected with HIV, or of a disgruntled fired employee kissing co-workers good-bye with the words "I just gave you AIDS."[23] (We now know, of course, that AIDS cannot be communicated by casual contact.) Even if we did not get AIDS or know someone who did, it seemed we were all somehow indelibly marked by it, should we wish to remain in any way sexually active. It seemed cruel when my mother, echoing surgeon general C. Everett Koop, warned me that "if you sleep with someone, you're sleeping with all their other past partners," which certainly did not make the venture very appealing. If AIDS was a punishment for "deviant" behaviors, then we were all in bed together, gay as well as straight. I resented the earlier generation that got to enjoy a guilt- and worry-free sexual revolution, while I felt that I now had to pay for the pleasures of my parents' generation. At the same time, I almost envied the old, who with their diminished sex drives and stable relationships, could no longer be touched by AIDS.

Later, when I finished grad school and started my first teaching job in the mid- to late 1990s, I noticed a dramatic shift occurring in cultural attitudes toward AIDS within my local community here in Vermont. When I mentioned AIDS to my students, their eyes glazed over as if they had no idea what I was talking about (as they do so even more now). I tried to draw parallels in my history classes between Giovanni Boccaccio's three psychological responses to the Black Death in

Florence of isolation, denial, or moderation and sexual responses to AIDS of either abstinence, unprotected sex, or wearing a condom, but the analogy seemed to fall flatter and flatter as the years went by. I must confess that I myself had unprotected intercourse with a few (female) sexual partners, but later my future wife did insist that we both get tested before we commenced intimate relations. (Both of us tested HIV-negative. A couple of states such as Illinois and Louisiana have in fact tried, and ultimately failed, to make AIDS testing mandatory before marriage.) When I had the campus nurse come in to my first-year seminar class at a local Vermont college to talk about sex education, she dwelled on the dangers posed by STDs such as genital warts and herpes, but not AIDS. Meanwhile, my local church wrestled with becoming an "open and affirming" congregation that would allow for civil unions to be performed by our pastor.

Nowadays, it seems our society has come to a stalemate, or a kind of equilibrium, with AIDS. It remains stubbornly incurable, unlike syphilis, but then what viral disease, even the common cold, has been cured? Instead, we seem reconciled to just living with it, both collectively and individually, as just another chronic, largely sexually transmitted disease that, like herpes, forever marks one with the taint of a moral lapse, however undeserved, but that refuses to kill its victims outright and keeps them in an agonizing pathogenic limbo. For most of us in the West, AIDS now exists on the margins of our consciousness—a disease of the "other" that perpetually hovers but never quite fully emerges into the light of day.

The other tale of AIDS that we need to tell is set primarily in sub-Saharan Africa and other unfortunate theaters of the third world. Even though awareness of the existence of AIDS in Africa came after its discovery in the United States, it is now thought that an epidemic had been incubating on that continent for far longer, since at least the late 1950s, with an epidemic fully emerging at the virus's most likely place of origin, west equatorial Africa, during the 1970s. To be even more specific, one can point to the year 1975 in Kinshasa, the capital city of the Democratic Republic of Congo, where hospital records point to large numbers of case definition conditions of AIDS, such as Kaposi's sarcoma and severe wasting disease, occurring at this time.[24] Currently, sub-Saharan Africa contains the vast majority of AIDS cases and newly emerging HIV infections, to the point that AIDS is now widely regarded as a distinctly "African disease." As of 2008, two-thirds of people living with AIDS and three-quarters of AIDS-related deaths occurred in Africa; 2 million Africans were newly infected with HIV in that year out of 2.7 million worldwide (bringing its total to approximately 22.4 million out of 33.4 million worldwide), and 1.4 million Africans died that year of the disease out of 2 million worldwide. Out of the twenty-five million deaths to date around the world from AIDS, most of these are thought to have occurred in Africa. Africa also had fourteen million "AIDS orphans" or children who lost one or both parents to the disease, as of 2008, and considerably more women than men in the region are infected by HIV, at a ratio of 60 to 40 percent, or 1.5 to 1. However, there are also signs that Africa's AIDS epidemic is by now maturing or leveling off. For example, in the worst-hit part of the continent, southern Africa, country after country is reporting substantially lower HIV prevalence rates in their adult populations as of 2007, compared to four years earlier, in 2003. Among the most dramatic drops are those in Swaziland at 26.1 percent, down from 38.8 percent in 2003; Botswana at 23.9 percent, down from 37.3 percent; Lesotho at 23.2 percent compared to 28.9 percent; South Africa at 18.1 percent from 21.5 percent; Zimbabwe at 15.3 percent from 24.6 percent; Namibia at 15.3 percent from 21.3 percent; and Malawi at 11.9 percent from 14.2 percent. Overall, HIV prevalence throughout Africa has declined slightly from 5.8 percent in 2001 to 5.2 percent in 2008. Since newly emerging infections continue to outpace deaths, these declining prevalence rates seem to be due primarily to the slowly declining infection rates that have been achieved in sub-Saharan Africa—as of 2008, new HIV infections throughout the continent declined 25 percent from the height of the epidemic in the mid-1990s. Greater access to antiretroviral treatment has meant that fewer people in Africa are now dying of AIDS, but this also means they are living longer, so that in absolute numbers the figure of people living with AIDS continues to rise, despite declining infection rates or prevalence. Indeed, the fact that such high proportions of the population in some countries continue to live with the disease means that the AIDS epidemic will persist as a major health crisis in Africa for some time to come. South Africa, with nearly six million people living with AIDS as of 2007, remains the country with the largest AIDS population in the world.[25]

Aside from the sheer scale of its epidemic, Africa's AIDS crisis also differs from the West's in terms of how the disease is thought to be transmitted—primarily through heterosexual intercourse in Africa as opposed to homosexual intercourse and drug use in Pattern I countries—although some would argue that anal sex is vastly underestimated in Africa largely due to homophobia, underreported incidence among heterosexual couples, or cultural misunderstandings as to what constitutes such an act.[26] Yet, this bare, banal fact alone, that AIDS in Africa is a widespread disease among the general population spread by a common and, one might almost say, biologically necessitated behavior among humans, namely, (unprotected) heterosexual intercourse, is precisely what makes the African AIDS epidemic so different from that in the West and comprises perhaps the most controversial statement in the AIDS discourse today. For it naturally implies that, in order for both epidemiological models in Pattern I and II countries to be valid, heterosexual sex must be of a radically different sort in sub-Saharan Africa as opposed to what is practiced in the United States or Europe, and indeed this is exactly what we get in much of the early literature on the African AIDS epidemic, such as that published by the Australian researchers John and Pat Caldwell and which continues to be repeated in some form among certain publications. But all too often assumptions about sexual promiscuity in Africa are based on outdated or strictly anecdotal evidence that play into centuries-old racial stereotypes about the exotic, hypersexed African.[27] However, some recent observers of the African AIDS crisis continue to insist, on the basis of focused surveys and mathematical models, that African sexual behaviors do differ in significant ways from those in the West and other countries around the world, particularly in terms of maintaining multiple concurrent partners (as opposed to serial relationships) that in turn make Africans substantially more susceptible to HIV infection.[28] And yet to make broad-based generalizations and comparisons about intensely personal behaviors is difficult and dangerous. If African culture does sanction sex outside marriage, early teenage sexual initiation, and sexual predation of younger females by older males, then very similar observations are also generally made of Western culture. This does not mean, of course, that, as in the West, sexual behaviors among certain "high-risk" groups in Africa—such as commercial sex workers, migrant populations, and urban dwellers displaced from their traditional rural environments—have not historically contributed to Africa's AIDS epidemic and continue to do so.[29] For example, the transient mining community in Carletonville, South Africa, some 65 percent of whom were found to be HIV-positive in 1999, the highest seroprevalence rate at that time anywhere in the world, undoubtedly played an incubating role in the spread of AIDS within their familial and social networks that was akin to what the bathhouses did for the gay community in San Francisco in the United States, among whom HIV infection rates likewise reached 65 percent by 1984.[30] Anecdotal reports of exotic sexual activities in Africa contributing to AIDS—such as "dry sex" (inserting drying agents into the vagina in order to increase male sexual pleasure), genital mutilation, and "widow inheritance" (a sexual "cleansing" ritual in which a widow must have sex with her husband's nearest male relative)—all might have some basis in reality within select groups in certain regions. These groups include commercial sex workers in South Africa, Muslim communities in east Africa, and tribal communities in the Rakai district of Uganda and in southern Zambia, but these can hardly be extrapolated to the general population throughout the entire continent.[31] In the end, it is important to keep in mind that heterosexual intercourse is no longer sufficient as the *sole* explanation of Africa's unprecedented and atypical AIDS epidemic; it is certainly a factor, and a very important one, but it is still just one among many that cannot be so easily disentangled from each other.

More recent studies of the African AIDS epidemic are now placing greater emphasis on poverty, famine and malnutrition, and opportunistic or coexisting diseases with AIDS, namely, tuberculosis; STDs such as syphilis, gonorrhea, chlamydia, and chancroid; and a host of parasitic illnesses that include malaria, leishmaniasis, schistosomiasis or bilharzia, filariasis, typanosomiasis or sleeping sickness, and helminth infections. Some of these diseases, such as malaria, schistosomiasis, and typanosomiasis, are well known to have a long, endemic history on the African continent, and their prevalence there, alongside extensive poverty and malnutrition, could be said to be an important distinguishing feature that makes Africa's situation different from the West's. What is more, all these cofactors have a synergistic relationship with HIV and AIDS. The link between STDs and HIV infection is a rather obvious and well-established article of faith, since both are sexually transmitted and the former produce inflammation or lesions in the genital area that facilitate (by as much as five times the norm) transmission of HIV. STDs also concentrate CD4 immune cells—the target of the AIDS virus—in the genital area and increase viral shedding in seminal fluids. There is also much evidence from prenatal clinics that STDs are quite common in Africa even as they go untreated or undiagnosed, particularly in female patients. What is not so well known, however, is that other diseases as well as malnutrition that are not normally associated with AIDS can likewise contribute in a direct, *biological* way to HIV transmission, just like STDs. For example, schistosomiasis, a parasitic worm disease carried by snails living in natural and artificial bodies of water, infects the genital tract and causes the same lesions and immune cell concentrations that facilitate HIV transmission in STDs; moreover, it is highly endemic to Africa, which hosts the vast majority of the world's second-most common tropical disease, and its prevalence has only become worse in recent decades with new dam construction and other projects that create surface water sites and that have spread the disease from rural to urban areas. Other parasitic diseases that are especially prevalent and acute in equatorial Africa, such as malaria, can greatly increase HIV viral loads in AIDS patients or trigger latent viruses into replication by stimulating the immune system. Malnutrition and vitamin deficiencies can also promote viral replication, weaken epithelial barriers to the virus, and increase the likelihood of MTCT. Tuberculosis, the leading cause of death of people with AIDS in Africa, may in turn increase susceptibility to the disease in HIV-negative populations due to its impact upon the immune system; most of the widely prevalent cases of TB in Africa in fact exist independently of AIDS and are especially rampant among young people. While both TB and AIDS are latent diseases, either can easily be reactivated by coinfection with the other. In addition to TB, AIDS can likewise make patients more vulnerable to all the above diseases. Like AIDS and TB, some of these diseases are asymptomatic, and their presence has been equally overlooked by researchers searching for more typical behavioral risk factors of HIV.[32]

Poverty also has a synergistic relationship with AIDS but in a more indirect way, by forcing people to engage in risky behaviors such as commercial sex work or migrancy (where a "survival strategy" becomes a "death strategy"), and in turn AIDS can amplify poverty or malnutrition by diverting scarce resources to health care or funerals and by incapacitating or removing wage earners and care givers.[33] Even though the scale of Africa's poverty dwarfs that of the West, poverty's connection with AIDS is nonetheless something that both Africa and the United States share, for one of the highest risk groups for AIDS in America today are poor minorities. Instead of AIDS being primarily a behavioral problem for Africans, therefore, poverty, climactic-related famines, and contingent diseases all make it more of an ecological or environmental one, with far less of the moralistic and cultural complications and judgmental comparisons that go with the former. On these grounds, there are now calls for a complete rethinking of international AIDS policy, particularly in Africa, as coordinated (since 1996) by the United Nations agency, UNAIDS. Since, it is argued, poverty all too often removes individual autonomy in choosing risky social behaviors, which are of course also impacted by cultural expectations, especially in terms of male-female relationships, intervention efforts should instead focus on the root cause of such behaviors (namely, poverty) or on biological cofactors such as malnutrition and other diseases besides AIDS—especially when, provided distribution mechanisms and political stability are adequate, these are more easily addressed through food aid or existing antibiotics (except for MDRTB). In this scenario, a whole decade or more has been lost to inappropriate and largely ineffective AIDS prevention strategies, which are now also being superseded by more effective antiretroviral (ARV) treatment programs. In response, some will point to the success of behavioral modification programs in places like Uganda (where it was famously called "ABC"—abstinence, be careful, use condoms) and Zimbabwe in reducing HIV prevalence rates, or that education and counseling programs have at least been proven effective in reducing risk behaviors and increasing condom use in countries like Tanzania, Kenya, Trinidad, and South Africa.[34] However, considerable debate still exists as to whether behavioral modifications are due to government programs or rather to simple fear and community awareness of AIDS, while others question how much of the decline in HIV prevalence is due to changes in behavior or instead to an inevitable maturing of the epidemic? But an even more apropos concern with an overly narrow or exclusive focus on poverty and malnutrition in AIDS strategy is the fact that these factors alone will not explain the unique severity of Africa's AIDS epidemic. Within Africa, for example, how do we account for a high HIV prevalence rate in the richest country on the continent, South Africa, but an exceptionally low one in a poor country like Senegal (where a third of the population lives on less than a dollar a day);

how do we explain why in other regions of the world that are just as poor as Africa, such as India or parts of Southeast Asia, AIDS infections and deaths have yet to reach the levels seen in Pattern II countries?[35] We also have to be mindful of the fact that some, such as former South African president Mbeki, have used poverty as a cover for denying the existence of AIDS or for abrogating their responsibilities in providing all possible treatments for the disease. In actuality, most historians are quick to point out that they are arguing for poverty having an intimate, synergistic relationship with HIV and AIDS, rather than that there is no relation or that poverty is an independent cause altogether.[36]

Despite all the attention being paid to poverty or sexual behaviors as the cause of AIDS in Africa, comparatively little notice has been taken of the actual history of the epidemic on the continent, for a third, and perhaps decisive, contributory factor to why Africa has the worst AIDS epidemic in the world is the simple reason that "it had the first AIDS epidemic."[37] This rather obvious fact has been somewhat obscured, however, by the controversy surrounding the origins of HIV in Africa, where some scholars have accused the theory of having an underlying racial prejudice that would naturally associate black Africans with monkeys, even though there is a sound scientific basis for doing so in terms of the specific disease of AIDS.[38] Granted there may really be some discrimination in this regard that is part of human nature and has always been a part of the history of disease, but this still doesn't obviate the necessity of arriving at a true understanding of the history of AIDS in Africa, if only to better understand how to draw up the right policy in treating the disease on the continent. Africa's early history with AIDS was largely determined by the latent, asymptomatic, and slow-to-progress qualities of the disease, which made it difficult to identify and target on a continent whose medical technology and health care system remain far behind those of the West; oftentimes AIDS' silent insidiousness was aided and abetted by attitudes of studied ignorance or outright denial, at both a local or individual level (reflected in a widespread reluctance to get an AIDS test) and even at the level of official government policy in some countries, such as the Democratic Republic of Congo and Zimbabwe. Whereas AIDS was confined fairly quickly in the United States to certain high-risk groups such as homosexuals and intravenous drug users, the epidemic in Africa was allowed to fester for a decade or more and was not fully addressed in most places on the continent until the late 1980s and 1990s. Thus, AIDS managed to insinuate itself deeply and broadly into African society, afflicting many more sectors of the population than just one or two "high-risk" groups, as in the United States. And just like its synergistic relationship with poverty and other diseases, AIDS also has a mutual, two-way dynamic with African history: at the same time that AIDS is having a unique impact upon the continent by virtue of the kind of disease it is, so modern trends in Africa during the twentieth century have paved the way for AIDS to make a tenacious home there, which include the political and socioeconomic legacies of colonialism; soaring populations after successful eradication of some deadly diseases, such as smallpox; rampant urbanization and displacement facilitated by new, transnational highway networks; ecological infringement upon previously isolated animal habitats; and widespread medicalization, including greater use of blood transfusions and injections, all of which contributed to the spread of AIDS in both direct and indirect ways. Rather like the Black Death, the current pandemic of AIDS in Africa seems destined to endure for quite some time, though what the end will be and how it will ultimately affect the history of the continent is still a mystery.[39]

Another way in which Africa differs from the rest of the world in its experience with AIDS is the sheer variety of circumstances and contexts in which the disease has historically evolved and currently exists in its status quo on the continent. In western equatorial Africa, where the disease most likely began, the epidemic matured early and has for the moment stabilized at seroprevalence rates of around 6 percent or less. Factors that have facilitated AIDS' spread there are thought to include widespread poverty, prevalent tropical diseases, wide sexual networks in some urban areas, such as Kinshasa, and the popular use of blood transfusions and syringe injections; on the other hand, the almost universal practice of circumcision (thought to limit the spread of STDs), as well as the difficulty of travel in the region and transport disruptions caused by war, are likely to have helped curb the scope of the epidemic.[40] In east Africa, where the disease migrated next, HIV prevalence rates are likewise currently stable at 6 percent or less, which represents a dramatic decline from highs in the teens and twenties in some countries, such as Uganda, during the 1990s. Transmission factors in this region include transient populations—such as truck drivers and migrant laborers—who traveled along the trans-Africa highway, an associated service economy of commercial sex workers, soldiers and refugees dispersed by civil wars, networks linking urban and rural areas, and a patriarchal and prudish culture (especially toward condoms and circumcision) in Christian communities. Uganda under President Yoweri Museveni is often held up as an example of the beneficial results of an enlightened AIDS policy, where as early as 1981 the government embarked on an open and frank discussion of the epidemic and took a "multisectoral" approach to changing high-risk behaviors, such as by advocating "zero grazing," or monogamy, on billboard signs. This was not entirely smooth sailing, as Museveni for a time opposed condom distribution and had a nasty tendency to stigmatize commercial sex workers (stereotyped as "Africa's urban witches") for spreading AIDS; he also displayed a willingness to privilege traditional, homegrown healing methods despite the fact that some healers and their clients attributed the disease to witchcraft.[41] In West Africa, the AIDS epidemic almost from the very beginning has been contained in many countries at low seroprevalence rates of 1 to 2 percent or even less, due largely, it seems, to Islamic cultural restraints on sexual promiscuity (despite sanctioning of polygamy), high rates of circumcision, less mobility and concentration of populations in large urban areas, greater economic opportunities for women (hence obviating the need to become commercial sex workers), and the endemic presence of HIV-2, a strain that is apparently far less virulent and infectious than HIV-1. Highest seroprevalence rates in the region, currently at 3 to 4 percent, are in Côte d'Ivoire, Nigeria, and Chad, where there are higher populations of migrant laborers, wider client networks patronizing commercial sex workers, and greater economic instability and poverty.[42]

We have already seen how many countries in southern Africa are currently laboring under the highest HIV prevalence rates on the continent, which were even higher just a few years ago. Many see this as chiefly due to the region's legacy of white domination, which lasted the longest of anywhere on the continent. The apartheid regime in South Africa, for example, was not toppled until 1994. Others view the epidemic's severity here as a product of the silent insidiousness of AIDS, which perhaps has been allowed to incubate unnoticed, whether deliberately or not, for an inordinately lengthy period of time when compared with other regions. But in a way this is not so different from the political question, for the two are closely linked: the dysfunctional regimes that emerged in much of southern Africa after independence were poorly equipped to tackle AIDS. Zimbabwe, for instance, has been ruled dictatorially under Robert Mugabe since 1980 and in addition has been racked by civil war; one-party rule has likewise characterized much of the recent history of Zambia, Malawi, and Tanzania. Swaziland is still anachronistically in the grip of a ruling monarch, King Mswati III.[43] And yet democracy is no guarantee of a more enlightened AIDS policy. While the response to the disease under the former apartheid regime in South Africa was characterized by neglect, prudishness, and distrust, under the democratically elected rule of the African National Congress (ANC), the country is still struggling to come fully to grips with its AIDS epidemic. Other factors amplifying AIDS's presence in southern Africa include migrant labor associated with the region's diamond, gold, and copper mines; female poverty and lack of economic opportunity that drive women to resort to commercial sex work; rapid urbanization and population growth, as well as a mutually infective relationship between rural and urban areas; and the severe social and economic disparities that persist throughout the general population.[44] AIDS, in turn, has only fed into all these social and economic problems that are helping to drive the disease crisis in southern Africa. Because of its extraordinarily high infection and death rates, AIDS has substantially lowered life expectancies in the region (by as much as twenty to thirty years), shifted the age distribution of the population to extremes at either end of the spectrum (AIDS typically targets those between fifteen and forty-nine years of age), and has artificially lowered, and in some cases even reversed, rates of population growth and economic expansion. Some would even argue that AIDS poses a threat to national security in certain countries.[45] Since the forces of disease and socioeconomic causes are thereby mutually reinforcing in southern Africa, this has created an almost self-perpetuating epidemic.

South Africa under the former ANC presidency of Thabo Mbeki (1999–2008), aided and abetted by two successive health ministers, presents a unique, some would say indeed bizarre, case of an AIDS policy that has been not only counterproductive but even quite harmful to the cause of AIDS patients in the country.[46] This is an excellent example of how just the way in which humans think about and define a disease can have significant and very real biological impacts. The world first learned of Mbeki's skepticism about HIV being the cause of AIDS in a remarkable public letter to world leaders that he sent out in April 2000, just before hosting the thirteenth international AIDS conference in his home country, where he provided a forum for dissident scientists like Peter Duesberg. Mbeki's letter was also noteworthy for its harnessing of antiapartheid rhetoric in support of the dissidence cause and for declaring that, since the African AIDS crisis was so different from that in the West in terms of its heterosexual transmission and sheer scale, this in turn necessitated a uniquely "African solution," a position that, for all the contrasts drawn between their respective responses, was actually quite close to that of Museveni of Uganda as gleaned from his own speeches about AIDS.[47] Some of Mbeki's positions can indeed be said to have some validity, such as that poverty has played a greater role in Africa's AIDS crisis than previously thought or at least admitted, but in the end these have only served as political cover or posturing for a blanket rejection of Western drugs and vaccines, which Mbeki perceived as being proffered by a pharmaceutical industry that was out to profit from an overhyped epidemic as a new form of racist imperialism. This is in spite of the fact that antiretrovirals had long been proven to not only prolong the lives of AIDS patients but also significantly reduce MTCT, and that they were now being offered by pharmaceutical companies at cut-rate or at-cost prices (some as low as one hundred dollars or less for a year's treatment, down from about twelve thousand dollars), after they had unsuccessfully pursued a lawsuit (dropped in 2001) in the South African courts to try to protect their drug patents from generic manufacturing. Ironically, by denying or delaying delivery of badly needed ARVs, Mbeki was in fact creating a new apartheid in South Africa, in which AIDS treatment was affordable only to some few thousands while the rest of the millions of people living with AIDS were in effect condemned to an early death. Many also observed hypocrisy in Mbeki's distrust of ARVs as potentially harmful to AIDS patients while at the same time promoting a home-grown drug, Virodene, which *was* shown to be actually toxic, or in his protests of lack of funds to finance ARV administration even as the government was pouring millions of rands into unnecessary defense spending. Mbeki's argument was also undercut by the fact that neighboring countries in southern Africa, including Botswana, Namibia, Swaziland, and Zambia, were concurrently implementing successful ARV programs that were reaching thousands of patients, representing 13 percent to as much as half of all those eligible for treatment; such programs were also being pioneered in several countries in West Africa, while in Uganda, the government was able to supply 40 percent of its need-based patients in 2004 by relying on free drugs supplied by international donors (mostly in the United States), whom it actively courted.[48] Other aspects of South Africa's AIDS policy, such as health minister Manto Tshabalala-Msimang's contention that AIDS was a nutritional disease (an idea she seems to have gotten from her adviser, Giraldo) that could be treated with an herbal concoction of lemon, ginger, olive oil, garlic, and beetroot, would be simply laughable if so many lives were not at stake. The silver lining in all this tragic denial has been that it sparked a political activism among AIDS sufferers in Africa who are demanding greater access to treatment, which can be compared to what the gay community achieved a decade earlier in the United States. It started in South Africa with the Treatment Action Campaign (TAC), led by the AIDS activist Zackie Achmat, which forced the Mbeki government to reverse course in 2003 and give at least a verbal commitment to making ARVs more available, and such political mobilization on behalf of AIDS victims has since spread to other countries including Ethiopia, Nigeria, Namibia, and Kenya. HAART has also been helped along in Africa by generic drug manufacturers, such as the Cipla corporation of India, which have made drug combinations much more affordable as well as easier to take in a single pill format (thus reducing the likelihood of drug resistance emerging from incomplete adherence to regimens) and by philanthropic nongovernmental organizations (NGOs) such as the Bill Gates Foundation and Médecins Sans Frontières (Doctors without Borders) that have provided funds and distribution mechanisms to help administer the drugs.[49] The latest UNAIDS report is that, as of 2008, antiretroviral therapy is available to 44 percent of all Africans living with AIDS, up from just 2 percent five years ago.[50] This has greatly lengthened the life expectancies of AIDS victims, reduced the number of AIDS orphans and MTCT transmissions, and probably helped to reduce AIDS stigma and reluctance to be tested for HIV, but some worry that it will not do much to reduce new HIV infections since there will now be longer windows of opportunity for transmissions, and that the cost of drugs will divert resources needed to address other health and socioeconomic problems, some of which are cofactors of AIDS.[51] Most recently, as of 2010, it has also been observed that ART programs in many African countries such as Uganda have stalled or flatlined due to caps placed on outside donations in the wake of a global recession and a shift in priorities toward treating less expensive diseases than AIDS, such as pneumonia, diarrhea, malaria, measles, and tetanus. This raises the dispiriting prospect that hard-won gains made in the fight against AIDS in Africa will be reversed in the near future.[52]

A final factor that distinguishes Africa's AIDS crisis from the rest of the world's, particularly in the West, is the unique vulnerability of the continent's women and children to the disease.[53] We have already seen that HIV infection rates in Africa are heavily skewed in favor of women, in contrast to what we find in Pattern I countries, and UNAIDS reports that young, teenaged women are particularly vulnerable to the disease in some African countries, such as Kenya, where they are three times as likely to be infected as their male counterparts.[54] Aside from their greater biological susceptibility to HIV, women caught up in Africa's AIDS crisis are also said to be victims of the patriarchal culture and gender inequality prevalent throughout much of the continent, which has not known the feminist liberation movements that have characterized much of modern history in the West, although some would argue that in any case Western-style feminism is simply inappropriate or inapplicable to the different culture of Africa.[55] In such an environment, it is claimed, women, both commercial sex workers with many partners and married women with only one, find it difficult to negotiate safe sex strategies, such as using condoms, for both economic reasons (the need to find clients) and social ones (that asking a partner to wear a condom signals a lack of trust). Women, particularly commercial sex workers and widows, have also borne the brunt of the stigmatizing and scapegoating tendencies associated with AIDS in Africa. And yet, being married is of course no guarantee against not being infected by a promiscuous partner, so that marriage itself can be a "high-risk" behavior for women in some circumstances, while the lack of economic opportunities for women in many African countries places single females and widows in conditions of poverty that tend to lead to another high-risk behavior for AIDS, namely, commercial sex work, or casual sex in exchange for "gifts." Early ages for marriage and sexual initiation, economic pressures to pay for necessities such as school fees, and even alleged rumors that sex with a virgin can cure AIDS have all placed younger women at greater risk. Women in Africa are also disproportionately burdened in terms of nursing and caring for AIDS patients, which can further restrict their economic and educational opportunities. Particularly heartbreaking has been the psychological and economic stress upon older women, such as grandmothers, who must care for their grandchildren orphaned by the disease at the same time that they mourn their children.[56] When familial networks prove unequal to the task of caring for Africa's numerous "AIDS orphans," their upbringing poses a challenge to state institutions, and there is a danger that, due to stigma or poverty, these children will then grow up to become alienated from their societies. Still, there is hope for women and children in Africa in the age of AIDS: greater access to antiretroviral treatments is allowing AIDS parents to live longer, while the disease is also driving various cultural changes and opportunities that can benefit women. For example, in Tanzania it is anecdotally reported that the AIDS epidemic has strengthened family bonds and partner fidelity, increased acceptance of condoms, improved women's access to education and legal ability to inherit, facilitated formation of women's clubs and other female-oriented community groups and organizations, and generally made society more aware of the special issues faced by women as a result of the disease.[57] In South Africa, a grassroots feminism movement seems to have been galvanized by the 2005 rape trial of the current president, Jacob Zuma, who was acquitted but whose testimony during the trial underscored some of the larger issues at stake in oppressive attitudes toward women that make them particularly vulnerable to AIDS. Zuma testified that he felt himself "obligated" to have sex with his alleged victim by her provocative dress and demeanor (his further claim that denying an aroused women is "tantamount to rape" defies logic), and that he was not concerned about contracting AIDS despite his alleged victim's HIV-positive status because he had showered afterward. Above all, the case demonstrated a need to address gender inequalities and sexual violence, even in a country with the most liberal democratic constitution in Africa, which nonetheless is reputed to have the highest incidence of rape in the world.[58]

Within the Caribbean, AIDS scholarship has naturally focused on Haiti and Cuba, even though AIDS has established a presence throughout the region. Because the epidemic here is primarily driven by heterosexual transmission, it has been classified as among Pattern II countries, along with those in sub-Saharan Africa. But there are other reasons for linking the Caribbean with Africa in terms of AIDS incidence: poverty, malnutrition, lack of safe drinking water, STDs, and other coexistent diseases are likewise prevalent throughout the region and are important cofactors of AIDS. Many Caribbean countries are also plagued by low ratios of doctors and poor availability of health services among the general population, and, as in Africa, commercial sex workers and migrant laborers are among the leading members of the "high-risk" population for AIDS. For instance, UNAIDS reports that, as of 2008, 27 percent of commercial sex workers in Guyana are infected, and in the Dominican Republic, the *bateye* migrants from neighboring Haiti who work on the country's sugarcane plantations are particularly vulnerable. Compared to other regions except for Africa, the Caribbean also has a high AIDS incidence among women, who currently make up about half of all infections, and as in Africa HIV prevalence is especially high among younger women; the Caribbean also ranks just behind Africa in terms of its overall seroprevalence rate, which currently stands at 1 percent of its general population, even though this is still a fifth of Africa's.[59] The spread of and response to AIDS in the Caribbean is heavily impacted by its long legacy of having been subjected to imperialist domination, which during the twentieth century prior to the epidemic came from the United States, just as Africa was likewise emerging from under European rule in the decades leading up to AIDS.

There are, however, circumstances that are unique to the Caribbean's experience with AIDS, which are best illustrated by the oft-cited case studies of Haiti and Cuba. Owing to its international sex tourism trade, including child prostitution (which is also prevalent throughout Latin America), the Caribbean, and Haiti in particular, is thought by many observers to have served as the key nexus, or Bermuda triangle if you will, of the global AIDS pandemic. It is possible, for example, that AIDS was imported to Haiti by French-speaking guest workers in the Belgian Congo or Zaire, as it was known then, during the 1960s and 1970s; the virus would then, in this scenario, have been imported to the United States and Europe through the gay sex tours that had long operated in impoverished Haiti.[60] Others point out, however, that AIDS did not emerge in Haiti until after 1980, at exactly the same time as in the United States, so that it is just as likely that the United States *exported* the disease to Haiti. (The five Caribbean basin nations with the most AIDS cases in 1986—Haiti, the Dominican Republic, the Bahamas, Trinidad/Tobago, and Mexico—also happen to be those most economically linked to the United States in terms of tourism and trade.)[61] In any case, because the CDC in the United States early on in the epidemic identified Haitians as one of its four "high-risk" groups for AIDS, in spite of the fact that they allegedly did not admit to engaging in gay sex or IV drug use, Haitian immigrants in the United States suffered terrible discrimination throughout much of the 1980s. Stories were told of taxi drivers hiding their identities, schoolchildren abused and beaten up, employees fired or refused work, and so on. This was most unjust, as subsequent research and reinterviewing of subjects revealed that, early on at least, HIV transmission in Haiti closely paralleled that in Pattern I countries such as the United States, namely, that the vast majority of victims were men having sex with men or who were bisexual, with the disease gradually spreading into the heterosexual population. (High HIV prevalence rates among men who have sex with men are still found in Trinidad/Tobago and Jamaica.) Outside the capital of Port-au-Prince, seroprevalence in Haiti was actually quite low in comparison with elsewhere in Latin America and even compared with some American cities, such as New York. Racial prejudice and misunderstandings abounded on both sides, in the United States and Haiti. Americans took seriously ridiculous rumors of exotic voodoo blood rituals and cannibalistic practices that allegedly spread AIDS in Haiti, while Haitians were willing to believe conspiracy theories that their powerful neighbor to the north had deliberately devised and exported the disease in an effort to further subjugate them.[62] Even though the Catholic culture prevalent throughout Latin America since the time of Columbus has impeded preventative efforts such as increasing condom use, HIV infection rates in Haiti have declined dramatically since the late 1980s, when they peaked at around 12 percent of some sampled populations; next door in the Dominican Republic, UNAIDS reports that recent reductions in HIV infections are due to sexual behavioral modifications, such as increased condom use and reduced partner exchange. Nonetheless, Haiti remains the region's epicenter for the epidemic. Haiti has by far the most people living with AIDS in the region, currently numbering 120,000, which represents half of the entire AIDS population in the Caribbean, and its seroprevalence rate is double that of the neighboring Dominican Republic.[63] Haiti's tourism economy has also taken a beating from AIDS. When the disease first became known in 1981–1983, the number of visitors to Haiti dropped by as much as 75 percent, and discrimination against Haitians has also been slow to die, since as late as 1990 they were still forbidden to donate blood in the United States.[64] And even though the Caribbean has benefited from the fifteen billion dollars in Emergency AIDS Relief pledged by the United States under former president George W. Bush, this has come at the price of enforced emphasis upon abstinence-only programs instead of more proven prevention techniques, such as condom distribution and education.[65]

The other anomaly in the Caribbean AIDS epidemic is, of course, Cuba. Owing to a decades-long trade embargo imposed by the United States against the Communist regime of Fidel Castro, some might think that Cuba's low incidence of AIDS might be due to its diplomatic isolation, but that is not actually the case. (To date, there are just over six thousand people living with AIDS in Cuba, for a seroprevalence rate of 0.1 percent, six times lower than that of the United States.) The first AIDS cases in Cuba are thought to have occurred among the hundreds of thousands who served as soldiers on military duty in Africa, such as Ethiopia and Angola, or those who participated in cultural exchange programs abroad. Rather, most scholars agree that Cuba's success in containing AIDS has been chiefly due to its mass testing program, which was first applied to high-risk groups such as expatriates and tourism industry workers but which was gradually extended to almost the entire population, and to its policy of quarantining all HIV-positive persons in special "sanatoriums" distributed throughout every province of Cuba.[66] Although Cuba's approach was unique in all the world, it was not developed in isolation, as its main motivating factor seems to have been a propagandistic desire to outperform the United States in terms of health care, for which AIDS provided a golden opportunity from the Cuban point of view, since it seemed to be a product of American "decadent" behaviors, such as homosexuality—nor was the Cuban response without historical precedent, as the sanatorium system was obviously pioneered during the era of tuberculosis in the nineteenth century, and quarantine was indeed adopted on a small scale during New York City's tuberculosis epidemic during the 1990s. But Cuba's policy was a direct contradiction of the privileging of individual rights over society's welfare, for which AIDS proved to be a turning point in the United States, and human rights organizations criticized Cuba's sanatoriums on the grounds that quarantine detention was for an indefinite period, despite the fact that its victims were otherwise healthy and could only infect others through conscious, intimate behaviors, and for inhumanely separating couples or even separating parents from their children if only one family member tested HIV-positive. While the Los Cocos sanatorium just outside Havana, which had originally been a rest and recreation center for military officers and therefore was easily transitioned into a facility servicing returning HIV-positive soldiers, showcased the apparent humanity of the system, with medical and housing facilities that, it was pointed out to visitors, were superior to those available to most Cubans on the outside, some inmates told a different tale that included homophobic beatings by guards, attempted suicides, and prisonlike surroundings.[67] By the early 1990s, Cuba began modifying its sanatorium regime, at the same time as placing greater emphasis on AIDS education, which some argue it should have done from the very beginning. These changes were partly in response to international pressure; partly in response to a growing economic crisis caused by the collapse of Cuba's leading economic and political partner, the Soviet Union, in 1991; and finally in response to a home-grown protest movement, known as the *roqueros* or "rockers," a music subculture of young people who self-injected themselves with HIV-tainted blood as an act of political defiance but whose numbers were also swelled by spouses who wished to join their loved ones sequestered in the sanatoriums. Though their numbers were relatively small, about two hundred by 1992, the *roqueros* grabbed some international media attention even if Cuban Americans in the United States were loath to embrace such a bizarre, some would say almost perverse, method of protest. At the present time, it is reported that most AIDS patients in Cuba reside in their local communities and receive care at outpatient clinics, while the sanatoriums now function as educational or training centers for an initial three-month period or else as a home base for those who otherwise live and work on the outside. Cuba has also stepped up its antiretroviral program, whose drugs are manufactured internally due to the embargo and which Cuba offers at low prices to other Caribbean nations.[68] In contrast to elsewhere in the region, homosexual intercourse, long a taboo subject in the country, may now be driving a rising incidence of AIDS in Cuba. One other territory that is bucking the trend in the Caribbean is Puerto Rico, where most HIV transmissions are due to intravenous drug use, accounting for 40 percent of new infections among men and 27 percent among women as of 2006.[69]

In Central and South America, AIDS has generally followed the transmission patterns that have also held true in the United States and other Pattern I countries, namely, being largely driven by homosexual intercourse and IV drug use, although there are exceptions, such as Honduras, which early on became the epicenter of the AIDS epidemic in Central America and where infections were attributed to heterosexual behaviors, especially among commercial sex workers.[70] As in the United States, men outnumber women in terms of those infected and living with AIDS, but again this may change due, it is said, to the possibility that bisexual behaviors may be underreported owing to the different ways in which gay sexuality is defined and understood in Latin America, where only transvestites and receptive partners are perceived as actually engaging in homosexual sex. Latin America also mirrors the United States in terms of its low seroprevalence rate, currently at 0.6 percent, almost exactly that of the United States, and in its higher than average provision of antiretroviral treatment to its HIV-positive population, which was 54 percent as of 2008. And yet, Latin America has many of the same disadvantages and cofactors for AIDS that we have seen operating in Africa and the Caribbean, namely, widespread poverty and income disparities; malnutrition; predisposing disease environments, such as malaria; a large migrant labor population; and, associated with that, a high incidence of sexual exploitation and prostitution.[71] Some countries in Central America, particularly Nicaragua, El Salvador, Guatemala, and Panama, have also known recent military intervention from the United States or else civil unrest just prior to and during the AIDS epidemic, while in South America numerous countries have until quite recently experienced brutal dictatorial regimes or domestic violence from drug cartels and guerrilla groups, such as in Colombia and Peru.[72] How, then, do we explain the region's relative success in combating AIDS?

The answer seems to be found in the country that has attracted the disproportionate share of AIDS observers' attention to the region: Brazil. As the largest and most populous country in Latin America with a reputedly liberal sexual culture (both gay and straight), wide gaps in wealth distribution, prevalent drug use and a vulnerable population of street children in the city's *favelas* or slums, a recent history of military dictatorship, and an underfunded health system, Brazil's prognosis for beating the AIDS epidemic was not good. Moreover, beginning in the second half of the 1980s, Brazil embarked on an AIDS policy that emphasized treatment in addition or even in preference to prevention, which most said was beyond the means of poor, developing countries in the third world. In 1991, the government began distributing AZT to AIDS patients, and in 1996, the year that triple combination drug therapy was announced to the world at the international AIDS conference in Vancouver, it took the remarkable and unprecedented step of offering HAART free to all who needed it, the first program of its kind in the world. Brazil also proved that developing countries could achieve high rates of compliance, and thus low rates of drug resistance, in treatment therapy programs. Much of the initiative for the Brazilian law mandating ARV access came from hundreds of local AIDS NGOs, many of which had sprung up at first in the gay community whose members were relatively affluent and unstigmatized in Brazilian society. As the disease spread into more and more regions of the country and affected not only high-risk groups but also all sectors of the population, especially the poor, political pressure began building on Brazil's politicians to take a more proactive approach to the epidemic. But even as the NGOs were organizing demonstrations and sponsoring lawsuits on behalf of its AIDS constituency, state and federal governments did prove responsive and headed off much of the confrontation through its bold ARV program. In a sense this was already predetermined by the country's 1988 constitution, which enshrined a universal right of access to health care for all its citizens, and AIDS proved to be the first big test of the young democracy (established in 1985). Despite the cost, antiretrovirals were also a good investment, as they kept patients out of hospitals (where treatment would be even more expensive), reduced viral loads and therefore the risk of new infections, and allowed patients to remain active members of society, whereas otherwise their lost productivity would be another drain on the country's economy.[73]

Yet, an even bigger challenge was to come from outside Brazil. In 1994, Brazil had signed the international Agreement on Trade-Related Aspects of Intellectual Property Rights (TRIPS), and in 1996, the country passed its own industrial property law recognizing pharmaceutical patents. In order to be able to afford its free drug distribution program, Brazil began manufacturing generic versions of antiretrovirals in its own manufacturing facilities and administering them through a home-grown network of dispensaries, in itself no mean feat. Brazil justified its generics program in legal terms on the grounds of an exception clause in TRIPS that allowed for violations in cases of "national emergency" and that its drugs were those manufactured prior to 1997, when its national patent law went into effect. Nonetheless, the pharmaceutical industry, with the backing of the U.S. government and the World Trade Organization (WTO), threatened a legal challenge and tariff sanctions since it perceived the Brazilian program as simply the start of a domino effect whereby other third world countries would seek to mimic Brazil's end run around the prohibitive cost of ARVs at Western prices. The end result of this standoff was that U.S. drug companies such as Bristol-Myers Squibb, Merck, Roche, and Abbott negotiated drastic price reductions (down to about $140 for a year's worth of treatment) in exchange for a suspension and notification of compulsory licensing of patented drugs. This was a clear victory for the third world's right to access the same "miracle" treatments for AIDS that were enjoyed by the affluent West, which in some ways could be considered a natural extension of political AIDS activism that had emerged in the early 1980s in the United States. Brazil won in part because it was able to mobilize world opinion on its side, even to the point of securing World Bank loans for its program. However, there is ongoing conflict about Brazil's efforts to export its logistical and technical expertise to other poor nations seeking to start their own generic drug programs, particularly elsewhere in Latin America and the Caribbean and in sub-Saharan Africa.[74] On one side of the debate is the argument that "Big Pharma," by the very nature of its business of health care, has a moral and social obligation to help sick people in need, especially when its companies are some of the most profitable on earth and many of its products are developed with the aid of public money or institutions, such as the National Cancer Institute; on the other hand, it is pointed out that drug companies will have little financial incentive to develop new antiretrovirals and protease inhibitors that are much needed in the fight against AIDS unless there is a sufficient profit motive to do so, and the industry itself claims that it needs to charge high prices in order to recoup the millions of dollars that are invested in research and development of new drugs, most of which do not end up being marketable.[75] Some also question whether Brazil's success story can be imitated around the world, given its unique context. It could be said that Brazil at this point in time had a most fortuitous combination of circumstances, including democratic reform, an existing (if poorly endowed) health infrastructure, biomedical knowhow, a mobilized and tolerant civil sector on behalf of AIDS victims, and the economic wherewithal, political will, and diplomatic credentials to bring its program to fruition. But Brazil, by its very example of beating great odds to show that Western-style treatments for citizens with AIDS can be done in a developing country, is a powerful counterargument to naysayers and has given hope and inspiration to other activists who have had to prod their governments into providing similar antiretroviral programs, such as we have seen in South Africa. What is more, Brazil has adopted a leadership role in this effort to expand access to HAART around the world, and not just in terms of lending advice and support already mentioned but also in the very act of making bulk purchases of the active ingredients of drugs and negotiating price reductions from drug manufacturers, by means of which it has made antiretrovirals that much more affordable for other countries.[76]

One other success story in Latin America that we should mention is Mexico, which aside from Cuba has one of the lowest HIV prevalence rates in the region, currently at 0.3 percent of the adult population (half of Brazil's 0.6 percent). Mexico has achieved this in part by means of a network of proactive AIDS NGOs, free distribution of antiretrovirals, and an educational program that operates with the tacit complicity (or benign neglect) of the Catholic Church, just like in Brazil. But Mexico also has a policy of closely monitoring and regulating its (legal) prostitution population, which has reduced cofactors such as STDs, decreased drug use, and increased availability and acceptance of condoms, placing it more in the mold of Thailand.[77] As a consequence, married housewives are said to be as much as ten times more likely to get AIDS than commercial sex workers in Mexico; thus, the country still faces a threat of AIDS spreading into the wider heterosexual population and into rural areas, largely through migrant labor, hidden bisexual behaviors, and drug use, especially along the U.S. border.[78]

Finally, let us briefly address the Pattern III countries, where the AIDS pandemic is still emerging and much of whose history with the disease is yet to be written. In Asia, dire predictions of a "second wave" of HIV infection, particularly in India and China, that would catapult the region ahead of sub-Saharan Africa with tens of millions of AIDS victims by 2010 have so far failed to materialize.[79] As of 2008, there were 4.7 million people living with AIDS in the region, about half of whom were in India alone. This still places Asia second only to Africa in terms of numbers of people living with AIDS (which is perhaps inevitable given that the region is home to 60 percent of the world's population), but the epidemic there does seem to be stabilizing. Overall, new HIV infections and AIDS-related deaths have so far been on the decline during the twenty-first century, with some notable exceptions such as China, Pakistan, and Bangladesh, and adult seroprevalence rates are below 1 percent everywhere except Thailand.[80] Nonetheless, Thailand is widely touted as one of the greatest success stories in the region and a model that has influenced adjacent countries such as Cambodia and Laos. An epidemic that was rampaging in the 1990s, fueled by the country's commercial sex industry intertwined with IV drug use, was contained by means of a targeted program that promoted AIDS education and universal condom use in brothels and which was led at the highest levels by government officials such as Senator Mechai Viravaidya (affectionately nicknamed "Mr. Condom"). Thailand has also benefited from hundreds of proactive AIDS NGOs which, as in Brazil, have lobbied for increased access to antiretrovirals and manufacturing of cheap generic drugs in spite of patent protections such as TRIPS, and which have also helped administer ARV distribution through district hospitals and gain acceptance and tolerance of people with AIDS in Thai society.[81] Thailand's seroprevalence rate and AIDS population has been brought down from 2 percent and nearly eight hundred thousand, respectively, during the 1990s to current levels of 1.4 percent and just over six hundred thousand, while the number of AIDS deaths has been cut in half from over sixty thousand per year between 2000 and 2003 to just thirty-one thousand today. Equally impressive are containment efforts in Japan and South Korea, where HIV prevalence rates are practically zero—each country as of 2008 reported only several thousand cases of people living with AIDS (most of whom got the disease through homosexual and heterosexual contact) out of total populations in the tens of millions. Such results have apparently been achieved through a combination of AIDS education and awareness programs, free voluntary HIV testing and counseling, and public health support networks that provide access to antiretrovirals and other medical services.[82]

Prevention programs targeted at commercial sex workers have also proven effective in stabilizing the epidemic in south India, mainly by increasing condom use and reducing STDs, even though there is a history of discrimination and violence against high-risk groups for AIDS in the country. Meanwhile, another area where the epidemic has been localized for the present is northeastern India, where the disease is mainly fueled by intravenous drug use, as is likewise the case for neighboring Pakistan and Bangladesh.[83] The extent of China's AIDS epidemic is still somewhat of a mystery. As of 2008, its population of people living with AIDS was reported to be three-quarters of a million, for a seroprevalence rate of 0.1 percent, but credible figures on annual rates of HIV infection and progression to AIDS have been released only in the last few years, and the first admission of transmission among men having sex with men was not made until 2005. Initially, China's epidemic was said to be almost exclusively confined to IV drug users, but lately heterosexual transmission—primarily through the country's underground network of commercial sex workers—has overtaken drug use as the leading risk behavior for AIDS, according to the most recent UNAIDS report.[84] While China has adopted some harm reduction measures such as methadone maintenance and needle exchange programs, these are undermined by oppressive actions by the Communist government, such as condemning drug users and sex workers, both officially classed as criminals, into undergoing "reeducation" or "rehabilitation" in forced labor camps. Hence, needle sharing remains high and condom use low owing to victims' fear of prosecution and police crackdowns; criminalization and stigmatization of AIDS victims has also hampered efforts at HIV testing, as was likewise true until recently in India. China and India also share a high level of ignorance or misconceptions about AIDS (such as that healthy looking people are not infective) among the general population. Some of China's epidemic has been self-inflicted. During the 1990s, a "bloodhead" scandal erupted in Henan province in east-central China, when whole villages and as many as fifty thousand people were infected with HIV owing to a business scheme whereby blood plasma was donated and then the remaining blood cells from different donors was mixed all together and reinjected into "blood sellers" (using reused needles) in order to allow them to keep donating on a continual basis; those who have not died are currently being treated with antiretrovirals.[85]

Elsewhere around the world, another region of concern is Eastern Europe and Central Asia, where the AIDS epidemic has grown rapidly in the twenty-first century, increasing by 66 percent since 2001 and currently afflicting one and a half million persons throughout the region. Ukraine, Russia, and Estonia all currently lead the region in HIV prevalence rates, which are over 1 percent of the adult population in each country.[86] Intravenous drug use has to date been the main engine of the epidemic here, although heterosexual intercourse has been steadily on the rise as an associated risk behavior, especially among commercial sex workers. Facilitating transmission of the disease have been an economic and social collapse in the aftermath of the disintegration of the former Soviet Union and its satellite states, high rates of migration in search of work, rise of a criminal mafia controlling drug and sex trafficking, and a concurrent tuberculosis epidemic, including MDRTB, which is especially prevalent in Russia and its prison population. The only hope for the region seems to be an expansion of ARV treatment and harm reduction programs, access to which is currently below the global average.[87]

A very different picture emerges of the Oceania region, encompassing Australia, New Zealand, and the Pacific Islands, where HIV prevalence rates are close to zero and a total of fifty-nine thousand people living with AIDS were counted as of 2008. The one exception is Papua New Guinea, which accounts for the vast majority of AIDS cases in the region and whose seroprevalence rate currently stands at 1.5 percent of the population. Here, heterosexual transmission seems to be behind the epidemic, but its true nature and extent is largely unknown due to the lack of good information available in a country that is highly rural and diverse.[88] (Over 850 different languages and tribal societies have been identified in Papua New Guinea.) Reliable epidemiological data is also in short supply in the Middle East and North Africa, where HIV testing and access to ARV therapy remains low and the disease is associated with certain marginalized "high-risk" groups such as drug users, gay men, prostitutes, and migrant laborers.[89] However, what information we have does suggest that the region's epidemic is on the rise, increasing by about 65 percent during the first decade of the twenty-first century, with thirty-five thousand new AIDS cases, representing 11 percent of the total, in 2008 alone.[90]

To conclude, AIDS has always been a ripe disease for drawing historical parallels and analogies. At first, we naturally compared it to other, terrifyingly deadly infectious diseases of the past, such as the medieval Black Death or plague, because it seemed to be all encompassing of our society, but as we learned of its continued entrenchment in certain high-risk behaviors, the relevance of this comparison seemed to fade. Now, AIDS seems to lend itself to being compared with other chronic diseases like syphilis, cancer, or tuberculosis, at least in their untreatable forms.[91] AIDS is thus a kind of catchall for every social issue associated with disease. For example, transmission of AIDS involves some morally stigmatizing behaviors that have also informed syphilis and some types of cancers. In its late, full-blown state it can be as disfiguring as leprosy or smallpox. Conditions of poverty, especially in the third world, seem every bit as conducive to its spread as tuberculosis, with which it is opportunistically linked. And AIDS in sub-Saharan Africa seems to be operating under the same victim dynamic as the influenza pandemic of 1918, in that it mainly targets people in the prime and most productive part of their lives while leaving the very young and the very old relatively unscathed. AIDS at times inspires fitful efforts at quarantine or ostracization, contact tracing, and other public health measures that conflict with individual liberties and that likewise were tried with plague, cholera, tuberculosis, and syphilis.

The late author Susan Sontag drew upon a rich array of these historical analogies in her famous book *AIDS and Its Metaphors*, but the counterintuitive lesson she took from it was that AIDS and other comparable diseases like cancer should be divorced from their social context and ideally approached in biological isolation in order to strip away their debilitating stigmas.[92] The problem is we have already seen how apparently biologically neutral statements about heterosexual transmission or epidemiological origins of AIDS can nonetheless be charged with their own political and social agendas. From the very beginning, it was nearly impossible to disentangle the social construction of AIDS from whatever independently objective, biological reality it had. Its name and even very existence has been a matter of some debate and dissidence, while its origins, transmission, and spread are deeply rooted in our society's variable trends and behaviors, on both a communal and a personal level.[93] And yet, while AIDS does act as a kind of grand summation of all the diseases of the past, it also possesses some unique and distinctive qualities of its own. AIDS is less easily spread than other latent diseases such as tuberculosis and syphilis (although this can change depending on various cofactors), and this fact can affect how urgently measures to protect the public welfare should be implemented. Meanwhile, AIDS is perhaps more asymptomatic or else more easily masked by opportunistic infections than these other diseases during its long, slowly progressing incubation and dormant periods, allowing it to silently worm its way into a target population until it becomes endemic, despite the difficulty with which it is transmitted. It is a disease of the blood as well as of seminal fluids, and blood has always had a singular fascination for society as the precious bodily fluid of life. At least initially, AIDS was intimately associated with a particular subgroup of society, the gay community, that until then had not received much attention in disease history, or for that matter in human history in general. The timing of AIDS came right after the sexual revolution of the 1960s and 1970s, mixing sex and death in a particularly potent and frightening combination. Above all, AIDS forever changed the way historians view the history of disease, coming as it did right after victory had been declared against major infectious diseases like smallpox and as the medical community began to shift its focus toward more chronic conditions like cancer and heart disease. Even though AIDS at last seems to be joining the ranks of these latter, chronic diseases, the damage has already been done and historians can now never go back to the assumptions of the past: that human society will inevitably triumph over and find a cure for its ills, especially when concurrently or fast in AIDS' wake has come other, exotic diseases like Ebola, bovine spongiform encephalopathy ("mad cow disease"), and hantavirus pulmonary syndrome. AIDS indeed changed the very definition of what a disease is, forcing recent historians to take a much more relativist approach to disease history. For teachers, it has likewise proved very useful for posing all sorts of questions with respect to disease, even as it has withheld all its answers, since its mysteries are still unfolding. AIDS has thus been a boon for people morbidly fascinated with disease like me. But even so, I fervently wish it had never come among us.

Conclusion

Toward the end of the second millennium, in 1994, two books were published that both warned of a "coming plague" apocalypse. The Pulitzer-prize-winning author Laurie Garrett, after chronicling over a dozen frightful diseases that were "newly emerging" in a "world out of balance," declared in her last chapter that our microbe predators now had the advantage over their macro hosts and would emerge victorious unless we changed our environmentally destructive ways.[1] Similarly, Richard Preston, in his best-selling book *The Hot Zone*, which tells the story of an outbreak of Ebola and Marburg hemorrhagic fevers in central sub-Saharan Africa and at an army research lab in Reston, Virginia (which served as the inspiration for the 1995 film *Outbreak*), concluded in his final pages that "the earth is mounting an immune response against the human species." By this he means that, as humans are destroying ecological environments such as the tropical rainforest, so does the earth, in a kind of role reversal, attempt "to rid itself of an infection by the human parasite" with the emergence of deadly new diseases, particularly the worldwide plague of AIDS.[2] Continuing this theme, a new study relates our heightened disease environment specifically to the loss of biodiversity and natural habitat destruction, which increases our exposure to exotic pathogens by "homogenizing" or spreading them around the world, where they displace complex local species varieties.[3] Such biodiversity loss would also deprive us of potential cures such as new antibiotic drugs that are desperately needed now more than ever, with the advent of hospital-raised "superbugs" such as methicillin-resistant staphylococcus aureus (MRSA) as well as drug-resistant strains of established diseases like tuberculosis and malaria. A good example of the consequences of our habitat encroachment is the sudden appearance of the deadly Hendra virus in Australia in 1994, around the same time as Ebola was wreaking havoc in Africa. In both cases, it seems these never-before-seen diseases were the result of destruction of or intrusion upon bat habitat, which allowed for once exotic pathogens harbored in a remote host environment to homogenize and jump species. Perhaps this is simply the Gaia effect, whereby mother nature on a global scale is simply correcting the imbalance of an exploding human population, which as of 2010 is approaching seven billion.[4] The last time there was a major correction was during the Black Death in the late Middle Ages; since population has been growing largely unchecked ever since, it could be argued we are overdue for another one.

But in addition to failing to respect the boundaries of the wildlife ecosystem, which is an especially big problem because it is estimated that 60 percent of all diseases crossover from animals to humans, there are other large-scale factors at work, both environmental and otherwise, that will affect our epidemiological history: global warming, poverty, warfare, and so forth. It seems we are locked in a never-ending war with microbes, a war that has gone on ever since humans began altering their natural surroundings for their own purposes with the advent of agriculture and settled communities at the start of the Neolithic era some twelve thousand years ago. In some scholars' schema, this was but the "first transition" to a new disease ecology, in which humans now had to live with a far greater prevalence and virulence of disease in their lives; a "second transition" is understood to have occurred with the advent of the agricultural and industrial revolutions during the eighteenth and nineteenth centuries, when populations, at least in the West, commenced a rapid expansion and began concentrating in urban environments as well as establishing colonies of themselves around the world, all of which were made possible by the more efficient production of food and creation of wealth and factory employment in the cities. The "third transition" currently under way is the product of globalization of disease environments, as already mentioned. But whereas most texts portray the emergence of so many new diseases since the 1980s and 1990s (such as AIDS, Ebola, mad cow's disease, Lyme disease, Legionnaire's disease, hantavirus pulmonary syndrome, SARS, and avian flu, to name just a few) as well as the reemergence of some old ones (such as tuberculosis, malaria, yellow fever, schistosomiasis, cholera) as being an unprecedented and alarmingly new phenomenon, it could actually be argued that all this is really just a natural extension of some ancient forces going back thousands of years, which include changing modes of subsistence, shifting populations, environmental disruptions, social inequalities, and so on. We are simply entering a new stage in our age-old struggle with disease, one that now combines the worst of both prior transitions: more contact with new disease environments and greater ease and speed of their spread among large numbers of people around the globe—nor ought all of these transitions be necessarily accompanied by a worsening of human health across the board. During the second transition, for instance, incidences of tuberculosis, smallpox, and cholera began to dramatically decline, helped partly but not exclusively by new medical advances, such as vaccination and the germ theory, although such benefits came considerably later to the developing world.[5]

At this point, we should remind ourselves that the germ of many of these ideas goes back to a notion first advanced by the historian William McNeill in *Plagues and Peoples*, and which has informed disease studies ever since: humans are "macroparasites" on their environments in a way that is analogous, and yet also mutually dependent upon, the relationship that "microparasites," or disease microbes, have with us. Even should we be successful in our medical fight against disease, McNeill argues that this would only be a temporary victory, as the "galloping increases" in human population as a result would then put enormous pressures on our food supply and other resources that inevitably need to be corrected, a kind of global neo-Malthusianism.[6] Although the rate of population growth seems to have slowed in recent years, estimates are that the world's population will reach eight to nine billion people by 2050 and nine to ten billion by the end of the twenty-first century, unless unforeseen catastrophic pandemics (or any number of other natural or man-made disasters) intervene.[7] The chance that we will self-impose limits or even reverse reproduction of our numbers seems remote. (Communist China's "one-child" policy has so far had limited success.) Therefore, it seems assured that disease will play an inevitable part of human history for the foreseeable future.

The main themes of our future history with disease are ones that I identified already in the first chapter on plague. Travel, which now exists in the form of relatively cheap airfare that makes possible the reaching of almost every corner of the globe from almost any other within a day, will continue to spread disease just as Mongol trade routes spread the Black Death, although the process has been speeded up so much that exotic diseases once confined to remote places are now practically in our backyard. The winners and losers of disease will continue to fall along the fault lines of wealthier countries mainly in the West—which are better able to weather the storms of pandemics and, with their pharmaceutical conglomerates, might even economically benefit from them—and poorer nations in the third world of Africa, Asia, and Latin America, which will bear the brunt of most disease mortalities, as India did, for example, during the Third Pandemic of plague and the 1918–1919 influenza outbreak. And medicine will find its limits in successfully preventing and treating infectious diseases, especially in this day and age with the emergence of so many new ills on nearly a daily basis.

Nevertheless, I mentioned in the introduction that I personally am more hopeful, optimistic, sanguine, or however you wish to call it, than probably most other authors about humans' future at the hands of disease.[8] Perhaps this is partly because I live in Vermont, where over the course of little more than a century, deforestation and biodiversity loss have actually been reversed, to the point where today 80 percent of the state is carpeted with trees, whereas in 1880 only 20 percent was, and many wild animal species—such as moose, whitetail deer, black bear, and turkey—have been reintroduced to the state and are now quite commonly sighted. But the principal reason for my positive outlook goes back to one of the main theses I identified at the start of this book: humans have proven throughout history their power to alter the course of epidemics and pandemics, simply through their cultural conceptions about disease. To my mind, too many histories of disease still focus on the biomedical fight against microbes with our impressive and continually evolving technologies, such as genetic engineering. But the even faster evolution of microbes means that the dream of a "gorillacillin" superdrug to match the superbugs is probably unrealistic.[9] It is likely then that we will forever have to fall back on our own cultural devices as at least some part of our future response to disease. This is why the history of that response such as we have been tracing in this book is so important and instructive. The SARS outbreak in 2003 is a good example of how a pandemic in the making was successfully contained, despite the fearfully fast pace of its spread, using tried and true methods of quarantine and information sharing among countries (after initial efforts at suppression in China); we perhaps benefited from our heightened state of readiness toward global terrorism. (In the event, the SARS scare was over in just a few months, but the stakes involved were demonstrated by the fact that in that brief time over eight thousand people in thirty-seven countries were infected, of whom eight hundred died.) And yet, I cannot help feeling that the focus in too many books with disease bioterrorism is rather overblown, given that most diseases through their natural modes of dissemination are terrifying enough.[10] It should be of some comfort to us that humanity was able to survive even the horrors of the plague, with its average mortality of 50 to 60 percent during the medieval Black Death. Europe's low-grade quarantines are still thought to have had some effect in helping to eventually end the plague by the eighteenth century, and our ancestors' widespread belief in the afterlife may have helped psychologically "inoculate" them against the mass death due to disease. The British physician John Snow demonstrated how good old-fashioned detective work could provide the tools for tracing and conquering cholera in the mid-nineteenth century, well before the germ theory heralded our modern biological approach to disease. Some of our current difficulties, such as multi-drug-resistant tuberculosis or new strains of avian flu, are entirely of our own making, whether by not taking the prescribed course of antibiotics or by mishandling our mass consumption of domestic poultry, and only behavioral changes will correct them. If a current disease like AIDS remains beyond our biomedical ability to cure it, then perhaps we should approach it as primarily a function of poverty, as the former South African president and AIDS denier, Thabo Mbeki, has argued. Only, the poverty we need to channel our ingenuity into combating is the poverty of third world sufferers to afford antiretroviral therapies by which they can still be functioning members of society, or the poverty of their economic ability to change risky social behaviors that are responsible for ever more people contracting the disease. Certainly, the decline of tuberculosis even before the age of antibiotics seems to support such an approach. We may have to resign ourselves to making our own cultural peace with our own, new plagues, such as AIDS.

The other main thesis I have tried to emphasize in this book is to take a comparative approach to the study of plagues, which can draw out both the commonalities and distinctive features among different diseases. Plague and cholera, for example, acquired the reputation of being particularly horrible diseases to die from, owing to the suddenness of their onslaught and the revolting nature of their symptoms. Societies responded to the uniquely terrifying aspects of these diseases with fevered campaigns against filth or hysterical accusations of poisoning. Tuberculosis and influenza, on the other hand, perhaps bred a certain degree of complacency as a result of the slow, latent progress the disease could take in the body or the relative mildness and ephemeral nature of the symptoms. The shock was then all the greater when fulminant forms of these diseases took hold, defying normal expectations to the point that perhaps societies simply denied their existence or else stigmatized and shunned their sufferers. Today, this denial or complacency has a real impact with the low completion rates of antibiotic treatments or low participation in vaccination programs, which only helps increase the virulence and propagation of these diseases. Smallpox demonstrated how a disease could wreak terrible havoc in a "virgin soil" population but also how other societies that were immune or less affected by the disease could use it as both a cultural and biological weapon. AIDS, much like syphilis in the past, has become a metaphor for all sorts of moral and ethical stigmas attached to a disease spread primarily (but in the case of AIDS not exclusively) by socially unacceptable behaviors, such as promiscuous heterosexual and homosexual intercourse and intravenous drug use.[11] Yet, some would argue instead that this moral and sexual dimension to AIDS has blinded us to its underlying causes in poverty and that our ethical obligation is to combat such causes, rather than attempt to change "risky" social behaviors such as by encouraging greater condom use or sexual abstinence, especially in countries that have a cultural aversion to them.[12]

I have chosen all these diseases for discussion in this book because of the many, particular lessons they have to teach. And yet these are lessons that, despite their particularity, can nonetheless be applied broadly to other diseases, both now and in the future, that happen to come our way. Let us hope we can learn to be sufficient pupils of disease.

✳

Notes

Introduction

1. This identification seems to have first emerged in the seventeenth century and then became more definite at the turn of the twentieth century when the Third Pandemic sparked concerted scientific study of the disease. See Lawrence I. Conrad, "Plague in the Early Medieval Near East" (PhD diss., Princeton University, 1981), 41.

2. Michael W. Dols, *The Black Death in the Middle East* (Princeton, N.J.: Princeton University Press, 1977), 315. Comparable terminology can be found in Arabic and Hebrew.

3. E. Fuller Torrey and Robert H. Yolken, *Beasts of the Earth: Animals, Humans, and Disease* (New Brunswick, N.J.: Rutgers University Press, 2005), 15–20, 28–30.

4. Torrey and Yolken, *Beasts of the Earth*, 38–43, 49–52; William H. McNeill, *Plagues and Peoples*, updated ed. (New York: Anchor Books, 1998), 54–93; Robert Sallares, *The Ecology of the Ancient Greek World* (Ithaca, N.Y.: Cornell University Press, 1991), 227–44.

5. McNeill, *Plagues and Peoples*, 62, 84–92; Sheldon Watts, *Disease and Medicine in World History* (New York: Routledge, 2003), 56.

6. Watts, *Disease and Medicine in World History*, 16.

7. Donald R. Hopkins, "Ramses V: Earliest Known Victim?" World Health Organization, May 1980, at http://whqlibdoc.who.int/smallpox/WH_5_1980_p22.pdf (accessed June 24, 2010).

8. Kenneth F. Kiple, *The Cambridge World History of Human Disease* (Cambridge: Cambridge University Press, 1993), 345–47.

9. A variety of words in the original Hebrew were used in the Bible when referring to disease epidemics. See Conrad, "Plague," 43–44.

10. James Orr, "Plague," Bible History Online, at www.bible-history.com/isbe/P/PLAGUE (accessed June 24, 2010).

11. Conrad, "Plague," 42–63.

12. Jo N. Hays, *Epidemics and Pandemics: Their Impacts on Human History* (Santa Barbara, Calif.: ABC–CLIO, 2005), 5.

13. Kiple, *Cambridge World History of Human Disease*, 408–9.

14. Kiple, *Cambridge World History of Human Disease*, 347–53; Carol Benedict, *Bubonic Plague in Nineteenth-Century China* (Stanford, Calif.: Stanford University Press, 1996), 101–5.

15. Kiple, *Cambridge World History of Human Disease*, 263–69, 347–53, 373–75, 390–92, 409–12.

16. For discussions of the issues involved, see J. C. F. Poole and A. J. Holladay, "Thucydides and the Plague of Athens," *Classical Quarterly* 29 (1979): 282–300; Sallares, *Ecology of the Ancient Greek World*, 245–46; and James Longrigg, "Epidemic, Ideas and Classical Athenian Society," in *Epidemics and Ideas: Essays on the Historical Perception of Pestilence*, ed. T. Ranger and P. Slack, 21–44 (Cambridge: Cambridge University Press, 1992), 33–36.

17. For works that attempt to identify the Plague of Athens with a specific disease, see those cited in Conrad, "Plague," 64n59, to which should be added the article by James Longrigg, "The Great Plague of Athens," *History of Science* 18 (1980): 209–25, and Sallares, *Ecology of the Ancient Greek World*, 244–51. Discussion of the Plague of Athens as smallpox will be resumed in chapter 2.

18. Thucydides, *The History of the Peloponnesian War*, II:53, available in English translation by R. Crawley (London: Longmans, Green, 1874).

19. Sallares, *Ecology of the Ancient Greek World*, 246; Longrigg, "Epidemic," 41–43.

20. Longrigg, "Epidemic," 32–33.

21. See, for example, J. V. A. Fine, *The Ancient Greeks: A Critical History* (Cambridge, Mass.: Harvard University Press, 1983), 464; McNeill, *Plagues and Peoples*, 121; D. Kagan, *The Peloponnesian War* (New York: Viking Press, 2003), 78–79; Victor Davis Hanson, *A War Like No Other: How the Athenians and Spartans Fought the Peloponnesian War* (New York: Random House, 2005), 65–88.

22. Thucydides, *History of the Peloponnesian War*, III:87; Sallares, *Ecology of the Ancient Greek World*, 258–59; Hanson, *A War Like No Other*, 79–80.

23. Hanson, *A War Like No Other*, 77–78.

24. For Thucydides' influence upon other classical authors who wrote about disease, see Longrigg, "Epidemic," 27.

25. General works on disease representative of the "positivist" approach include the following: Hans Zinsser, *Rats, Lice and History* (Boston: Little, Brown, 1934); Henry E. Sigerist, *Civilization and Disease* (Chicago: University of Chicago Press, 1943); and Frederick F. Cartwright, *Disease and History* (New York: Thomas Y. Crowell Co., 1972).

26. See especially Charles-Edward Amory Winslow, *The Conquest of Epidemic Disease: A Chapter in the History of Ideas* (Princeton, N.J.: Princeton University Press, 1943); and

L. Fabian Hirst, *The Conquest of Plague: A Study of the Evolution of Epidemiology* (Oxford, UK: Clarendon Press, 1953).

27. McNeill, *Plagues and Peoples*, 22–23.

28. William H. McNeill, *The Rise of the West: A History of the Human Community* (Chicago: University of Chicago Press, 1963).

29. McNeill, *Plagues and Peoples*, 19–21. The importance of the "Columbian exchange," not just in terms of disease pathogens, was first explored by Alfred W. Crosby, *The Columbian Exchange: Biological and Cultural Consequences of 1492* (Westport, Conn.: Greenwood Press, 1972). Crosby later explored this theme on a global scale in *Ecological Imperialism: The Biological Expansion of Europe, 900–1900* (Cambridge: Cambridge University Press, 1986), in which disease plays but one part of the story.

30. McNeill, *Plagues and Peoples*, 24–27.

31. For works in the relativist school, see Robert P. Hudson, *Disease and Its Control: The Shaping of Modern Thought* (Westport, Conn.: Greenwood Press, 1983); Claudine Herzlich and Janine Pierret, *Illness and Self in Society*, trans. E. Forster (Baltimore: Johns Hopkins University Press, 1987); Allan M. Brandt, "AIDS and Metaphor: Toward the Social Meaning of Epidemic Disease," in *In Time of Plague: The History and Social Consequences of Lethal Epidemic Disease*, ed. A. Mack, 91–110 (New York: New York University Press, 1991); and Charles E. Rosenberg, *Explaining Epidemics and Other Studies in the History of Medicine* (Cambridge: Cambridge University Press, 1992), esp. 278–318.

32. Hudson, *Disease and Its Control*, x.

33. McNeill, *Plagues and Peoples*, 291–95.

34. McNeill, *Plagues and Peoples*, 9–17.

35. See, in particular, Richard Preston, *The Hot Zone* (New York: Random House, 1994); and Laurie Garrett, *The Coming Plague: Newly Emerging Diseases in a World Out of Balance* (Harmondsworth, UK: Penguin, 1994). These have been joined by such films as *Outbreak* (1995) and *I Am Legend* (2007). A far more balanced and temperate view of the topic is taken up in Jo N. Hays, *The Burdens of Disease: Epidemics and Human Response in Western History* (New Brunswick, N.J.: Rutgers University Press, 1998), esp. 240–77; and Arno Karlen, *Man and Microbes: Disease and Plagues in History and Modern Times* (New York: Putnam, 1995), esp. 1–11, 215–30.

36. Sallares, *Ecology of the Ancient Greek World*, 224.

37. For classic works in this vein, see David Arnold, *Colonizing the Body: State Medicine and Epidemic Disease in Nineteenth-Century India* (Berkeley: University of California Press, 1993); O. A. Bushnell, *The Gifts of Civilization: Germs and Genocide in Hawaii* (Honolulu: University of Hawaii Press, 1993); Sheldon Watts, *Epidemics and History: Disease, Power and Imperialism* (New Haven, Conn.: Yale University Press, 1997); and Suzanne Austin Alchon, *A Pest in the Land: New World Epidemics in a Global Perspective* (Albuquerque: University of New Mexico Press, 2003). McNeill specifically rejects the colonialist/imperialist argument (albeit even before it was made by the above champions) in *Plagues and Peoples*, 215.

38. See especially P. D. Curtin, *Death by Migration: Europe's Encounter with the Tropical World in the Nineteenth Century* (Cambridge: Cambridge University Press, 1989).

39. McNeill, *Plagues and Peoples*, 194; William H. McNeill, "Migration Patterns and Infection in Traditional Societies," in *Changing Disease Patterns and Human Behavior*, ed. N. F. Stanley and R. A. Joske, 27–36 (London: Academic Press, 1980), 34.

40. David Herlihy, *The Black Death and the Transformation of the West*, ed. S. K. Cohn Jr. (Cambridge, Mass.: Harvard University Press, 1997); and Samuel K. Cohn Jr., *The Black Death Transformed: Disease and Culture in Early Renaissance Europe* (London: Arnold, 2002). For a reevaluation of this "silver lining" thesis about the Black Death, see John Aberth, *From the Brink of the Apocalypse: Confronting Famine, War, Plague and Death in the Later Middle Ages*, 2nd ed. (London: Routledge, 2010), 206–10.

41. Sallares, *Ecology of the Ancient Greek World*, 262.

42. See, for example, Brian Fagan, *The Little Ice Age: How Climate Made History, 1300–1850* (New York: Basic Books, 2000), and Brian Fagan, *The Great Warming: Climate Change and the Rise and Fall of Civilizations* (New York: Bloomsbury Press, 2008).

43. It is perhaps a significant sign of the shift in disease studies that Alfred Jay Bollet, in the second, 2004 edition of his book, *Plagues and Poxes*, changed the subtitle from *The Rise and Fall of Epidemic Disease* to *The Impact of Human History on Epidemic Disease*, albeit the main thrust of his new focus is on disease as a weapon of bioterrorism. See Alfred Jay Bollet, *Plagues and Poxes: The Impact of Human History on Epidemic Disease* (New York: Demos, 2004), 1–13.

44. Sallares, *Ecology of the Ancient Greek World*, 262.

45. Jo N. Hays, "Historians and Epidemics: Simple Questions, Complex Answers," in *Plague and the End of Antiquity: The Pandemic of 541–750*, ed. L. K. Little, 33–58 (Cambridge: Cambridge University Press, 2007), 42–46.

46. This argument is made with particular reference to identifying the three pandemics of plague as all caused by the same disease: See A. Cunningham, "Transforming Plague: The Laboratory and the Identity of Infectious Disease," in *The Laboratory Revolution in Medicine*, ed. A. Cunningham and P. Williams, 209–44 (Cambridge: Cambridge University Press, 1992), 209; D. Harrison, "Plague, Settlement and Structural Changes at the Dawn of the Middle Ages," *Scandia* 59 (1993): 19; and Jon Arrizabalaga, "Facing the Black Death: Perceptions and Reactions of University Medical Practitioners," in *Practical Medicine from Salerno to the Black Death*, ed. L. García-Ballester, R. French, J. Arrizabalaga, and A. Cunningham, 237–88 (Cambridge: Cambridge University Press, 1994), 239. This position is refuted by C. J. Duncan and S. Scott, *Biology of Plagues: Evidence from Historical Populations* (Cambridge: Cambridge University Press, 2001), 53; and Robert Sallares, "Ecology, Evolution, and Epidemiology of Plague," in *Plague and the End of Antiquity: The Pandemic of 541–750*, ed. L. K. Little, 231–89 (Cambridge: Cambridge University Press, 2007), 255–56.

47. Cohn, *Black Death Transformed*, 83–95.

48. For example, in 1998–2000, a French team announced it had isolated *Yersinia pestis* DNA from the dental pulp of fourteenth- and sixteenth-century plague victims at Montpellier, which they offered as conclusive evidence that the Black Death was true plague: see Michel Drancourt et al., "Detection of 400-Year-Old *Yersinia pestis* DNA in Human Dental Pulp: An Approach to the Diagnosis of Ancient Septicemia," *Proceedings*

of the National Academy of Science 95 (1998): 12637–40; and Michel Drancourt et al., "Molecular Identification by 'Suicide PCR' of *Yersinia pestis* as the Agent of Medieval Black Death," *Proceedings of the National Academy of Science* 97 (2000): 12800–803. While their identification still remains controversial, the French team's results have now been duplicated in London and Germany: see essays by Lester K. Little, Robert Sallares, and Michael McCormick in *Plague and the End of Antiquity: The Pandemic of 541–750*, ed. L. K. Little (Cambridge: Cambridge University Press, 2007), 19–20, 254, and 294–97, as well as references cited there in footnotes.

49. For example, William McNeill, even though he acknowledged the role that Native American attitudes toward disease played in the Spanish conquest of the Americas, failed to draw any contrasts between the native view of disease and that of Europeans that could explain that role. Instead, he simply noted that both sides saw disease as coming from divine sources and put any differences in response down to immunity (or lack thereof). See McNeill, *Plagues and Peoples*, 20–21, 215–17.

50. See especially Hays, *Burdens of Disease*, esp. 1–7; and Hays, "Historians and Epidemics," 33–36, 52–56.

Chapter 1: Plague

1. Lawrence I. Conrad, "Plague in the Early Medieval Near East" (PhD diss., Princeton University, 1981), 488.

2. Based on personal telephone interview conducted with John Tull and Lucinda Marker on February 20, 2004.

3. For a comprehensive, up-to-date summary of fleas' role in spreading bubonic plague, see Kenneth L. Gage and Michael Y. Kosoy, "Natural History of Plague: Perspectives from More than a Century of Research," *Annual Review of Entomology* 50 (2005): 505–28. Older works still worth consulting on this topic include the following: Wu Lien-Teh, J. W. H. Chun, R. Pollitzer, and C. Y. Wu, *Plague: A Manual for Medical and Public Health Workers* (Shanghai, China: Weishengshu National Quarantine Service, 1936), 265–70; R. Pollitzer, *Plague* (Geneva: World Health Organization, 1954), 346–55; Graham Twigg, *The Black Death: A Biological Reappraisal* (New York: Schocken Books, 1984), 16–17.

4. Many of these statistics were collected during the Third Pandemic in India and Egypt and presented in the *Journal of Hygiene*, but they are conveniently summarized in Ole J. Benedictow, *Plague in the Late Medieval Nordic Countries: Epidemiological Studies* (Oslo, Norway: Middelalderforlaget, 1992), 164; and Robert Sallares, "Ecology, Evolution, and Epidemiology of Plague," in *Plague and the End of Antiquity: The Pandemic of 541–750*, ed. L. K. Little, 231–89 (Cambridge: Cambridge University Press, 2007), 278.

5. Personal telephone interview conducted with John Tull, February 20, 2004.

6. Wu Lien-Teh (Liande), *A Treatise on Pneumonic Plague* (Geneva: Publications of the League of Nations, 1926), 162–64, 252–55, 296–306.

7. W. F. Gatacre, *Report on the Bubonic Plague in Bombay, 1896–97* (Bombay, India: Times of India Steam Press, 1897), 138–39; J. K. Condon, *The Bombay Plague, Being a History of the Progress of Plague in the Bombay Presidency from September 1896 to June 1899*

(Bombay, India: Education Society's Steam Press, 1900), 72–73; Lien-Teh, *Treatise on Pneumonic Plague*, 245; Lien-Teh et al., *Plague*, 309–16; Pollitzer, *Plague*, 411–18, 441. Marker noted an inexplicable sense of foreboding or "doom" that accompanied what she otherwise thought were symptoms typical of the flu at the onset of her case of plague.

8. Samuel K. Cohn Jr., "The Black Death: End of a Paradigm," *American Historical Review* 107 (2002): 716–17; Sallares, "Ecology," 240–41.

9. Condon, *The Bombay Plague*, 73; Lien-Teh et al., *Plague*, 158, 311, 314, 322; Pollitzer, *Plague*, 420–21, 424–27.

10. Gatacre, *Report on the Bubonic Plague*, 50; Sallares, "Ecology," 236.

11. Procopius of Caesarea, *History of the Wars*, II:xxii.17, trans. H. B. Dewing (London: W. Heinemann and Macmillan, 1914–1940); John of Ephesus' description is available in English translation in Pseudo-Dionysius of Tel-Mahre, *The Chronicle of Zuqnīn, Parts III and IV*, trans. A. Harrak (Toronto: Pontifical Institute of Mediaeval Studies, 1999), 104; and Pseudo-Dionysius of Tel-Mahre, *Chronicle, Part III*, trans. Witold Witakowski, Translated Texts for Historians 22 (Liverpool, UK: Liverpool University Press, 1996), 87. This was by no means the first occurrence of *boubon* as a term for bubonic swellings; the symptom was discussed centuries earlier in the Hippocratic *Epidemics*, which record Greek doctors' case histories from the end of the fifth and first half of the fourth centuries B.C.E.

12. Medieval testimony comes from the fifteenth-century German treatise of a "Master Berthold," printed in Karl Sudhoff, "Pestschriften aus den ersten 150 Jahren nach der Epidemie des 'schwarzen Todes' 1348," *Archiv für Geschichte der Medizin* 16 (1925): 93. For modern diagnosis, see Condon, *The Bombay Plague*, 73; Pollitzer, *Plague*, 421–23. Marker also noted this same phenomenon in her bout with bubonic plague in November 2002.

13. Gatacre, *Report on the Bubonic Plague*, 141, 223; Condon, *The Bombay Plague*, 73–74; Pollitzer, *Plague*, 423.

14. Condon, *The Bombay Plague*, 77; Lien-Teh, *Treatise on Pneumonic Plague*, 241–59; Pollitzer, *Plague*, 441–42; Ole J. Benedictow, *The Black Death, 1346–1353: The Complete History* (Woodbridge, UK: Boydell Press, 2004), 28.

15. Gatacre, *Report on the Bubonic Plague*, 138, 223; Condon, *The Bombay Plague*, 76–77; Pollitzer, *Plague*, 439–40.

16. Conrad, "Plague," 73–76; Sallares, "Ecology," 251.

17. Robert Sallares, *The Ecology of the Ancient Greek World* (Ithaca, N.Y.: Cornell University Press, 1991), 252–53; Sallares, "Ecology," 245–54.

18. Most recently, a collection of essays on the First Pandemic was published as Little, *Plague and the End of Antiquity*, but other general works that should be consulted include Conrad's "Plague" and Dionysios Stathakopoulos, *Famine and Pestilence in the Late Roman and Early Byzantine Empire: A Systematic Survey of Subsistence Crises and Epidemics* (Burlington, Vt.: Ashgate, 2004).

19. For an overview of the debate as to the origins of the First Pandemic in Africa, see Peter Sarris, "Bubonic Plague in Byzantium: The Evidence of Non-Literary Sources," in *Plague and the End of Antiquity: The Pandemic of 541–750*, ed. L. K. Little, 119–34 (Cambridge: Cambridge University Press, 2007), 120–23.

20. For more detailed chronologies, see Dionysios Stathakopoulos, "Crime and Punishment: The Plague in the Byzantine Empire, 541–749," in *Plague and the End of Antiquity: The Pandemic of 541–750*, ed. L. K. Little, 99–118 (Cambridge: Cambridge University Press, 2007), 99–105; Stathakopoulos, *Famine and Pestilence*, 113–24, 278–386; Conrad, "Plague," 91–311; Jean-Noël Biraben, *Les Hommes et la Peste en France et dans les Pays Européens et Méditerranéens*, 2 vols. (Paris: Mouton, 1975–1976), 1:27–32; Jean-Noël Biraben and Jacques Le Goff, "The Plague in the Early Middle Ages," in *Biology of Man in History: Selections from the Annales: Économies, Sociétés, Civilisations*, ed. and trans. E. Forster, R. Forster, O. Ranum, and P. M. Ranum, 48–80 (Baltimore: Johns Hopkins University Press, 1975), 58–60.

21. Procopius, *History of the Wars*, II:22.17; Pseudo-Dionysius of Tel-Mahre, *Chronicle of Zuqnīn*, 104; Pseudo-Dionysius of Tel-Mahre, *Chronicle*, 87–88. Bubonic symptoms are also mentioned in contemporary saints' lives, cited in Stathakopoulos, *Famine and Pestilence*, 136n119.

22. Evagrius Scholasticus, *Ecclesiastical History*, IV:29, translated as *A History of the Church* (London: S. Bagster and Sons, 1846).

23. Michael G. Morony, "'For Whom Does the Writer Write?': The First Bubonic Plague Pandemic According to Syriac Sources," in *Plague and the End of Antiquity: The Pandemic of 541–750*, ed. L. K. Little, 59–86 (Cambridge: Cambridge University Press, 2007), 60–61; Lawrence I. Conrad, "*Tā'ūn* and *Wabā*: Conceptions of Plague and Pestilence in Early Islam," *Journal of the Economic and Social History of the Orient* 25 (1982): 291–301; Michael W. Dols, *The Black Death in the Middle East* (Princeton, N.J.: Princeton University Press, 1977), 315–19.

24. John Maddicott, "Plague in Seventh-Century England," in *Plague and the End of Antiquity: The Pandemic of 541–750*, ed. L. K. Little, 171–214 (Cambridge: Cambridge University Press, 2007), 183.

25. Procopius, *History of the Wars*, II:22.10–14.

26. Pseudo-Dionysius of Tel-Mahre, *Chronicle of Zuqnīn*, 95–97; Pseudo-Dionysius of Tel-Mahre, *Chronicle*, 76–77; Morony, "'For Whom Does the Writer Write?'" 82.

27. Pseudo-Dionysius of Tel-Mahre, *Chronicle of Zuqnīn*, esp. 95–96, 100–103, 107; Pseudo-Dionysius of Tel-Mahre, *Chronicle*, 75–76, 81–85, 90.

28. Compare Procopius, *History of the Wars*, II:23.14–16 with Thucydides, *The History of the Peloponnesian War*, trans. R. Crawley (London: Longmans, Green, 1874), II:53.

29. Procopius, *History of the Wars*, II:22.27, 33–34; Thucydides, *History of the Peloponnesian War*, II:51.

30. Pseudo-Dionysius of Tel-Mahre, *Chronicle of Zuqnīn*, 97–98; 109–10; Pseudo-Dionysius of Tel-Mahre, *Chronicle*, 77–78, 93–94.

31. Thucydides, *History of the Peloponnesian War*, II:52.

32. For instance, many readers may bring to mind the U.S. government's shameful handling of the aftermath of Hurricane Katrina in New Orleans in 2005.

33. Procopius, *History of the Wars*, II:23.6–13; Pseudo-Dionysius of Tel-Mahre *Chronicle of Zuqnīn*, 107–8, 110; Pseudo-Dionysius of Tel-Mahre, *Chronicle*, 91–92, 94.

34. Pseudo-Dionysius of Tel-Mahre, *Chronicle of Zuqnīn*, 108, 111; Pseudo-Dionysius of Tel-Mahre, *Chronicle*, 91, 95–96.

35. Pseudo-Dionysius of Tel-Mahre, *Chronicle of Zuqnīn*, 106–8; Pseudo-Dionysius of Tel-Mahre, *Chronicle*, 89–92.

36. Pseudo-Dionysius of Tel-Mahre, *Chronicle of Zuqnīn*, 106–7; Pseudo-Dionysius of Tel-Mahre, *Chronicle*, 90.

37. Pseudo-Dionysius of Tel-Mahre, *Chronicle of Zuqnīn*, 109; Pseudo-Dionysius of Tel-Mahre, *Chronicle*, 93. See also Procopius, *History of the Wars*, II:23.12.

38. Pseudo-Dionysius of Tel-Mahre, *Chronicle of Zuqnīn*, 99–100, 105, 109; Pseudo-Dionysius of Tel-Mahre, *Chronicle*, 81, 88, 93; Procopius, *History of the Wars*, II:23.17–19.

39. Procopius, *History of the Wars*, II:22.29, 32–34.

40. Pseudo-Dionysius of Tel-Mahre, *Chronicle of Zuqnīn*, 112–13; Pseudo-Dionysius of Tel-Mahre, *Chronicle*, 97–98.

41. Pseudo-Dionysius of Tel-Mahre, *Chronicle of Zuqnīn*, 98–99; Pseudo-Dionysius of Tel-Mahre, *Chronicle*, 79; Scholasticus, *Ecclesiastical History*, VI:23.

42. Stathakopoulos, "Crime and Punishment," 113–14.

43. See especially the text of Justinian's Novella 141 against homosexuals, issued in 559, a year after a second outbreak of plague had struck the capital. The text is available in English through the online publication of Fred H. Blume and Timothy Kearley, *Annotated Justinian Code*, 2nd ed. (Laramie: University of Wyoming College of Law, 2009), at http://uwacadweb.uwyo.edu/blume&justinian (accessed August 3, 2010).

44. Josiah Cox Russell, "That Earlier Plague," *Demography* 5 (1968): 181–82.

45. See Guy Halsall, *Barbarian Migrations and the Roman West, 376–568* (Cambridge: Cambridge University Press, 2007), 507–15, for a discussion of the various issues involved. Russell's monocausal explanation is criticized by Stathakopoulos, "Crime and Punishment," 116–17.

46. Conrad, "Plague," 121–22, 134.

47. Procopius, *The Secret History*, trans. G. A. Williamson (London: Folio Society, 1990), 83–88. In an earlier chapter, Procopius cites the testimony of several witnesses, including the emperor's own mother, who alleged that they had personally experienced the demonic origins or character of the emperor (58–60). The fact that Justinian himself came down with bubonic plague, and survived, could be taken as evidence either for or against a theory that was considered not implausible for its time.

48. Gregory of Tours, *History of the Franks*, X:1, trans. Lewis Thorpe (Harmondsworth, UK: Penguin, 1974).

49. 1 Chronicles 21:14–27, discussed in Lester K. Little, "Life and Afterlife of the First Plague Pandemic," in *Plague and the End of Antiquity: The Pandemic of 541–750*, ed. L. K. Little, 3–32 (Cambridge: Cambridge University Press, 2007), 31–32.

50. Michael Kulikowski, "Plague in Spanish Late Antiquity," in *Plague and the End of Antiquity: The Pandemic of 541–750*, ed. L. K. Little, 150–70 (Cambridge: Cambridge University Press, 2007), 155–56, 160–70.

51. Kulikowski, "Plague in Spanish Late Antiquity," 167–68.

52. For a detailed history of the Plague of 'Amwâs, see Conrad, "Plague," 167–246.

53. Conrad, "Plague," 169–76; Lawrence I. Conrad, "Umar at Sargh: The Evolution of an Umayyad Tradition on Flight from the Plague," in *Story-telling in the Framework of Non-fictional Arabic Literature*, ed. S. Leder, 488–528 (Wiesbaden, Germany: Harrassowitz, 1998); Dols, *Black Death*, 21–25.

54. Conrad, "Plague," 460–65.

55. Michael W. Dols, "The Comparative Communal Responses to the Black Death in Muslim and Christian Societies," *Viator* 5 (1974): 272–73, 279, 285.

56. Kulikowski, "Plague in Spanish Late Antiquity," 164–65.

57. Stathakopoulos, "Crime and Punishment," 107–8; John Haldon, "The Works of Anastasius of Sinai: A Key Source for the History of Seventh-Century East Mediterranean Society and Belief," in *The Byzantine and Early Islamic Near East, Volume I: Problems in the Literary Source Material*, ed. A. Cameron and L. I. Conrad, 107–47 (Princeton, N.J.: Darwin Press, 1992), 143–44.

58. Paul the Deacon, *History of the Lombards*, II:4, trans. William Dudley Foulke (Philadelphia: University of Pennsylvania Press, 1974).

59. S. P. Brock, "North Mesopotamia in the Late Seventh Century: Book XV of John Bar Penkāyē's *Rīš Mellē*," *Jerusalem Studies in Arabic and Islam* 9 (1987): 68–69; Morony, "'For Whom Does the Writer Write?'" 76–77.

60. Stathakopoulos, "Crime and Punishment," 116–18.

61. Russell, "That Earlier Plague," 178–84. Russell bases his argument on the assumption that plague mortality during the First Pandemic can be modeled on that of the Second, but there simply is not enough evidence to justify his position. For a more subtle version of this thesis, arguing for the rise of Western Europe on the basis of plague's differential mortality, see Biraben and Le Goff, "Plague in the Early Middle Ages," 63.

62. Conrad, "Plague," 293–94, 329–38, 415–89.

63. Richard Hodges and David Whitehouse, *Mohammed, Charlemagne and the Origins of Europe: Archaeology and the Pirenne Thesis* (Ithaca, N.Y.: Cornell University Press, 1983), 20–76; Michael McCormick, *Origins of the European Economy: Communications and Commerce, A.D. 300–900* (Cambridge: Cambridge University Press, 2001), 27–119.

64. McCormick, *Origins of the European Economy*, 40–41.

65. Conrad, "Plague," 449–89; Hodges and Whitehouse, *Mohammed, Charlemagne*, 52–53, 75–76.

66. Michael McCormick, "Toward a Molecular History of the Justinianic Pandemic," in *Plague and the End of Antiquity: The Pandemic of 541–750*, ed. L. K. Little, 290–312 (Cambridge: Cambridge University Press, 2007), 310–12.

67. John Norris, "East or West? The Geographic Origin of the Black Death," *Bulletin of the History of Medicine* 51 (1977): 10.

68. Michael W. Dols, "Ibn al-Wardi's *Risalah al-Naba' 'an al-Waba'*, a Translation of a Major Source of the History of the Black Death in the Middle East," in *Near Eastern Numismatics, Iconography, Epigraphy and History: Studies in Honor of George C. Miles*, ed. D. K. Kouymjian, 443–55 (Beirut, Lebanon: American University of Beirut, 1974), 448.

69. J. B. Hinnebusch, "Bubonic Plague: A Molecular Genetic Case History of the Emergence of an Infectious Disease," *Journal of Molecular Medicine* 75 (1997): 645–52; Sallares, "Ecology," 245–54.

70. Norris, "East or West?" 7–16; Benedictow, *Black Death*, 44–54.

71. Another contemporary commentator on the Black Death, the Moorish physician Ibn Khātima, who, like al-Wardī, claims to have received information on the plague's origins from merchant sources, writes from Almería, Spain, in February 1349 that the Genoese in Caffa were "besieged by an army of Turks and Romans." This would imply that Greek Byzantines from Constantinople had joined the Mongols in the siege.

72. H. H. Lamb, *Climate, History and the Modern World*, 2nd ed. (London: Routledge, 1995), 200; Dols, *Black Death*, 41; Norris, "East or West?" 4.

73. Dols, *Black Death*, 39.

74. Rosemary Horrox, trans. and ed., *The Black Death* (Manchester, UK: Manchester University Press, 1994), 17.

75. For the geographical spread of the Black Death in Europe and the Middle East, readers are advised to consult the detailed work of Benedictow, *Black Death*, 57–224, which has now supplanted Biraben's chronology in *Les Hommes et la Peste*, 1:71–85.

76. The one article devoted to this topic mainly addresses whether the First Pandemic was bubonic or pneumonic plague but never really questions that it was plague. See T. L. Bratton, "The Identity of the Plague of Justinian: Part 1," *Transactions and Studies of the College of Physicians of Philadelphia* 3 (June 1981): 113–24.

77. My greatest contempt, however, is reserved for those who refuse to enter into the debate at all but argue that medieval and modern diseases simply can't be compared, which strikes me as an attempt, unintentional or not, to suppress historical enquiry. See the introduction.

78. For instance, Samuel K. Cohn Jr., in his revisionist history, *The Black Death Transformed: Disease and Culture in Early Renaissance Europe* (London: Arnold, 2002), 247, refuses to propose any alternative at all to plague, while the revisionist authors, Susan Scott and Christopher J. Duncan, in *Biology of Plagues: Evidence from Historical Populations* (Cambridge: Cambridge University Press, 2001), 384–89, make up their own disease to replace plague, which they call "hemorrhagic plague," which seems akin to Ebola (caused by a virus). But one can't even engage in debate over a fictional illness.

79. The original French results, their detractors, and the new evidence are all cited by Little, "Life and Afterlife," 19–21, and McCormick, "Toward a Molecular History," 294–97.

80. See, in particular, William M. Bowsky, ed., *The Black Death: A Turning Point in History?* (New York: Holt, Rinehart and Winston, 1971).

81. See Benedictow, *Black Death*, 245–384.

82. Massimo Livi Bacci, *The Population of Europe: A History*, trans. C. De Nardi and C. Ipsen (Oxford: Blackwell, 2000), 74; Stathakopoulos, "Crime and Punishment," 105.

83. Carlo M. Cipolla, *Miasmas and Disease: Public Health and the Environment in the Pre-Industrial Age*, trans. E. Potter (New Haven, Conn.: Yale University Press, 1992), 68.

84. John Aberth, *From the Brink of the Apocalypse: Confronting Famine, War, Plague and Death in the Later Middle Ages*, 2nd ed. (London: Routledge, 2010), 96–99; C. N. Fabbri, "Continuity and Change in Late Medieval Plague Medicine: A Survey of 152 Plague Tracts from 1348 to 1599" (PhD diss., Yale University, 2006), 126; Cipolla, *Miasmas and Disease*, 6.

85. A much fuller study of the medical response to the Black Death will be forthcoming in my *Doctoring the Black Death: The Late Medieval Medical Response to Epidemic Disease*, to be published by Rowman & Littlefield.

86. Dols, "Comparative Communal Responses," 275; Dols, *Black Death*, 109; Lawrence I. Conrad, "Epidemic Disease in Formal and Popular Thought in Early Islamic Society," in *Epidemics and Ideas: Essays on the Historical Perception of Pestilence*, ed. T. Ranger and P. Slack, 77–99 (Cambridge: Cambridge University Press, 1992).

87. A point made most cogently by Justin Stearns with regard to contagion in his dissertation, "Infectious Ideas: Contagion in Medieval Islamic and Christian Thought" (PhD diss., Princeton University, 2007), but one that is also made by Marie-Hélène Congourdeau and Mohamed Melhaoui, "La Perception de la Peste en Pays Chrétien, Byzantine, et Musulman," *Revue des Études Byzantines* 59 (2001): 95–124.

88. Stearns, "Infectious Ideas," 182–99; Conrad, "Epidemic Disease," 86–91.

89. Stearns, "Infectious Ideas," 204–9; John Aberth, *The Black Death: The Great Mortality of 1348–1350. A Brief History with Documents* (Boston: Bedford/St. Martin's, 2005), 62–63.

90. Stearns, "Infectious Ideas," 32–43, 182–211; Aberth, *The Black Death*, 56.

91. Stearns, "Infectious Ideas," 204.

92. M. Isabel Calero Secall, "El Proceso de Ibn al-Jatīb," *Al-Qantas: Arab Studies Journal* 22 (2001): 437–38.

93. Gentile da Foligno, *Consilium contra Pestilentiam* (Colle di Valdelsa, c. 1479), 4–5.

94. Horrox, *The Black Death*, 182–84.

95. Sudhoff, "Pestschriften aus den ersten 150 Jahren nach der Epidemie des 'schwarzen Todes' 1348," *Archiv für Geschichte der Medizin* 4 (1911): 422.

96. Stearns, "Infectious Ideas," 208.

97. Aberth, *The Black Death*, 45, 51.

98. Sudhoff, "Pestschriften aus den ersten 150 Jahren nach der Epidemie des 'schwarzen Todes' 1348," *Archiv für Geschichte der Medizin* 16 (1925): 170.

99. Sudhoff, "Pestschriften aus den ersten 150 Jahren nach der Epidemie des 'schwarzen Todes' 1348," *Archiv für Geschichte der Medizin* 11 (1919): 44–47.

100. Sudhoff, "Pestschriften aus den ersten 150 Jahren nach der Epidemie des 'schwarzen Todes' 1348," *Archiv für Geschichte der Medizin* 5 (1912): 341–48.

101. Sudhoff, "Pestschriften aus den ersten 150 Jahren nach der Epidemie des 'schwarzen Todes' 1348," *Archiv für Geschichte der Medizin* 14 (1923): 159.

102. Stearns, "Infectious Ideas," 112–13.

103. Aberth, *The Black Death*, 115.

104. Aberth, *The Black Death*, 115.

105. Stearns, "Infectious Ideas," 204–5.

106. Stearns, "Infectious Ideas," 116–30.

107. Stearns, "Infectious Ideas," 138–41, 218.

108. Galen's original aphorism was "I urge you, go far away and don't come back soon." However, it is unclear which of Galen's works, if any, this is from. See Stathakopoulos, "Crime and Punishment," 111n93.

109. Sudhoff, "Pestschriften aus den ersten 150 Jahren nach der Epidemie des 'schwarzen Todes' 1348," *Archiv für Geschichte der Medizin* 16 (1925): 26.

110. Horrox, *The Black Death*, 203.

111. Foligno, *Consilium contra Pestilentiam*, 3.

112. Sudhoff, "Pestschriften aus den ersten 150 Jahren nach der Epidemie des 'schwarzen Todes' 1348," *Archiv für Geschichte der Medizin* 5 (1912): 333.

113. Horrox, *The Black Death*, 184.

114. Aberth, *The Black Death*, 77.

115. S. K. Wray, "Boccaccio and the Doctors: Medicine and Compassion in the Face of the Plague," *Journal of Medieval History* 30 (2004): 301–22.

116. Aberth, *The Black Death*, 76.

117. Aberth, *The Black Death*, 77.

118. Horrox, *The Black Death*, 28.

119. MS Vatic. Lat. 4589, fols. 138r–155v.

120. Aberth, *The Black Death*, 112–13.

121. Aberth, *The Black Death*, 110–14.

122. Stearns, "Infectious Ideas," 116–26, 189–97, 212–18.

123. Dols, "Comparative Communal Responses," 276–77; Dols, *Black Death*, 112–13.

124. Sudhoff, "Pestschriften aus den ersten 150 Jahren nach der Epidemie des 'schwarzen Todes' 1348," *Archiv für Geschichte der Medizin* 16 (1925): 26.

125. Aberth, *The Black Death*, 73.

126. MS Vatic. Lat. 4589, fols. 146r.–149r.

127. Sudhoff, "Pestschriften aus den ersten 150 Jahren nach der Epidemie des 'schwarzen Todes' 1348," *Archiv für Geschichte der Medizin* 11 (1919): 150.

128. Julian of Norwich, *Revelations of Divine Love*, in *A Book of Showings to the Anchoress Julian of Norwich*, ed. Edmund Colledge and James Walsh, chap. 27 (Toronto: Pontifical Institute of Mediaeval Studies, 1978).

129. Aberth, *The Black Death*, 123–24.

130. See, especially, Norman Cohn, *The Pursuit of the Millennium: Revolutionary Messianism in Medieval and Reformation Europe and Its Bearing on Modern Totalitarian Movements* (New York: Harper, 1961), 124–48.

131. Dols, "Comparative Communal Responses," 273, 283–84; Dols, *Black Death*, 287–88, 294–95.

132. Dols, "Comparative Communal Responses," 285; Dols, *Black Death*, 296–97.

133. I argue that the Flagellant movement was mainly motivated by a desire to ward off or take away the plague, which I elaborate on in more detail in *From the Brink of the Apocalypse*, 133–56.

134. See, for example, Ibn Kathīr's description of Muslim prayers and processions during the Black Death in Damascus, Syria, available in Aberth, *The Black Death*, 110–12.

135. The issue is raised in Dols, "Comparative Communal Responses," 274–75; and Dols, *Black Death*, 288–89.

136. For a fuller discussion of the supposed connection between the Jewish pogroms and the Flagellants, see Aberth, *From the Brink of the Apocalypse*, 153–56.

137. See Aberth, *From the Brink of the Apocalypse*, 156–91, for a more detailed explanation of this argument.

138. Sudhoff, "Pestschriften aus den ersten 150 Jahren nach der Epidemie des 'schwarzen Todes' 1348," *Archiv für Geschichte der Medizin* 4 (1911): 215.

139. Congourdeau and Melhaoui, "La Perception," 124; Stearns, "Infectious Ideas," 238.

140. Stearns, "Infectious Ideas," 236–37.

141. Dols, "Comparative Communal Responses," 286–87.

142. Joseph-Jean de Smet, ed., *Recueil des Chroniques de Flandre*, 4 vols. (Brussels, 1837–1865), 2:280; Ibn Battūta, *Travels, A.D. 1325–1354*, trans. H. A. R. Gibb, 5 vols. (Cambridge, UK: Hakluyt Society, 1958–2000), 4:919.

143. Aberth, *The Black Death*, 115.

144. Escorial MS 1785, fols. 107r–v. This manuscript was translated for me from the Arabic by Russell Hopley of Bowdoin College.

145. Escorial MS 1785, fol. 107r.

146. Cohn, *The Black Death Transformed*, 49.

147. Carlo M. Cipolla, *Public Health and the Medical Profession in the Renaissance* (Cambridge: Cambridge University Press, 1976), 36–44; Carlo M. Cipolla, *Faith, Reason, and the Plague in Seventeenth-Century Tuscany*, trans. M. Kittel (Ithaca, N.Y.: Cornell University Press, 1979), 1–14; Paul Slack, *The Impact of Plague in Tudor and Stuart England* (London: Routledge and Kegan Paul, 1985), 228–32; Paul Slack, "Responses to Plague in Early Modern Europe: The Implications of Public Health," in *In Time of Plague: The History and Social Consequences of Lethal Epidemic Disease*, ed. A. Mack, 111–32 (New York: New York University Press, 1991), 123; Brian Pullan, "Plague and Perceptions of the Poor in Early Modern Italy," in *Epidemics and Ideas: Essays on the Historical Perception of Pestilence*, ed. T. Ranger and P. Slack, 101–23 (Cambridge: Cambridge University Press, 1992).

148. Nancy Elizabeth Gallagher, *Medicine and Power in Tunisia, 1780–1900* (Cambridge: Cambridge University Press, 1983), 24–32.

149. Andrew Appleby, "The Disappearance of Plague: A Continuing Puzzle," *Economic History Review* 33 (1980): 167–69; Paul Slack, "The Disappearance of Plague: An Alternative View," *Economic History Review* 34 (1981): 469–76; Sheldon Watts, *Epidemics and History: Disease, Power and Imperialism* (New Haven, Conn.: Yale University Press, 1997), 34–39.

150. Aberth, *The Black Death*, 85.

151. Marchionne di Coppo Stefani, *Cronaca Fiorentina*, ed. Niccolò Rodolica, Rerum Italicarum Scriptores 30/1 (Città di Castello, 1903), 230.

152. Dols, *Black Death*, 248.

153. Aberth, *The Black Death*, 85; Pullan, "Plague and Perceptions of the Poor," 117.

154. Samuel K. Cohn Jr., *The Cult of Remembrance and the Black Death: Six Renaissance Cities in Central Italy* (Baltimore: Johns Hopkins University Press, 1992); Samuel K. Cohn Jr., "The Place of the Dead in Flanders and Tuscany: Towards a Comparative History of the Black Death," in *The Place of the Dead: Death and Remembrance in Late Medieval and Early Modern Europe*, ed. B. Gordon and P. Marshall, 17–43 (Cambridge: Cambridge University Press, 2000).

155. See Aberth, *From the Brink of the Apocalypse*, 210–75, for a more detailed presentation of this argument.

156. Stuart J. Borsch, *The Black Death in Egypt and England: A Comparative Study* (Austin: University of Texas Press, 2005), 19–20.

157. Dols, *Black Death*, 212–23; Borsch, *Black Death in Egypt and England*, 15, 24–25.

158. Dols, *Black Death*, 256–80.

159. Borsch, *Black Death in Egypt and England*, 10–11.

160. Borsch, *Black Death in Egypt and England*, 40–112.

161. Borsch, *Black Death in Egypt and England*, 24–39.

162. Borsch, *Black Death in Egypt and England*, 115.

163. Sudhoff, "Pestschriften aus den ersten 150 Jahren nach der Epidemie des 'schwarzen Todes' 1348," *Archiv für Geschichte der Medizin* 11 (1919): 144.

164. Sudhoff, "Pestschriften aus den ersten 150 Jahren nach der Epidemie des 'schwarzen Todes' 1348," *Archiv für Geschichte der Medizin* 11 (1919): 147–48, and 17 (1925): 82.

165. Aberth, *The Black Death*, 16–18, 112–14.

166. Carol Benedict, *Bubonic Plague in Nineteenth-Century China* (Stanford, Calif.: Stanford University Press, 1996), 17–71.

167. Myron Echenberg, *Plague Ports: The Global Urban Impact of Bubonic Plague, 1894–1901* (New York: New York University Press, 2007).

168. In addition to David Arnold's *Colonizing the Body: State Medicine and Epidemic Disease in Nineteenth-Century India* (Berkeley: University of California Press, 1993), a useful summary of the issues involved with the Third Pandemic in India is available in Rajnarayan Chandavarkar, "Plague Panic and Epidemic Politics in India, 1896–1914," in *Epidemics and Ideas: Essays on the Historical Perception of Pestilence*, ed. T. Ranger and P. Slack, 203–40 (Cambridge: Cambridge University Press, 1992); and John Aberth, *The First Horseman: Disease in Human History* (Upper Saddle River, N.J.: Pearson/Prentice Hall, 2007), 76–85, 88–92, 96–97.

169. Aberth, *The First Horseman*, 85–87, 102–9.

170. Aberth, *The First Horseman*, 111.

171. Lien-Teh, *Treatise on Pneumonic Plague*, 421–26.

172. Arnold, *Colonizing the Body*, 70–77; Chandavarkar, "Plague Panic," 223–26.

173. Lien-Teh, *Treatise on Pneumonic Plague*, 112.

174. Myron Echenberg, *Black Death, White Medicine: Bubonic Plague and the Politics of Public Health in Colonial Senegal, 1914–1945* (Portsmouth, N.H.: Heinemann, 2002), 58–89.

175. Echenberg, *Black Death, White Medicine*, 106–9.

176. Appleby, "The Disappearance of Plague," 169–73. Appleby explains the persistence of plague in the Middle East beyond its terminal date in Europe as due to different strains of *Yersinia pestis* being present in each region. However, one should also read the response by Slack, "The Disappearance of Plague," 469–73.

177. Aberth, *The First Horseman*, 89.

178. Aberth, *The First Horseman*, 94.

179. Aberth, *The First Horseman*, 78–79.

180. Chandavarkar, "Plague Panic," 206, 218–20, 232.

181. W. C. Rand, *Draft of Report to Government of Bombay* (n.p., n.d.), 3.

182. Chandavarkar, "Plague Panic," 91.

183. Chandavarkar, "Plague Panic," 99.

184. Chandavarkar, "Plague Panic," 91, 94.

185. Chandavarkar, "Plague Panic," 112.

186. Chandavarkar, "Plague Panic," 84–85.

187. Chandavarkar, "Plague Panic," 88–89.

188. Chandavarkar, "Plague Panic," 93.

189. Chandavarkar, "Plague Panic," 226–32.

190. Echenberg, *Plague Ports*, 16–107, 131–302.

191. Pullan, "Plague and Perceptions of the Poor," 120–21.

192. Arnold, *Colonizing the Body*, 211.

193. Chandavarkar, "Plague Panic," 232–33.

Chapter 2: Smallpox

1. Donald R. Hopkins, *The Greatest Killer: Smallpox in History* (Chicago: University of Chicago Press, 1983), 15.

2. Hopkins, *The Greatest Killer*, 15–16.

3. Hopkins, *The Greatest Killer*, 16–17.

4. E. Fuller Torrey and Robert H. Yolken, *Beasts of the Earth: Animals, Humans, and Disease* (New Brunswick, N.J.: Rutgers University Press, 2005), 41–42.

5. John Aberth, *From the Brink of the Apocalypse: Confronting Famine, War, Plague, and Death in the Later Middle Ages*, 2nd ed. (London: Routledge, 2010), 229–37.

6. Victor Davis Hanson, *A War Like No Other: How the Athenians and Spartans Fought the Peloponnesian War* (New York: Random House, 2005), 66, 70–71, 77–78.

7. Jo N. Hays, *Epidemics and Pandemics: Their Impacts on Human History* (Santa Barbara, Calif.: ABC–CLIO, 2005), 17–20.

8. Hopkins, *The Greatest Killer*, 168.

9. Suzanne Austin Alchon, *A Pest in the Land: New World Epidemics in a Global Perspective* (Albuquerque: University of New Mexico Press, 2003), 63–105.

10. A good overview of the debate is available in Alchon, *A Pest in the Land*, 147–77.

11. David Noble Cook, *Born to Die: Disease and New World Conquest, 1492–1650* (Cambridge: Cambridge University Press, 1998), 13.

12. Their major works include the following: John Duffy, *Epidemics in Colonial America* (Baton Rouge: Louisiana State University Press, 1953); Alfred W. Crosby, *The Columbian Exchange: Biological and Cultural Consequences of 1492* (Westport, Conn.: Greenwood Press, 1972); Alfred W. Crosby, *Ecological Imperialism: The Biological Expansion of Europe, 900–1900* (Cambridge: Cambridge University Press, 1986); William McNeill, *Plagues and Peoples*, updated ed. (New York: Anchor Books, 1998).

13. Hays, *Epidemics and Pandemics*, 84–85; Alchon, *A Pest in the Land*, 68–79.

14. Thomas M. Whitmore, *Disease and Death in Early Colonial Mexico: Simulating Amerindian Depopulation* (Boulder, Colo.: Westview, 1992), 208.

15. Alfred W. Crosby, "Conquistador y Pestilencia: The First New World Pandemic and the Fall of the Great Indian Empires," *Hispanic American Historical Review* 47 (1967): 321–37; McNeill, *Plagues and Peoples*, 208–41; Cook, *Born to Die*, 60–94.

16. Alchon, *A Pest in the Land*, 81–82.

17. John Hatcher, "Mortality in the Fifteenth Century: Some New Evidence," *Economic History Review* 39 (1986): 19–38.

18. Robert Hoeniger, *Der Schwarze Tod in Deutschland* (Berlin: Grosser, 1882), 176.

19. Alchon, *A Pest in the Land*, 110; Bernard R. Ortiz de Montellano, *Aztec Medicine, Health, and Nutrition* (New Brunswick, N.J.: Rutgers University Press, 1990), 37–38.

20. Ortiz de Montellano, *Aztec Medicine*, 129–92.

21. Alchon, *A Pest in the Land*, 109–45.

22. William P. Caferro, "Warfare and Economy in Renaissance Italy, 1350–1450," *Journal of Interdisciplinary History* 39 (2008): 173.

23. Aberth, *From the Brink of the Apocalypse*, 79–275.

24. *The Annals of the Cakchiquels*, trans. A. Recinos and D. Goetz (Norman: University of Oklahoma Press, 1953), 116.

25. David E. Stannard, "Disease and Infertility: A New Look at the Demographic Collapse of Native Populations in the Wake of Western Contact," *Journal of American Studies* 24 (1990): 325–50; Alfred W. Crosby, "Hawaiian Depopulation as a Model for the Amerindian Experience," in *Epidemics and Ideas: Essays on the Historical Perception of Pestilence*, ed. T. Ranger and P. Slack, 175–201 (Cambridge: Cambridge University Press, 1992).

26. McNeill, *Plagues and Peoples*, 216–17.

27. Kark Sudhoff, "Pestschriften aus den ersten 150 Jahren nach der Epidemie des 'schwarzen Todes' 1348," *Archiv für Geschichte der Medizin* 8 (1915): 247–52, and 17 (1925): 63–64.

28. Daniel T. Reff, *Disease, Depopulation, and Culture Change in Northwestern New Spain, 1518–1764* (Salt Lake City: University of Utah Press, 1991), 260–64.

29. Hopkins, *The Greatest Killer*, 29–41.

30. Elizabeth Fenn, *Pox Americana: The Great Smallpox Epidemic of 1775–1782* (New York: Hill and Wang, 2001).

31. Hopkins, *The Greatest Killer*, 46–96.

32. David Arnold, *Colonizing the Body: State Medicine and Epidemic Disease in Nineteenth-Century India* (Berkeley: University of California Press, 1993), 116–58; David Arnold, "Smallpox and Colonial Medicine in Nineteenth-Century India," in *Imperial*

Medicine and Indigenous Societies, ed. D. Arnold, 45–65 (Manchester, UK: Manchester University Press, 1988).

33. Arnold, *Colonizing the Body*, 116–58; Myron Echenberg, *Plague Ports: The Global Urban Impact of Bubonic Plague, 1894–1901* (New York: New York University Press, 2007), 174–77.

34. Hopkins, *The Greatest Killer*, 304–10.

35. Lawrence K. Altman, "W.H.O. Panel Backs Gene Manipulation in Smallpox Virus," *New York Times*, November 12, 2004.

Chapter 3: Tuberculosis

1. E. Fuller Torrey and Robert H. Yolken, *Beasts of the Earth: Animals, Humans, and Disease* (New Brunswick, N.J.: Rutgers University Press, 2005), 42–43.

2. B. Rothschild et al., "Mycobacterium Tuberculosis Complex DNA from an Extinct Bison Dated 17,000 Years before the Present," *Clinical Infectious Diseases* 33 (2001): 305–11.

3. John Hatcher, "Mortality in the Fifteenth Century: Some New Evidence," *Economic History Review* 39 (1986): 30.

4. Rene Dubos and Jean Dubos, *The White Plague: Tuberculosis, Man and Society* (Boston: Little, Brown, 1952), 8; T. M. Daniel, *Captain of Death: The Story of Tuberculosis* (Rochester, N.Y.: University of Rochester Press, 1997), 27.

5. Dubos and Dubos, *White Plague*, 8; Daniel, *Captain of Death*, 30; F. B. Smith, *The Retreat of Tuberculosis, 1850–1950* (London: Croom Helm, 1988), 4–9; Jo N. Hays, *Epidemics and Pandemics: Their Impacts on Human History* (Santa Barbara, Calif.: ABC–CLIO, 2005), 201.

6. Thomas Dormandy, *The White Death: A History of Tuberculosis* (New York: New York University Press, 2000), 139–46; Smith, *Retreat of Tuberculosis*, 56–62.

7. Frank Ryan, *The Forgotten Plague: How the Battle against Tuberculosis Was Won—and Lost* (Boston: Little, Brown, 1992), 31–48, 209–23.

8. Dubos and Dubos, *White Plague*, 154–72; Dormandy, *White Death*, 339–49; Lee B. Reichman and Janice Hopkins Tanne, *Timebomb: The Global Epidemic of Multi-Drug Resistant Tuberculosis* (New York: McGraw-Hill, 2002), 30–35.

9. Dubos and Dubos, *White Plague*, 28–43, 94–128; Smith, *Retreat of Tuberculosis*, 166–211; David S. Barnes, *The Making of a Social Disease: Tuberculosis in Nineteenth-Century France* (Berkeley: University of California Press, 1995), 23–47, 138–73; Dormandy, *White Death*, 73–84.

10. Reichman and Tanne, *Timebomb*, 87–107.

11. Barnes, *Making of a Social Disease*, 74–111.

12. Reichman and Tanne, *Timebomb*, 43–62.

13. Dubos and Dubos, *White Plague*, 69–76.

14. Dubos and Dubos, *White Plague*, 173–81; Mark Caldwell, *The Last Crusade: The War on Consumption, 1862–1954* (New York: Atheneum, 1988), 40–151; Smith, *Retreat of Tuberculosis*, 97–135; Dormandy, *White Death*, 147–86.

15. Smith, *Retreat of Tuberculosis*, 142–45; Dormandy, *White Death*, 249–63, 351–60.

16. Hays, *Epidemics and Pandemics*, 208–9.

17. Dubos and Dubos, *White Plague*, 197–207; Smith, *Retreat of Tuberculosis*, 212–35; Barnes, *Making of a Social Disease*, 112–37.

18. Dormandy, *White Death*, 13–25. See also Susan Sontag's *Illness as Metaphor* (New York: Picador/Farrar, Straus and Giroux, 1977), where she discusses tuberculosis as a "metaphor" for the myth of a romantic death, in contrast to cancer.

19. Dubos and Dubos, *White Plague*, 11–27, 44–66; Dormandy, *White Death*, 13–25, 85–100.

20. Paul Barber, *Vampires, Burial, and Death* (New Haven, Conn.: Yale University Press, 1988), 115.

21. Michael E. Bell, *Food for the Dead: On the Trail of New England's Vampires* (New York: Carroll and Graf, 2001); Joseph A. Citro, *Passing Strange: True Tales of New England Hauntings and Horrors* (Boston: Houghton Mifflin, 1996), 204–19; Joseph A. Citro, *Green Mountain Ghosts, Ghouls and Unsolved Mysteries* (Boston: Houghton Mifflin, 1994), 68–72.

22. This information is available at the WHO website, www.who.int/mediacentre/factsheets/fs104/en.

23. This epidemic is discussed at some length in the following works: Ryan, *Forgotten Plague*, 389–411; Richard Coker, *From Chaos to Coercion: Detention and the Control of Tuberculosis* (New York: St. Martin's Press, 2000); Reichman and Tanne, *Timebomb*, 139–54; Deborah Wallace and Rodrick Wallace, "The Recent Tuberculosis Epidemic in New York City: Warning from the De-Developing World," in *The Return of the White Plague: Global Poverty and the "New" Tuberculosis*, ed. M. Gandy and A. Zumla, 125–46 (London: Verso, 2003).

24. Reichman and Tanne, *Timebomb*, 142–53.

25. Reichman and Tanne, *Timebomb*, 149.

26. Coker, *From Chaos to Coercion*, 83–119, 141–89.

27. Judith Walzer Leavitt, *Typhoid Mary: Captive to the Public's Health* (Boston: Beacon Press, 1996), esp. 39–125.

28. Reichman and Tanne, *Timebomb*, 63–125.

29. Information available on USAID website, at www.usaid.gov/our_work/global_health/id/tuberculosis/countries/eande/russia_profile.html. See also Vivien Stern, "*The House of the Dead* Revisited: Prisons, Tuberculosis and Public Health in the Former Soviet Bloc," in *The Return of the White Plague: Global Poverty and the "New" Tuberculosis*, ed. M. Gandy and A. Zumla, 178–91 (London: Verso, 2003).

30. Coker, *From Chaos to Coercion*, 6–11.

31. Reichman and Tanne, *Timebomb*, 176–77.

32. Reichman and Tanne, *Timebomb*, 181–86. Trials are currently under way for one such vaccine developed by the Aeras Global TB Vaccine Foundation in Rockville, Maryland.

33. Léopold Blanc and Mukund Uplekar, "The Present Global Burden of Tuberculosis," in *The Return of the White Plague: Global Poverty and the "New" Tuberculosis*, ed. M. Gandy and A. Zumla, 95–111 (London: Verso, 2003), 106–7.

Chapter 4: Cholera

1. Robert D. Morris, *The Blue Death: Disease, Disaster, and the Water We Drink* (New York: HarperCollins, 2007), 120–30; Christopher Hamlin, *Cholera: The Biography* (Oxford: Oxford University Press, 2009), 19–23.

2. Jo N. Hays, *Epidemics and Pandemics: Their Impacts on Human History* (Santa Barbara, Calif.: ABC–CLIO, 2005), 230.

3. Hays, *Epidemics and Pandemics*, 214; R. J. Morris, *Cholera 1832: The Social Response to an Epidemic* (New York: Holmes and Meier, 1976), 15–16; Michael Durey, *The Return of the Plague: British Society and the Cholera, 1831–2* (Dublin: Gill and Macmillan, 1979), 216–18; Morris, *The Blue Death*, 80–81.

4. Hays, *Epidemics and Pandemics*, 193–200, 211–38, 267–79, 303–14, 321–29, 345–54, 369–75, 421–26.

5. Morris, *The Blue Death*, 257–92.

6. I am indebted to Jo N. Hays and his historiographical essay, "Nineteenth-Century Cholera in Twentieth-Century Historical Writing," page 2, which he presented at my panel on "Plagues in World History" at the 2008 annual meeting of the American Historical Association, Washington, D.C., January 3–6. But see also Roderick E. McGrew, *Russia and the Cholera, 1823–1832* (Madison: University of Wisconsin Press, 1965), 7–9; Morris, *Cholera 1832*, 170–84; Durey, *Return of the Plague*, 107–20; François Delaporte, *Disease and Civilization: The Cholera in Paris, 1832* (Cambridge, Mass.: MIT Press, 1986), 139–95; Catherine J. Kudlick, *Cholera in Post-Revolutionary Paris: A Cultural History* (Berkeley: University of California Press, 1996), 75–81.

7. Delaporte, *Disease and Civilization*, 47–72; Kudlick, *Cholera in Post-Revolutionary Paris*, 31–64, 176–219; William Coleman, *Death Is a Social Disease: Public Health and Political Economy in Early Industrial France* (Madison: University of Wisconsin Press, 1982), 171–80; Richard J. Evans, "Epidemics and Revolutions: Cholera in Nineteenth-Century Europe," in *Epidemics and Ideas: Essays on the Historical Perception of Pestilence*, ed. T. Ranger and P. Slack, 149–73 (Cambridge: Cambridge University Press, 1992).

8. McGrew, *Russia and the Cholera*, esp. 98–158.

9. Durey, *Return of the Plague*, 155–84.

10. Richard J. Evans, *Death in Hamburg: Society and Politics in the Cholera Years, 1830–1910* (Oxford: Oxford University Press, 1987), esp. 470–568. Not even the "slum clearances" in Hamburg five years later, when allegedly unsanitary housing near the river was razed and the working-class residents forced to relocate, apparently elicited significant protests from this politically "dangerous" sector.

11. Frank M. Snowden, *Naples in the Time of Cholera, 1884–1911* (Cambridge: Cambridge University Press, 1995), 149–54, 285–59.

12. David Arnold, *Colonizing the Body: State Medicine and Epidemic Disease in Nineteenth-Century India* (Berkeley: University of California Press, 1993), 168–99; David Arnold, "Cholera and Colonialism in British India," *Past and Present* 113 (1986): 128–45; Hays, *Epidemics and Pandemics*, 267.

13. Arnold, *Colonizing the Body*, 179–89; Hays, *Epidemics and Pandemics*, 197–98.

14. Sheldon Watts, *Epidemics and History: Disease, Power and Imperialism* (New Haven, Conn.: Yale University Press, 1997), 200–212. Watts argues further that commercial interests promoted engineering projects, such as railways and canals, that actually made cholera worse in India.

15. Arnold, *Colonizing the Body*, 171–78.

16. Hays, *Epidemics and Pandemics*, 345, 349–50; Reynaldo C. Ileto, "Cholera and the Origins of the American Sanitary Order in the Philippines," in *Imperial Medicine and Indigenous Societies*, ed. D. Arnold, 125–48 (Manchester, UK: Manchester University Press, 1988); Rodney Sullivan, "Cholera and Colonialism in the Philippines, 1899–1903," in *Disease, Medicine, and Empire: Perspectives on Western Medicine and the Experience of European Expansion*, ed. R. M. MacLeod and M. J. Lewis, 284–300 (London: Routledge, 1988).

17. Nancy Elizabeth Gallagher, *Medicine and Power in Tunisia, 1780–1900* (Cambridge: Cambridge University Press, 1983), 40–64.

18. Morris, *Cholera 1832*, 206–10; Morris, *The Blue Death*, 75–95.

19. Alfred Jay Bollet, *Plagues and Poxes: The Impact of Human History on Epidemic Disease*, 2nd ed. (New York: Demos, 2004), 40, 62.

20. Charles E. Rosenberg, *The Cholera Years* (Chicago: University of Chicago Press, 1962), 192–212; Durey, *Return of the Plague*, 77–100.

21. Morris, *Cholera 1832*, 210; Morris, *The Blue Death*, 96–108.

22. Evans, *Death in Hamburg*, 490–507.

23. Hays, *Epidemics and Pandemics*, 426.

24. Morris, *Cholera 1832*, 166–70.

25. Hays, *Epidemics and Pandemics*, 424–26.

26. Norman Howard-Jones, "Cholera Therapy in the Nineteenth Century," *Journal of the History of Medicine and Allied Sciences* 27 (1972): 373–95.

Chapter 5: Influenza

1. Dorothy A. Pettit and Janice Bailie, *A Cruel Wind: Pandemic Flu in America, 1918–1920* (Murfreesboro, Tenn.: Timberland Books, 2008), 2–18. For a far more detailed and scientific discussion of influenza biology, readers will want to consult Edwin D. Kilbourne, *Influenza* (New York: Plenum Medical Book, 1987).

2. Paul Tambyah and Ping-Chung Leung, eds., *Bird Flu: A Rising Pandemic in Asia and Beyond?* (Singapore: World Scientific Publishing, 2006), 7–8, 60–62.

3. Pettit and Bailie, *A Cruel Wind*, 4.

4. This is indeed the basis for an alternative hypothesis as to how influenza epidemics arise and spread: see R. Edgar Hope-Simpson, *The Transmission of Epidemic Influenza* (New York: Plenum, 1992).

5. See, for example, Tom Quinn's discussion of the pre-eighteenth-century occurrence of the disease in *Flu: A Social History of Influenza* (London: New Holland Publishers, 2008), 39–57.

6. Howard Phillips and David Killingray, eds., *The Spanish Influenza Pandemic of 1918–19: New Perspectives* (New York: Routledge, 2003), 8–9, 40–41; Jo N. Hays, *Epidemics and Pandemics: Their Impacts on Human History* (Santa Barbara, Calif.: ABC-CLIO, 2005), 386–87.

7. Phillips and Killingray, *Spanish Influenza Pandemic*, 5–7; Hays, *Epidemics and Pandemics*, 385–88.

8. Kilbourne, *Influenza*, 268–70.

9. Alfred W. Crosby, *America's Forgotten Pandemic: The Influenza of 1918*, 2nd ed. (Cambridge: Cambridge University Press, 2003), esp. 311–28.

10. E. Fuller Torrey and Robert H. Yolken, *Beasts of the Earth: Animals, Humans, and Disease* (New Brunswick, N.J.: Rutgers University Press, 2005), 114–16.

11. Quinn, *Flu*, 39–57; W. I. B. Beveridge, *Influenza: The Last Great Plague: An Unfinished Story of Discovery* (New York: Prodist, 1977), 24–26.

12. Ken Albala, *Eating Right in the Renaissance* (Berkeley: University of California Press, 2002), 122–23.

13. Quinn, *Flu*, 59–83; K. David Patterson, *Pandemic Influenza, 1700–1900: A Study in Historical Epidemiology* (Totowa, N.J.: Rowman & Littlefield, 1986), 11–28.

14. Quinn, *Flu*, 85–121; Patterson, *Pandemic Influenza*, 29–82; Hays, *Epidemics and Pandemics*, 394.

15. Crosby's original title was *Epidemic and Peace, 1918* (Westport, Conn.: Greenwood Press, 1976), subsequently issued in a second edition in 2003 as *America's Forgotten Pandemic* with Cambridge University Press. Around this same time, a more popular, less historically rigorous account was published by Richard Collier, *The Plague of the Spanish Lady: The Influenza Pandemic of 1918–1919* (New York: Atheneum, 1974). Among the more notable of the recent narrative histories to appear are as follows: Gina Kolata, *Flu: The Story of the Great Influenza Pandemic of 1918 and the Search for the Virus that Caused It* (New York: Farrar, Straus and Giroux, 1999); John M. Barry, *The Great Influenza: The Epic Story of the Deadliest Plague in History* (New York: Viking Penguin, 2004); Pettit and Bailie, *A Cruel Wind*.

16. Hays, *Epidemics and Pandemics*, 387, 389; Quinn, *Flu*, 151; I. D. Mills, "The 1918–1919 Influenza Pandemic: The Indian Experience," *Indian Economic and Social History Review* 23 (1986): 1–40.

17. Phillips and Killingray, *Spanish Influenza Pandemic*, 221–29.

18. Phillips and Killingray, *Spanish Influenza Pandemic*, 86–98.

19. Phillips and Killingray, *Spanish Influenza Pandemic*, 110–31, 156–72; Hays, *Epidemics and Pandemics*, 387, 391; Crosby, *America's Forgotten Pandemic*, 227–63.

20. Pettit and Bailie, *A Cruel Wind*, 232–37; Phillips and Killingray, *Spanish Influenza Pandemic*, 39–46.

21. Mike Davis, *The Monster at Our Door: The Global Threat of Avian Flu* (New York: Owl Books, 2005), 50.

22. Quinn, *Flu*, 132–33, 156–59.

23. Felissa R. Lashley and Jerry D. Durham, eds., *Emerging Infectious Diseases: Trends and Issues*, 2nd ed. (New York: Springer, 2007), 133–57, 185–96, 325–36.

24. Crosby, *America's Forgotten Pandemic*, 295–308; Quinn, *Flu*, 140.

25. Pettit and Bailie, *A Cruel Wind*, 62–64, 231–32; Barry, *The Great Influenza*, 91–97, 453–56.

26. Alfred Jay Bollet, *Plagues and Poxes: The Impact of Human History on Epidemic Disease*, 2nd ed. (New York: Demos, 2004), 105–11; Quinn, *Flu*, 126–31.

27. Phillips and Killingray, *Spanish Influenza Pandemic*, 73–85, 132–55, 173–201.

28. Hays, *Epidemics and Pandemics*, 387.

29. Quinn, *Flu*, 195–96.

30. Phillips and Killingray, *Spanish Influenza Pandemic*, 139–41; 202–17.

31. Phillips and Killingray, *Spanish Influenza Pandemic*, 49–69.

32. Quinn, *Flu*, 140–45; June E. Osborn, ed., *History, Science and Politics: Influenza in America, 1918–1976* (New York: Prodist, 1977), 23.

33. Crosby, *America's Forgotten Pandemic*, 319–23; Kolata, *Flu*, 53–54.

34. Quinn, *Flu*, 161–71; Kilbourne, *Influenza*, 16–19.

35. Kilbourne, *Influenza*, 326–27; Bollet, *Plagues and Poxes*, 113; Osborn, *History, Science and Politics*, 24; Martin A. Levin and Mary Bryna Sanger, *After the Cure: Managing AIDS and Other Public Health Crises* (Lawrence: University Press of Kansas, 2000), 51–52.

36. Kilbourne, *Influenza*, 328–29; Bollet, *Plagues and Poxes*, 113–14; Osborn, *History, Science and Politics*, 25–51; Levin and Sanger, *After the Cure*, 52–55; Davis, *The Monster at Our Door*, 40–42.

37. Kilbourne, *Influenza*, 314–15, 329–31; Bollet, *Plagues and Poxes*, 115; Osborn, *History, Science and Politics*, 63–64.

38. Kilbourne, *Influenza*, 331.

39. Osborn, *History, Science and Politics*, 66–70.

40. Davis, *The Monster at Our Door*, 43–44.

41. Kilbourne, *Influenza*, 329; Bollet, *Plagues and Poxes*, 115–16; Levin and Sanger, *After the Cure*, 56–70.

42. www.who.int/csr/disease/avian_influenza.

43. Tambyah and Ping-Chung, *Bird Flu*, 7–8, 25–33, 64–66; Davis, *The Monster at Our Door*, 45–54; Quinn, *Flu*, 177–84.

44. Joseph Mercola and Pam Killeen, *The Great Bird Flu Hoax: The Truth They Don't Want You to Know about the "Next Big Pandemic"* (Nashville: Nelson Books, 2006), 1–55, 99–123.

45. Quinn, *Flu*, 188–89, 203–4.

46. Quinn, *Flu*, 182–85; Mercola and Killeen, *The Great Bird Flu Hoax*, 4–6.

47. Davis, *The Monster at Our Door*, 97–114; Mercola and Killeen, *The Great Bird Flu Hoax*, 56–98.

48. Tambyah and Ping-Chung, *Bird Flu*, 140–42; Quinn, *Flu*, 189, 199–202.

49. Tambyah and Ping-Chung, *Bird Flu*, 99–118, 127–146; Quinn, *Flu*, 173–77, 185–87, 190–95; Mercola and Killeen, *The Great Bird Flu Hoax*, 158–94.

50. Most information on the 2009 flu pandemic is available on the websites of WHO, the CDC, and the European CDC: www.who.int/csr/disease/swineflu; www.cdc.gov/H1N1FLU; www.ecdc.europa.eu/en/healthtopics/H1N1.

51. Richard Wenzel, "What We Learned from H1N1's First Year," *New York Times*, April 13, 2010.

52. Wenzel, "What We Learned."

Chapter 6: AIDS

1. For a more detailed description of the biology of HIV, see I. Edward Alcamo, *AIDS: The Biological Basis*, 3rd ed. (Sudbury, Mass.: Jones and Bartlett, 2003), 30–83; Hung Y. Fan, Ross F. Conner, and Luis P. Villarreal, *AIDS: Science and Society*, 5th ed. (Sudbury, Mass.: Jones and Bartlett, 2007), 17–54.

2. Alcamo, *AIDS*, 84–108; Fan, Conner, and Villarreal, *AIDS*, 67–84; James Chin, *The AIDS Pandemic: The Collision of Epidemiology with Political Correctness* (Oxford, UK: Radcliffe, 2007), 46–50.

3. Alcamo, *AIDS*, 120–34; Fan, Conner, and Villarreal, *AIDS*, 117–29; Chin, *The AIDS Pandemic*, 61–66; John Aberth, *The First Horseman: Disease in Human History* (Upper Saddle River, N.J.: Pearson/Prentice Hall, 2007), 119–20.

4. Alcamo, *AIDS*, 260–84; Jonathan Engel, *The Epidemic: A Global History of AIDS* (New York: HarperCollins, 2006), 63–66.

5. Alcamo, *AIDS*, 212–53; Fan, Conner, and Villarreal, *AIDS*, 84–92.

6. This theory was popularized by Edward Hooper's book, *The River: A Journey to the Source of HIV and AIDS* (Boston: Little, Brown, 1999). Despite the fact that it has now been conclusively disproved, Hooper has yet to retract his theory.

7. Alcamo, *AIDS*, 13–18; Helen Epstein, *The Invisible Cure: Africa, the West, and the Fight against AIDS* (New York: Farrar, Straus and Giroux, 2007), 39–48; John Iliffe, *The African AIDS Epidemic: A History* (Athens: Ohio University Press, 2006), 3–9; Jo N. Hays, *Epidemics and Pandemics: Their Impacts on Human History* (Santa Barbara, Calif.: ABC–CLIO, 2005), 446–47.

8. Alcamo, *AIDS*, 34, 73; Fan, Conner, and Villarreal, *AIDS*, 13–14; Chin, *The AIDS Pandemic*, 50–52.

9. Mirko D. Grmek, *History of AIDS: Emergence and Origin of a Modern Pandemic*, trans. R. C. Maulitz and J. Duffin (Princeton, N.J.: Princeton University Press, 1990), 108–9; Iliffe, *The African AIDS Epidemic*, 6.

10. On the 1980s decade of AIDS in the United States, see Randy Shilts, *And the Band Played On: Politics, People, and the AIDS Epidemic* (New York: St. Martin's Press, 1987); Engel, *The Epidemic*, 5–210; Martin A. Levin and Mary Bryna Sanger, *After the Cure: Managing AIDS and Other Public Health Crises* (Lawrence: University Press of Kansas, 2000), 119–40; Kenneth J. Doka, *AIDS, Fear, and Society: Challenging the Dreaded Disease* (Bristol, Pa.: Taylor and Francis, 1997), 61–81.

11. Michael Fumento, *The Myth of Heterosexual AIDS* (New York: Basic Books, 1991); Engel, *The Epidemic*, 197–201.

12. Most of the social, legal, and cultural issues surrounding AIDS in the United States and Europe are thoroughly vetted in the following works: Elizabeth Fee and Daniel M. Fox, eds., *AIDS: The Burdens of History* (Berkeley: University of California

Press, 1988); Peter Aggleton, Peter Davies, and Graham Hart, eds., *AIDS: Individual, Cultural and Policy Dimensions* (Basingstoke, UK: Falmer Press, 1990); Douglas A. Feldman, ed., *Culture and AIDS* (New York: Praeger, 1990); Dorothy Nelkin, David P. Willis, and Scott V. Parris, eds., *A Disease of Society: Cultural and Institutional Responses to AIDS* (Cambridge: Cambridge University Press, 1991); Elizabeth Fee and Daniel M. Fox, eds., *AIDS: The Making of a Chronic Disease* (Berkeley: University of California Press, 1992); Albert R. Jonsen and Jeff Stryker, eds., *The Social Impact of AIDS in the United States* (Washington, D.C.: National Academy Press, 1993); Virginia Berridge and Philip Strong, eds., *AIDS and Contemporary History* (Cambridge: Cambridge University Press, 1993); Brenda Almond, ed., *AIDS: A Moral Issue—The Ethical, Legal and Social Aspects*, 2nd ed. (New York: St. Martin's Press, 1996); Doka, *AIDS, Fear, and Society*, esp. 99–114; Lawrence O. Gostin, *The AIDS Pandemic: Complacency, Injustice, and Unfulfilled Expectations* (Chapel Hill: University of North Carolina Press, 2004).

13. Engel, *The Epidemic*, 76–86, 189–92, 233–34, 276–78.

14. Engel, *The Epidemic*, 240–49, 267–75.

15. Statistics pulled from the website of www.avert.org/. However, readers should compare the 2007 statistics with those from www.unaids.org/.

16. Susan Hunter, *AIDS in America* (New York: Palgrave Macmillan, 2006).

17. Statistics pulled from www.avert.org/.

18. The theory arose from an analysis of the DNA of descendents of the survivors of a plague in Eyam, England, in 1665, all of whom were found to have a genetic mutation in the chemokine receptor called "delta-32," although it is not clear if this granted immunity to plague. See Irwin W. Sherman, *The Power of Plagues* (Washington, D.C.: ASM Press, 2006), 97–99.

19. Engel, *The Epidemic*, 160–66, 282–87; Samuel V. Duh, *Blacks and AIDS: Causes and Origins* (Newbury Park, Calif.: Sage, 1991); Jacob Levenson, *The Secret Epidemic: The Story of AIDS and Black America* (New York: Pantheon Books, 2004); Dooley Worth, "Minority Women and AIDS: Culture, Race, and Gender," in *Culture and AIDS*, ed. D. A. Feldman, 111–35 (New York: Praeger, 1990).

20. Engel, *The Epidemic*, 202–3; Jeanine M. Buzy and Helene D. Gayle, "The Epidemiology of HIV and AIDS in Women," in *Women's Experiences with HIV/AIDS: An International Perspective*, ed. L. D. Long and E. M. Ankrah, 181–204 (New York: Columbia University Press, 1996); Hunter, *AIDS in America*, 69–85; Diane Richardson, "AIDS Education and Women: Sexual and Reproductive Issues," in *AIDS: Individual, Cultural and Policy Dimensions*, ed. P. Aggleton, P. Davies, and G. Hart, 169–79 (Basingstoke, UK: Falmer Press, 1990).

21. Engel, *The Epidemic*, 147–60; Hunter, *AIDS in America*, 133–47; Aggleton, Davies, and Hart, *AIDS*, 133–67; Anna Alexandrova, ed., *AIDS, Drugs and Society*, rev. ed. (New York: International Debate Education Association, 2004).

22. Benjamin Heim Shepard, "Shifting Priorities in US AIDS Policy," in *The Global Politics of AIDS*, ed. P. G. Harris and P. D. Siplon, 171–99 (Boulder, Colo.: Lynne Rienner, 2007); Gostin, *The AIDS Pandemic*, 185.

23. The monograph was prepared in 1985 as part of the briefing series for the American Management Association in New York.

24. Iliffe, *The African AIDS Epidemic*, 12.

25. Recent statistics were derived from the UNAIDS website, at www.unaids.org/. Statistics from 2003 were derived from Aberth, *The First Horseman*, 129.

26. This issue is extensively explored in Marc Epprecht, *Heterosexual Africa? The History of an Idea from the Age of Exploration to the Age of AIDS* (Athens: Ohio University Press, 2008); and Neville Hoad, *African Intimacies: Race, Homosexuality, and Globalization* (Minneapolis: University of Minnesota Press, 2007). However, the argument of the hidden African homosexual can be taken to extremes, as in William A. Rushing, *The AIDS Epidemic: Social Dimensions of an Infectious Disease* (Boulder, Colo.: Westview, 1995). The 2009 report from UNAIDS claims that "unprotected sex between men is probably a more important factor in sub-Saharan Africa's HIV epidemics than is commonly thought" and that, "although common in sub-Saharan Africa, homosexual behavior is highly stigmatized in the region." UNAIDS, at www.unaids.org/ (accessed February 6, 2010).

27. Eileen Stillwaggon, *AIDS and the Ecology of Poverty* (Oxford: Oxford University Press, 2006), 133–57; Nana K. Poku, *AIDS in Africa: How the Poor Are Dying* (Cambridge, UK: Polity Press, 2005), 57–58; Joseph R. Oppong and Ezekiel Kalipeni, "Perceptions and Misperceptions of AIDS in Africa," in *HIV and AIDS in Africa: Beyond Epidemiology*, ed. E. Kalipeni, S. Craddock, J. R. Oppong, and J. Ghosh, 47–57 (Oxford, UK: Blackwell, 2004), 48–50. A complete list of the Caldwells' publications is also given in Stillwaggon's bibliography on page 234.

28. Epstein, *The Invisible Cure*, 49–65; Iliffe, *The African AIDS Epidemic*, 62–63.

29. The 2009 UNAIDS report claims that "sex work continues to play a notable role in many national epidemics" in sub-Saharan Africa and cites that sex workers accounted for 14 percent and 10 percent of all new HIV infections in Kenya and Uganda, respectively, in 2008. UNAIDS, at www.unaids.org/ (accessed February 6, 2010).

30. Poku, *AIDS in Africa*, 76; Iliffe, *The African AIDS Epidemic*, 11–12.

31. Iliffe, *The African AIDS Epidemic*, 93–94; Aberth, *The First Horseman*, 121; S. S. Abdool Karim and Q. Abdool Karim, eds., *HIV/AIDS in South Africa* (Cambridge: Cambridge University Press, 2005), 291.

32. Stillwaggon, *AIDS and the Ecology of Poverty*, 31–78; Anthony De. Harries, Nicola J. Hargreaves, and Alimuddin Zumla, "Tuberculosis and HIV Infection in Sub-Saharan Africa," in *The Return of the White Plague: Global Poverty and the "New" Tuberculosis*, ed. M. Gandy and A. Zumla, 112–24 (London: Verso, 2003), 116–18.

33. Poku, *AIDS in Africa*, 69–123; Iliffe, *The African AIDS Epidemic*, 112–25; Alan Whiteside, "Poverty and HIV/AIDS in Africa," in *Global Health and Governance: HIV/AIDS*, ed. N. K. Poku and A. Whiteside, 123–42 (Basingstoke, UK: Palgrave Macmillan, 2004).

34. Catherine Mathews, "Reducing Sexual Risk Behaviours: Theory and Research, Successes and Challenges," in *HIV/AIDS in South Africa*, ed. S. S. Abdool Karim and Q. Abdool Karim, 143–65 (Cambridge: Cambridge University Press, 2005); Douglas A. Feldman, *Global AIDS Policy* (Westport, Conn.: Bergin and Garvey, 1994). See also UNAIDS report for 2009 at www.unaids.org/.

35. Iliffe, *The African AIDS Epidemic*, 63–64, 127–29.

36. See, for example, Stillwaggon, *AIDS and the Ecology of Poverty*, 3–17.

37. Iliffe, *The African AIDS Epidemic*, 58.

38. Richard Chirimuuta and Rosalind Chirimuuta, *AIDS, Africa, and Racism*, 2nd ed. (London: Free Association Books, 1989); Margaret Cerullo and Evelynn Hammonds, "AIDS in Africa: The Western Imagination and the Dark Continent," in *AIDS: Readings on a Global Crisis*, ed. E. R. Bethel, 45–54 (Boston: Allyn and Bacon, 1995).

39. Iliffe, *The African AIDS Epidemic*, 58–64; Susan Hunter, *Black Death: AIDS in Africa* (Basingstoke, UK: Palgrave Macmillan, 2003), esp. 49–146.

40. Iliffe, *The African AIDS Epidemic*, 10–18.

41. Iliffe, *The African AIDS Epidemic*, 19–32, 126–32; Maryinez Lyons, "Mobile Populations and HIV/AIDS in East Africa," in *HIV and AIDS in Africa: Beyond Epidemiology*, ed. E. Kalipeni, S. Craddock, J. R. Oppong, and J. Ghosh, 175–90 (Oxford, UK: Blackwell, 2004). Works with a focus on the Ugandan response to AIDS include Maj-Lis Follér and Håkan Thörn, eds., *The Politics of AIDS: Globalization, the State and Civil Society* (New York: Palgrave Macmillan, 2008), 87–137; Amy S. Patterson, *The Politics of AIDS in Africa* (Boulder, Colo.: Lynne Rienner, 2006), 29–34; Tony Barnett and Piers Blaikie, *AIDS in Africa: Its Present and Future Impact* (New York: Guilford Press, 1992); Maryinez Lyons, "The Point of View: Perspectives on AIDS in Uganda," in *AIDS in Africa and the Caribbean*, ed. G. Bond, J. Kreniske, I. Susser, and J. Vincent, 131–46 (Boulder, Colo.: Westview, 1997).

42. Iliffe, *The African AIDS Epidemic*, 48–57, 137; Joseph R. Oppong and Samuel Agyei-Mensah, "HIV/AIDS in West Africa: The Case of Senegal, Ghana, and Nigeria," in *HIV and AIDS in Africa: Beyond Epidemiology*, ed. E. Kalipeni, S. Craddock, J. R. Oppong, and J. Ghosh, 70–82 (Oxford, UK: Blackwell, 2004).

43. For case studies of Zimbabwe and Swaziland, see Patterson, *The Politics of AIDS in Africa*, 44–57; Jake Batsell, "AIDS, Politics, and NGOs in Zimbabwe," in *The African State and the AIDS Crisis*, ed. A. S. Patterson, 59–77 (Burlington, Vt.: Ashgate, 2005). Patterson's conclusions about the role of political leadership in the AIDS crisis are, however, rather ambivalent.

44. Good overviews of the AIDS crisis in southern Africa are available in Iliffe, *The African AIDS Epidemic*, 33–47; and Ezekiel Kalipeni, Susan Craddock, and Jayati Ghosh, "Mapping the AIDS Pandemic in Eastern and Southern Africa: A Critical Overview," in *HIV and AIDS in Africa: Beyond Epidemiology*, ed. E. Kalipeni, S. Craddock, J. R. Oppong, and J. Ghosh, 58–69 (Oxford, UK: Blackwell, 2004).

45. Poku, *AIDS in Africa*, 85–123; Follér and Thörn, *The Politics of AIDS*, 27–70; Doka, *AIDS, Fear, and Society*, 120–24; Robert L. Ostergard Jr., "Politics in the Hot Zone: AIDS and National Security in Africa," in *Global Health and Governance: HIV/AIDS*, ed. N. K. Poku and A. Whiteside, 143–60 (Basingstoke, UK: Palgrave Macmillan, 2004).

46. Works and articles that focus on the political context of the AIDS epidemic in South Africa include Didier Fassin, *When Bodies Remember: Experiences and Politics of AIDS in South Africa*, trans. A. Jacobs and G. Varro (Berkeley: University of California Press, 2007); Nawaal Deane, "The Political History of AIDS Treatment," in *HIV/AIDS in*

South Africa, ed. S. S. Abdool Karim and Q. Abdool Karim, 538–47 (Cambridge: Cambridge University Press, 2005); Patrick Furlong and Karen Ball, "The More Things Change: AIDS and the State in South Africa, 1987–2003," in *The African State and the AIDS Crisis*, ed. A. S. Patterson, 127–53 (Burlington, Vt.: Ashgate, 2005); Nicoli Nattrass, *The Moral Economy of AIDS in South Africa* (Cambridge: Cambridge University Press, 2004), 41–65; Virginia van der Vliet, "South Africa Divided against AIDS: A Crisis of Leadership," in *AIDS and South Africa: The Social Expression of a Pandemic*, ed. K. D. Kauffman and D. L. Lindauer, 48–96 (Basingstoke, UK: Palgrave Macmillan, 2004).

47. Aberth, *The First Horseman*, 131–44.

48. Iliffe, *The African AIDS Epidemic*, 148–54.

49. Iliffe, *The African AIDS Epidemic*, 142–54; Follér and Thörn, *The Politics of AIDS*, 177–232; Patterson, *The Politics of AIDS in Africa*, 95–129.

50. Pulled from the UNAIDS website, at www.unaids.org/ (accessed February 11, 2010).

51. Iliffe, *The African AIDS Epidemic*, 156–57; Nattrass, *Moral Economy of AIDS*, 132–49.

52. Donald G. McNeil Jr., "At Front Lines, AIDS War Is Falling Apart," *New York Times*, May 9, 2010.

53. Works on this topic include Geoff Foster, Carol Levine, and John Williamson, eds., *A Generation at Risk: The Global Impact of HIV/AIDS on Orphans and Vulnerable Children* (Cambridge: Cambridge University Press, 2005); Ezekiel Kalipeni, Susan Craddock, Joseph R. Oppong, and Jayati Ghosh, eds., *HIV and AIDS in Africa: Beyond Epidemiology* (Oxford, UK: Blackwell, 2004), 89–103, 133–43, 304–15; Emma Guest, *Children of AIDS: Africa's Orphan Crisis*, 2nd ed. (London: Pluto, 2003); Jeff Gow and Chris Desmond, eds., *Impacts and Interventions: The HIV/AIDS Epidemic and the Children of South Africa* (Pietermaritzburg, South Africa: University of Natal Press, 2002); Carolyn Baylies, Janet Bujra, et al., *AIDS, Sexuality and Gender in Africa: Collective Strategies and Struggles in Tanzania and Zambia* (London: Routledge, 2000); Long and Ankrah, *Women's Experiences with HIV/AIDS*; Felissa L. Cohen and Jerry D. Durham, eds., *Women, Children, and HIV/AIDS* (New York: Springer, 1993).

54. Pulled from UNAIDS website, at www.unaids.org/ (accessed February 11, 2010).

55. Suzanne Leclerc-Madlala, "Global Struggles, Local Contexts: Prospects for a Southern African AIDS Feminism," in *The Politics of AIDS: Globalization, the State and Civil Society*, ed. M. Follér and H. Thörn, 141–43 (New York: Palgrave Macmillan, 2008).

56. Aberth, *The First Horseman*, 144–54.

57. Patricia D. Siplon and Kristin M. Novotny, "Overcoming the Contradictions: Women, Autonomy, and AIDS in Tanzania," in *The Global Politics of AIDS*, ed. P. G. Harris and P. D. Siplon, 87–107 (Boulder, Colo.: Lynne Rienner, 2007); Anne Outwater, "The Socioeconomic Impact of AIDS on Women in Tanzania," in *Women's Experiences with HIV/AIDS: An International Perspective*, ed. L. D. Long and E. M. Ankrah, 112–22 (New York: Columbia University Press, 1996); Baylies, Bujra, et al., *AIDS, Sexuality and Gender in Africa*.

58. Follér and Thörn, *The Politics of AIDS*, 139–76.

59. Stillwaggon, *AIDS and the Ecology of Poverty*, 90–98; Shawn Smallman, *The AIDS Pandemic in Latin America* (Chapel Hill: University of North Carolina Press, 2007), 27–31; UNAIDS, at www.unaids.org/ (accessed February 12, 2010).

60. Chin, *The AIDS Pandemic*, 31–36; Engel, *The Epidemic*, 50–51.

61. Paul Farmer, *AIDS and Accusation: Haiti and the Geography of Blame* (Berkeley: University of California Press, 1992), esp. 125–50; Paul Farmer, "AIDS and Accusation: Haiti, Haitians, and the Geography of Blame," in *Culture and AIDS*, ed. D. A. Feldman, 67–91 (New York: Praeger, 1990).

62. Farmer, *AIDS and Accusation*, 193–251; Smallman, *The AIDS Pandemic in Latin America*, 23–32.

63. Pulled from UNAIDS website, at www.unaids.org/ (accessed February 12, 2010). Earlier figures are from Farmer, *AIDS and Accusation*, 130–31.

64. Smallman, *The AIDS Pandemic in Latin America*, 25–27.

65. Smallman, *The AIDS Pandemic in Latin America*, 33; Shepard, "Shifting Priorities in US AIDS Policy," 189.

66. Engel, *The Epidemic*, 94–95, is inclined to accept Cuban statistics at face value, but Doka, *AIDS, Fear, and Society*, 99, is more skeptical.

67. Smallman, *The AIDS Pandemic in Latin America*, 35–46; Doka, *AIDS, Fear, and Society*, 99.

68. Smallman, *The AIDS Pandemic in Latin America*, 46–66.

69. Pulled from UNAIDS website, at www.unaids.org/ (accessed February 12, 2010).

70. Smallman, *The AIDS Pandemic in Latin America*, 151–54.

71. Stillwaggon, *AIDS and the Ecology of Poverty*, 88–100.

72. Smallman, *The AIDS Pandemic in Latin America*, 146–57, 167–90.

73. Smallman, *The AIDS Pandemic in Latin America*, 67–92; Tim Frasca, *AIDS in Latin America* (Basingstoke, UK: Palgrave Macmillan, 2005), 187–209.

74. Smallman, *The AIDS Pandemic in Latin America*, 92–109; André de Mello e Souza, "Defying Globalization: Effective Self-Reliance in Brazil," in *The Global Politics of AIDS*, ed. P. G. Harris and P. D. Siplon, 37–49 (Boulder, Colo.: Lynne Rienner, 2007).

75. Anton A. Van Niekerk and Loretta M. Kopelman, eds., *Ethics and AIDS in Africa: The Challenge to Our Thinking* (Walnut Creek, Calif.: Left Coast Press, 2006), 111–40; Nana K. Poku and Alan Whiteside, eds., *Global Health and Governance: HIV/AIDS* (Basingstoke, UK: Palgrave Macmillan, 2004), 27–41, 61–74.

76. Mello e Souza, "Defying Globalization," 49–63; Smallman, *The AIDS Pandemic in Latin America*, 109–12.

77. According to the UNAIDS report, as of 2008, Mexico is one of the few countries in the region to have prevention programs that focus on the high-risk groups of commercial sex workers, men who have sex with men, and drug users. Pulled from www.unaids.org/ (accessed February 14, 2010).

78. Smallman, *The AIDS Pandemic in Latin America*, 117–46; Frasca, *AIDS in Latin America*, 71–99.

79. Marika Vicziany, "The Political Economy of HIV/AIDS in India," in *The Global Politics of AIDS*, ed. P. G. Harris and P. D. Siplon, 109–36 (Boulder, Colo.: Lynne

Rienner, 2007), 129; Susan Hunter, *AIDS in Asia: A Continent in Peril* (Basingstoke, UK: Palgrave Macmillan, 2005), 9–10.

80. Pulled from UNAIDS website, at www.unaids.org/ (accessed February 14, 2010).

81. Chris Lyttleton, "AIDS and Civil Belonging: Disease Management and Political Change in Thailand and Laos," in *The Politics of Aids: Globalization, the State and Civil Society*, ed. M. Follér and H. Thörn, 255–73 (New York: Palgrave Macmillan, 2008); Engel, *The Epidemic*, 256–64.

82. Pulled from UNAIDS website, at www.unaids.org/ (accessed February 15, 2010).

83. David Wilson and Mariam Claeson, "Dynamics of the HIV Epidemic in South Asia," in *HIV and AIDS in South Asia: An Economic Development Risk*, ed. M. Haacker and M. Claeson, 3–40 (Washington, D.C.: World Bank, 2009), 14–22, 27–32; Vicziany, "The Political Economy of HIV/AIDS in India," 109–36.

84. Pulled from UNAIDS website, at www.unaids.org/ (accessed February 15, 2010).

85. Susanne Y. P. Choi and Roman David, "Law Enforcement, Public Health, and HIV/AIDS in China," in *The Global Politics of AIDS*, ed. P. G. Harris and P. D. Siplon, 137–54 (Boulder, Colo.: Lynne Rienner, 2007); Neil Renwick, "The 'Nameless Fever': The HIV/AIDS Pandemic and China's Women," in *Global Health and Governance: HIV/AIDS*, ed. N. K. Poku and A. Whiteside, 187–203 (Basingstoke, UK: Palgrave Macmillan, 2004).

86. Pulled from UNAIDS website, at www.unaids.org/ (accessed February 15, 2010).

87. Stillwaggon, *AIDS and the Ecology of Poverty*, 105–29; Olusoji Adeyi, ed., *Averting AIDS Crises in Eastern Europe and Central Asia: A Regional Support Strategy* (Washington, D.C.: World Bank, 2003), 15–35; Joana Godinho et al., *Reversing the Tide: Priorities for HIV/AIDS Prevention in Central Asia* (Washington, D.C.: World Bank, 2005), 11–38.

88. Pulled from UNAIDS website, at www.unaids.org/ (accessed February 15, 2010).

89. Carol Jenkins and David A. Robalino, *HIV/AIDS in the Middle East and North Africa: The Costs of Inaction* (Washington D.C.: World Bank, 2003), 25–36.

90. Pulled from UNAIDS website, at www.unaids.org/ (accessed February 15, 2010).

91. Hays, *Epidemics and Pandemics*, 432; Doka, *AIDS, Fear, and Society*, 3–58.

92. Susan Sontag, *AIDS and Its Metaphors* (New York: Picador/Farrar, Straus and Giroux, 1989); Susan Sontag, *Illness as Metaphor* (New York: Picador/Farrar, Straus and Giroux, 1977).

93. Allan M. Brandt, "AIDS and Metaphor: Toward the Social Meaning of Epidemic Disease," in *In Time of Plague: The History and Social Consequences of Lethal Epidemic Disease*, ed. A. Mack, 91–110 (New York: New York University Press, 1991), 92–96.

Conclusion

1. Laurie Garrett, *The Coming Plague: Newly Emerging Diseases in a World Out of Balance* (Harmondsworth, UK: Penguin, 1994), 620.

2. Richard Preston, *The Hot Zone* (New York: Random House, 1994), 287–88.

3. Montira J. Pongsiri et al., "Biodiversity Loss Affects Global Disease Ecology," *BioScience* 59 (2009): 945–54.

4. Tom Quinn, *Flu: A Social History of Influenza* (London: New Holland Publishers, 2008), 173–77, 191.

5. These ideas will be more fully expounded upon in the forthcoming volume by Ron Barrett and George Armelagos, *An Unnatural History of Emerging Infections*, to be published by Rowman & Littlefield.

6. William H. McNeill, *Plagues and Peoples*, updated ed. (New York: Anchor Books, 1998), 23–32, 293–95.

7. Dorothy H. Crawford, *Deadly Companions: How Microbes Shaped Our History* (Oxford: Oxford University Press, 2007), 186.

8. Arno Karlen, in *Man and Microbes: Disease and Plagues in History and Modern Times* (New York: Putnam, 1995), 1–11, 215–30, also expresses a "cautious optimism" with regard to humankind's future history with disease.

9. Crawford, *Deadly Companions*, 212.

10. For instance, as I write today (February 20, 2010), the U.S. Justice Department has announced it is officially closing its case on the 2001 anthrax bioterrorism scare, which killed five people in the United States; evidence produced by the FBI suggests the incident was in fact a domestic one, perpetrated by an army microbiologist, Bruce Ivins, who later committed suicide.

11. See Susan Sontag's *AIDS and Its Metaphors* (New York: Picador/Farrar, Straus and Giroux, 1989), 93–183.

12. Eileen Stillwaggon, *AIDS and the Ecology of Poverty* (Oxford: Oxford University Press, 2006).

Bibliography

General Works

Aberth, John. *The First Horseman: Disease in Human History*. Upper Saddle River, N.J.: Pearson/Prentice Hall, 2007.

Albala, Ken. *Eating Right in the Renaissance*. Berkeley: University of California Press, 2002.

Arnold, David. *Colonizing the Body: State Medicine and Epidemic Disease in Nineteenth-Century India*. Berkeley: University of California Press, 1993.

———, ed. *Imperial Medicine and Indigenous Societies*. Manchester, UK: Manchester University Press, 1988.

Barber, Paul. *Vampires, Burial, and Death*. New Haven, Conn.: Yale University Press, 1988.

Bell, Michael E. *Food for the Dead: On the Trail of New England's Vampires*. New York: Carroll and Graf, 2001.

Bollet, Alfred Jay. *Plagues and Poxes: The Impact of Human History on Epidemic Disease*. 2nd ed. New York: Demos, 2004.

Bushnell, O. A. *The Gifts of Civilization: Germs and Genocide in Hawaii*. Honolulu: University of Hawaii Press, 1993.

Cartwright, Frederick F. *Disease and History*. New York: Thomas Y. Crowell Co., 1972.

Cipolla, Carlo M. *Miasmas and Disease: Public Health and the Environment in the Pre-Industrial Age*. Translated by E. Potter. New Haven, Conn.: Yale University Press, 1992.

———. *Public Health and the Medical Profession in the Renaissance*. Cambridge: Cambridge University Press, 1976.

Citro, Joseph A. *Green Mountain Ghosts, Ghouls and Unsolved Mysteries*. Boston: Houghton Mifflin, 1994.

———. *Passing Strange: True Tales of New England Hauntings and Horrors*. Boston: Houghton Mifflin, 1996.

215

Coleman, William. *Death Is a Social Disease: Public Health and Political Economy in Early Industrial France*. Madison: University of Wisconsin Press, 1982.

Crawford, Dorothy H. *Deadly Companions: How Microbes Shaped Our History*. Oxford: Oxford University Press, 2007.

Crosby, Alfred W. *Ecological Imperialism: The Biological Expansion of Europe, 900–1900*. Cambridge: Cambridge University Press, 1986.

Curtin, P. D. *Death by Migration: Europe's Encounter with the Tropical World in the Nineteenth Century*. Cambridge: Cambridge University Press, 1989.

Drexler, Madeline. *Secret Agents: The Menace of Emerging Infections*. Washington, D.C.: Joseph Henry Press, 2002.

Fagan, Brian. *The Great Warming: Climate Change and the Rise and Fall of Civilizations*. New York: Bloomsbury Press, 2008.

———. *The Little Ice Age: How Climate Made History, 1300–1850*. New York: Basic Books, 2000.

Fine, J. V. A. *The Ancient Greeks: A Critical History*. Cambridge, Mass.: Harvard University Press, 1983.

Gallagher, Nancy Elizabeth. *Medicine and Power in Tunisia, 1780–1900*. Cambridge: Cambridge University Press, 1983.

Garrett, Laurie. *The Coming Plague: Newly Emerging Diseases in a World Out of Balance*. Harmondsworth, UK: Penguin, 1994.

Gregory of Tours. *History of the Franks*. Translated by Lewis Thorpe. Harmondsworth, UK: Penguin, 1974.

Halsall, Guy. *Barbarian Migrations and the Roman West, 376–568*. Cambridge: Cambridge University Press, 2007.

Hanson, Victor Davis. *A War Like No Other: How the Athenians and Spartans Fought the Peloponnesian War*. New York: Random House, 2005.

Hatcher, John. "Mortality in the Fifteenth Century: Some New Evidence." *Economic History Review* 39 (1986): 19–38.

Hays, Jo N. *The Burdens of Disease: Epidemics and Human Response in Western History*. New Brunswick, N.J.: Rutgers University Press, 1998.

———. *Epidemics and Pandemics: Their Impacts on Human History*. Santa Barbara, Calif.: ABC–CLIO, 2005.

———. "Historians and Epidemics: Simple Questions, Complex Answers." In *Plague and the End of Antiquity: The Pandemic of 541–750*, edited by L. K. Little, 33–58. Cambridge: Cambridge University Press, 2007.

Herzlich, Claudine, and Janine Pierret. *Illness and Self in Society*. Translated by E. Forster. Baltimore: Johns Hopkins University Press, 1987.

Hodges, Richard, and David Whitehouse. *Mohammed, Charlemagne and the Origins of Europe: Archaeology and the Pirenne Thesis*. Ithaca, N.Y.: Cornell University Press, 1983.

Hudson, Robert P. *Disease and Its Control: The Shaping of Modern Thought*. Westport, Conn.: Greenwood Press, 1983.

Kagan, D. *The Peloponnesian War*. New York: Viking Press, 2003.

Karlen, Arno. *Man and Microbes: Disease and Plagues in History and Modern Times*. New York: Putnam, 1995.

Kiple, Kenneth F. *The Cambridge World History of Human Disease*. Cambridge: Cambridge University Press, 1993.

Lashley, Felissa R., and Jerry D. Durham, eds. *Emerging Infectious Diseases: Trends and Issues*. 2nd ed. New York: Springer, 2007.

Leavitt, Judith Walzer. *Typhoid Mary: Captive to the Public's Health*. Boston: Beacon Press, 1996.

Longrigg, James. "Epidemic, Ideas and Classical Athenian Society." In *Epidemics and Ideas: Essays on the Historical Perception of Pestilence*, edited by T. Ranger and P. Slack, 21–44. Cambridge: Cambridge University Press, 1992.

Mack, Arien, ed. *In Time of Plague: The History and Social Consequences of Lethal Epidemic Disease*. New York: New York University Press, 1991.

MacLeod, Roy M., and Milton James Lewis, eds. *Disease, Medicine, and Empire: Perspectives on Western Medicine and the Experience of European Expansion*. London: Routledge, 1988.

McCormick, Michael. *Origins of the European Economy: Communications and Commerce, A.D. 300–900*. Cambridge: Cambridge University Press, 2001.

McNeill, William H. "Migration Patterns and Infection in Traditional Societies." In *Changing Disease Patterns and Human Behavior*, edited by N. F. Stanley and R. A. Joske, 27–36. London: Academic Press, 1980.

———. *Plagues and Peoples*. Updated ed. New York: Anchor Books, 1998.

———. *The Rise of the West: A History of the Human Community* (Chicago: University of Chicago Press, 1963.

Oldstone, Michael B. A. *Viruses, Plagues, and History: Past, Present and Future*. Revised and updated ed. Oxford: Oxford University Press, 2010.

Pongsiri, Montira J., et al. "Biodiversity Loss Affects Global Disease Ecology." *BioScience* 59 (2009): 945–54.

Preston, Richard. *The Hot Zone*. New York: Random House, 1994.

Ranger, Terence, and Paul Slack, eds. *Epidemics and Ideas: Essays on the Historical Perception of Pestilence*. Cambridge: Cambridge University Press, 1992.

Rosenberg, Charles E. *Explaining Epidemics and Other Studies in the History of Medicine*. Cambridge: Cambridge University Press, 1992.

Sallares, Robert. *The Ecology of the Ancient Greek World*. Ithaca, N.Y.: Cornell University Press, 1991.

Scholasticus, Evagrius. *Ecclesiastical History*. Translated as *A History of the Church* (London: S. Bagster and Sons, 1846.

Sherman, Irwin W. *The Power of Plagues*. Washington, D.C.: ASM Press, 2006.

Sigerist, Henry E. *Civilization and Disease*. Chicago: University of Chicago Press, 1943.

Sontag, Susan. *Illness as Metaphor*. New York: Picador/Farrar, Straus and Giroux, 1977.

Stanley, N. F., and R. A. Joske, eds. *Changing Disease Patterns and Human Behavior*. London: Academic Press, 1980.

Torrey, E. Fuller, and Robert H. Yolken. *Beasts of the Earth: Animals, Humans, and Disease*. New Brunswick, N.J.: Rutgers University Press, 2005.

Watts, Sheldon. *Disease and Medicine in World History*. New York: Routledge, 2003.

————. *Epidemics and History: Disease, Power and Imperialism.* New Haven, Conn.: Yale University Press, 1997.

Winslow, Charles-Edward Amory. *The Conquest of Epidemic Disease: A Chapter in the History of Ideas.* Princeton, N.J.: Princeton University Press, 1943.

Zinsser, Hans. *Rats, Lice and History.* Boston: Little, Brown, 1934.

Plague

Aberth, John. *The Black Death: The Great Mortality of 1348–1350. A Brief History with Documents.* Boston: Bedford/St. Martin's, 2005.

————. *From the Brink of the Apocalypse: Confronting Famine, War, Plague and Death in the Later Middle Ages.* 2nd ed. London: Routledge, 2010.

Amasuna Sárraga, M. V. *La Peste en la Corona de Castilla durante la Segunda Mitad del Siglo XIV.* Valladolid, Spain: Junta de Castilla y León, Ministry of Education and Culture, 1996.

Appleby, Andrew. "The Disappearance of Plague: A Continuing Puzzle." *Economic History Review* 33 (1980): 161–73.

Arrizabalaga, Jon. "Facing the Black Death: Perceptions and Reactions of University Medical Practitioners." In *Practical Medicine from Salerno to the Black Death,* edited by L. García-Ballester, R. French, J. Arrizabalaga, and A. Cunningham, 237–88. Cambridge: Cambridge University Press, 1994.

Bacci, Massimo Livi. *The Population of Europe: A History.* Translated by C. De Nardi and C. Ipsen. Oxford: Blackwell, 2000.

Battūta, Ibn. *Travels, A.D. 1325–1354.* Translated by H. A. R. Gibb. 5 vols. Cambridge, UK: Hakluyt Society, 1958–2000.

Benedict, Carol. *Bubonic Plague in Nineteenth-Century China.* Stanford, Calif.: Stanford University Press, 1996.

Benedictow, Ole J. *The Black Death, 1346–1353: The Complete History.* Woodbridge, UK: Boydell Press, 2004.

————. *Plague in the Late Medieval Nordic Countries: Epidemiological Studies.* Oslo, Norway: Middelalderforlaget, 1992.

Biraben, Jean-Noël. *Les Hommes et la Peste en France et dans les Pays Européens et Méditerranéens.* 2 vols. Paris: Mouton, 1975–1976.

Biraben, Jean-Noël, and Jacques Le Goff. "The Plague in the Early Middle Ages." In *Biology of Man in History: Selections from the Annales: Économies, Sociétés, Civilisations,* edited and translated by E. Forster, R. Forster, O. Ranum, and P. M. Ranum, 48–80. Baltimore: Johns Hopkins University Press, 1975.

Blume, Fred H., and Timothy Kearley. *Annotated Justinian Code.* 2nd ed. Laramie: University of Wyoming College of Law, 2009. http://uwacadweb.uwyo.edu/blume&justinian (accessed August 3, 2010).

Borsch, Stuart J. *The Black Death in Egypt and England: A Comparative Study.* Austin: University of Texas Press, 2005.

Bowsky, William M. *The Black Death: A Turning Point in History?* New York: Holt, Rinehart and Winston, 1971.

Bratton, T. L. "The Identity of the Plague of Justinian: Part 1." *Transactions and Studies of the College of Physicians of Philadelphia* 3 (June 1981): 113–24.

Brock, S. P. "North Mesopotamia in the Late Seventh Century: Book XV of John Bar Penkāyē's *Rīš Mellē*." *Jerusalem Studies in Arabic and Islam* 9 (1987): 68–69.

Caferro, William P. "Warfare and Economy in Renaissance Italy, 1350–1450." *Journal of Interdisciplinary History* 39 (2008): 167–209.

Calero Secall, Maria Isabel. "El Proceso de Ibn al-Jaṭīb." *Al-Qantas: Arab Studies Journal* 22 (2001): 421–62.

Chandavarkar, Rajnarayan. "Plague Panic and Epidemic Politics in India, 1896–1914." In *Epidemics and Ideas: Essays on the Historical Perception of Pestilence*, edited by T. Ranger and P. Slack, 203–40. Cambridge: Cambridge University Press, 1992.

Cipolla, Carlo M. *Faith, Reason, and the Plague in Seventeenth-Century Tuscany*. Translated by M. Kittel. Ithaca, N.Y.: Cornell University Press, 1979.

Cohn, Norman. *The Pursuit of the Millennium: Revolutionary Messianism in Medieval and Reformation Europe and Its Bearing on Modern Totalitarian Movements*. New York: Harper, 1961.

Cohn, Samuel K., Jr. "The Black Death: End of a Paradigm." *American Historical Review* 107 (2002): 703–38.

———. *The Black Death Transformed: Disease and Culture in Early Renaissance Europe*. London: Arnold, 2002.

———. *The Cult of Remembrance and the Black Death: Six Renaissance Cities in Central Italy*. Baltimore: Johns Hopkins University Press, 1992.

———. "The Place of the Dead in Flanders and Tuscany: Towards a Comparative History of the Black Death." In *The Place of the Dead: Death and Remembrance in Late Medieval and Early Modern Europe*, edited by B. Gordon and P. Marshall, 17–43. Cambridge: Cambridge University Press, 2000.

Condon, J. K. *The Bombay Plague, Being a History of the Progress of Plague in the Bombay Presidency from September 1896 to June 1899*. Bombay, India: Education Society's Steam Press, 1900.

Congourdeau, Marie-Hélène, and Mohamed Melhaoui. "La Perception de la Peste en Pays Chrétien, Byzantine, et Musulman." *Revue des Études Byzantines* 59 (2001): 95–124.

Conrad, Lawrence I. "Epidemic Disease in Formal and Popular Thought in Early Islamic Society." In *Epidemics and Ideas: Essays on the Historical Perception of Pestilence*, edited by T. Ranger and P. Slack, 77–99. Cambridge: Cambridge University Press, 1992.

———. "Plague in the Early Medieval Near East." PhD diss., Princeton University, 1981.

———. "*Tāʿūn* and *Wabāʾ*: Conceptions of Plague and Pestilence in Early Islam." *Journal of the Economic and Social History of the Orient* 25 (1982): 268–307.

———. "Umar at Sargh: The Evolution of an Umayyad Tradition on Flight from the Plague." In *Story-telling in the Framework of Non-fictional Arabic Literature*, edited by S. Leder, 488–528. Wiesbaden, Germany: Harrassowitz, 1998.

Cunningham, A. "Transforming Plague: The Laboratory and the Identity of Infectious Disease." In *The Laboratory Revolution in Medicine*, edited by A. Cunningham and P. Williams, 209–44. Cambridge: Cambridge University Press, 1992.

Dols, Michael W. *The Black Death in the Middle East*. Princeton, N.J.: Princeton University Press, 1977.

———. "The Comparative Communal Responses to the Black Death in Muslim and Christian Societies." *Viator* 5 (1974): 269–87.

———. "Ibn al-Wardi's *Risalah al-Naba' 'an al-Waba'*, a Translation of a Major Source of the History of the Black Death in the Middle East." In *Near Eastern Numismatics, Iconography, Epigraphy and History: Studies in Honor of George C. Miles*, edited by D. K. Kouymjian, 443–55. Beirut, Lebanon: American University of Beirut, 1974.

Drancourt, Michel, et al. "Detection of 400-Year-Old *Yersinia pestis* DNA in Human Dental Pulp: An Approach to the Diagnosis of Ancient Septicemia." *Proceedings of the National Academy of Science* 95 (1998): 12637–40.

———. "Molecular Identification by 'Suicide PCR' of *Yersinia pestis* as the Agent of Medieval Black Death." *Proceedings of the National Academy of Science* 97 (2000): 12800–803.

Duncan, Christopher J., and Susan Scott. *Biology of Plagues: Evidence from Historical Populations*. Cambridge: Cambridge University Press, 2001.

Echenberg, Myron. *Black Death, White Medicine: Bubonic Plague and the Politics of Public Health in Colonial Senegal, 1914–1945*. Portsmouth, N.H.: Heinemann, 2002.

———. *Plague Ports: The Global Urban Impact of Bubonic Plague, 1894–1901*. New York: New York University Press, 2007.

Fabbri, C. N. "Continuity and Change in Late Medieval Plague Medicine: A Survey of 152 Plague Tracts from 1348 to 1599." PhD diss., Yale University, 2006.

Gage, Kenneth L., and Michael Y. Kosoy. "Natural History of Plague: Perspectives from More than a Century of Research." *Annual Review of Entomology* 50 (2005): 505–28.

Gatacre, W. F. *Report on the Bubonic Plague in Bombay, 1896–97*. Bombay, India: Times of India Steam Press, 1897.

Gentile da Foligno. *Consilium contra Pestilentiam*. Colle di Valdelsa, Italy, c. 1479.

Guilleré, Christian. "La Peste Noire a Gérone (1348)." *Annals de Institut d'Estudis Gironins* 27 (1984): 87–161.

Haldon, John. "The Works of Anastasius of Sinai: A Key Source for the History of Seventh-Century East Mediterranean Society and Belief." In *The Byzantine and Early Islamic Near East, Volume I: Problems in the Literary Source Material*, edited by A. Cameron and L. I. Conrad, 107–47. Princeton, N.J.: Darwin Press, 1992.

Harrison, D. "Plague, Settlement and Structural Changes at the Dawn of the Middle Ages." *Scandia* 59 (1993): 15–48.

Herlihy, David. *The Black Death and the Transformation of the West*, edited by S. K. Cohn Jr. Cambridge, Mass.: Harvard University Press, 1997.

———. "Population, Plague and Social Change in Rural Pistoia, 1201–1430." *Economic History Review* 18 (1965): 225–44.

Hinnebusch, J. B. "Bubonic Plague: A Molecular Genetic Case History of the Emergence of an Infectious Disease." *Journal of Molecular Medicine* 75 (1997): 645–52.

Hirst, L. Fabian. *The Conquest of Plague: A Study of the Evolution of Epidemiology*. Oxford, UK: Clarendon Press, 1953.

Hoeniger, Robert. *Der Schwarze Tod in Deutschland*. Berlin: Grosser, 1882.

Horrox, Rosemary, trans. and ed. *The Black Death*. Manchester, UK: Manchester University Press, 1994.

Kulikowski, Michael. "Plague in Spanish Late Antiquity." In *Plague and the End of Antiquity: The Pandemic of 541–750*, edited by L. K. Little, 150–70. Cambridge: Cambridge University Press, 2007.

Julian of Norwich. *Revelations of Divine Love*. In *A Book of Showings to the Anchoress Julian of Norwich*, edited by Edmund Colledge and James Walsh, chap. 27. Toronto: Pontifical Institute of Mediaeval Studies, 1978.

Lamb, H. H. *Climate, History and the Modern World*. 2nd ed. London: Routledge, 1995.

Lien-Teh (Liande), Wu. *A Treatise on Pneumonic Plague*. Geneva: Publications of the League of Nations, 1926.

Lien-Teh, Wu, J. W. H. Chun, R. Pollitzer, and C. Y. Wu. *Plague: A Manual for Medical and Public Health Workers*. Shanghai, China: Weishengshu National Quarantine Service, 1936.

Little, Lester K. "Life and Afterlife of the First Plague Pandemic," in *Plague and the End of Antiquity: The Pandemic of 541–750*, edited by L. K. Little, 3–32. Cambridge: Cambridge University Press, 2007.

———, ed. *Plague and the End of Antiquity: The Pandemic of 541–750*. Cambridge: Cambridge University Press, 2007.

Maddicott, John. "Plague in Seventh-Century England." In *Plague and the End of Antiquity: The Pandemic of 541–750*, edited by L. K. Little, 171–214. Cambridge: Cambridge University Press, 2007.

McCormick, Michael. "Rats, Communications, and Plague." *Journal of Interdisciplinary History* 34 (2003): 1–25.

———. "Toward a Molecular History of the Justinianic Pandemic." In *Plague and the End of Antiquity: The Pandemic of 541–750*, edited by L. K. Little, 290–312. Cambridge: Cambridge University Press, 2007.

Morony, Michael G. "'For Whom Does the Writer Write?': The First Bubonic Plague Pandemic According to Syriac Sources." In *Plague and the End of Antiquity: The Pandemic of 541–750*, edited by L. K. Little, 59–86. Cambridge: Cambridge University Press, 2007.

Norris, John. "East or West? The Geographic Origin of the Black Death." *Bulletin of the History of Medicine* 51 (1977): 1–24.

Paul the Deacon. *History of the Lombards*. Translated by William Dudley Foulke. Philadelphia: University of Pennsylvania Press, 1974.

Pollitzer, R. *Plague*. Geneva: World Health Organization, 1954.

Procopius. *History of the Wars*. Translated by H. B. Dewing. London: W. Heinemann and Macmillan, 1914–1940.

———. *The Secret History*. Translated by G. A. Williamson. London: Folio Society, 1990.

Pseudo-Dionysius of Tel-Mahre. *Chronicle, Part III*. Translated by Witold Witakowski. Translated Texts for Historians 22. Liverpool, UK: Liverpool University Press, 1996.

———. *The Chronicle of Zuqnīn, Parts III and IV*. Translated by A. Harrak. Toronto: Pontifical Institute of Mediaeval Studies, 1999.

Pullan, Brian. "Plague and Perceptions of the Poor in Early Modern Italy." In *Epidemics and Ideas: Essays on the Historical Perception of Pestilence*, edited by T. Ranger and P. Slack, 101–23. Cambridge: Cambridge University Press, 1992.

Rand, W. C. *Draft of Report to Government of Bombay*. n.p., n.d.

Russell, Josiah Cox. "That Earlier Plague." *Demography* 5 (1968): 174–84.

Sallares, Robert. "Ecology, Evolution, and Epidemiology of Plague." In *Plague and the End of Antiquity: The Pandemic of 541–750*, edited by L. K. Little, 231–89. Cambridge: Cambridge University Press, 2007.

Sarris, Peter. "Bubonic Plague in Byzantium: The Evidence of Non-Literary Sources." In *Plague and the End of Antiquity: The Pandemic of 541–750*, edited by L. K. Little, 119–34. Cambridge: Cambridge University Press, 2007.

Slack, Paul. "The Disappearance of Plague: An Alternative View." *Economic History Review* 34 (1981): 469–76.

———. *The Impact of Plague in Tudor and Stuart England*. London: Routledge and Kegan Paul, 1985.

———. "Responses to Plague in Early Modern Europe: The Implications of Public Health." In *In Time of Plague: The History and Social Consequences of Lethal Epidemic Disease*, edited by A. Mack, 111–32. New York: New York University Press, 1991.

Smet, Joseph-Jean de, ed. *Recueil des Chroniques de Flandre*. 4 vols. Brussels, 1837–1865.

Stathakopoulos, Dionysios. "Crime and Punishment: The Plague in the Byzantine Empire, 541–749." In *Plague and the End of Antiquity: The Pandemic of 541–750*, edited by L. K. Little, 99–118. Cambridge: Cambridge University Press, 2007.

———. *Famine and Pestilence in the Late Roman and Early Byzantine Empire: A Systematic Survey of Subsistence Crises and Epidemics*. Burlington, Vt.: Ashgate, 2004.

Stearns, Justin. "Infectious Ideas: Contagion in Medieval Islamic and Christian Thought." PhD diss., Princeton University, 2007.

Stefani, Marchionne di Coppo. *Cronaca Fiorentina*, edited by Niccolò Rodolica. Rerum Italicarum Scriptores 30/1. Città di Castello, 1903.

Sudhoff, Karl. "Pestschriften aus den ersten 150 Jahren nach der Epidemie des 'schwarzen Todes' 1348." *Archiv für Geschichte der Medizin* 4 (1911), 5 (1912), 8 (1915), 11 (1919), 14 (1923), 16 (1925), 17 (1925).

Twigg, Graham. *The Black Death: A Biological Reappraisal*. New York: Schocken Books, 1984.

Wray, S. K. "Boccaccio and the Doctors: Medicine and Compassion in the Face of the Plague." *Journal of Medieval History* 30 (2004): 301–22.

Smallpox

Alchon, Suzanne Austin. *A Pest in the Land: New World Epidemics in a Global Perspective*. Albuquerque: University of New Mexico Press, 2003.

Altman, Lawrence K. "W.H.O. Panel Backs Gene Manipulation in Smallpox Virus." *New York Times*, November 12, 2004.

The Annals of the Cakchiquels. Translated by A. Recinos and D. Goetz. Norman: University of Oklahoma Press, 1953.

Arnold, David. "Smallpox and Colonial Medicine in Nineteenth-Century India." In *Imperial Medicine and Indigenous Societies*, edited by D. Arnold, 45–65. Manchester, UK: Manchester University Press, 1988.

Cook, David Noble. *Born to Die: Disease and New World Conquest, 1492–1650*. Cambridge: Cambridge University Press, 1998.

Crosby, Alfred W. *The Columbian Exchange: Biological and Cultural Consequences of 1492*. Westport, Conn.: Greenwood Press, 1972.

———. "Conquistador y Pestilencia: The First New World Pandemic and the Fall of the Great Indian Empires." *Hispanic American Historical Review* 47 (1967): 321–37.

———. "Hawaiian Depopulation as a Model for the Amerindian Experience." In *Epidemics and Ideas: Essays on the Historical Perception of Pestilence*, edited by T. Ranger and P. Slack, 175–201. Cambridge: Cambridge University Press, 1992.

Duffy, John. *Epidemics in Colonial America*. Baton Rouge: Louisiana State University Press, 1953.

Fenn, Elizabeth. *Pox Americana: The Great Smallpox Epidemic of 1775–1782*. New York: Hill and Wang, 2001.

Hopkins, Donald R. *The Greatest Killer: Smallpox in History*. Chicago: University of Chicago Press, 1983.

Longrigg, James. "The Great Plague of Athens." *History of Science* 18 (1980): 209–25.

Ortiz de Montellano, Bernard R. *Aztec Medicine, Health, and Nutrition*. New Brunswick, N.J.: Rutgers University Press, 1990.

Poole, J. C. F., and A. J. Holladay. "Thucydides and the Plague of Athens." *Classical Quarterly* 29 (1979): 282–300.

Reff, Daniel T. *Disease, Depopulation, and Culture Change in Northwestern New Spain, 1518–1764*. Salt Lake City: University of Utah Press, 1991.

Stannard, David E. "Disease and Infertility: A New Look at the Demographic Collapse of Native Populations in the Wake of Western Contact." *Journal of American Studies* 24 (1990): 325–50.

Thucydides. *The History of the Peloponnesian War*. Translated by R. Crawley. London: Longmans, Green, 1874.

Whitmore, Thomas M. *Disease and Death in Early Colonial Mexico: Simulating Amerindian Depopulation*. Boulder, Colo.: Westview, 1992.

Tuberculosis

Barnes, David S. *The Making of a Social Disease: Tuberculosis in Nineteenth-Century France*. Berkeley: University of California Press, 1995.

Blanc, Léopold, and Mukund Uplekar. "The Present Global Burden of Tuberculosis." In *The Return of the White Plague: Global Poverty and the "New" Tuberculosis*, edited by M. Gandy and A. Zumla, 95–111. London: Verso, 2003.

Caldwell, Mark. *The Last Crusade: The War on Consumption, 1862–1954*. New York: Atheneum, 1988.

Coker, Richard. *From Chaos to Coercion: Detention and the Control of Tuberculosis*. New York: St. Martin's Press, 2000.

Daniel, T. M. *Captain of Death: The Story of Tuberculosis*. Rochester, N.Y.: University of Rochester Press, 1997.

Dormandy, Thomas. *The White Death: A History of Tuberculosis*. New York: New York University Press, 2000.

Dubos, Rene, and Jean Dubos. *The White Plague: Tuberculosis, Man and Society*. Boston: Little, Brown, 1952.

Gandy, Matthew, and Alimudden Zumla, eds. *The Return of the White Plague: Global Poverty and the "New" Tuberculosis*. London: Verso, 2003.

Harries, Anthony De., Nicola J. Hargreaves, and Alimuddin Zumla. "Tuberculosis and HIV Infection in Sub-Saharan Africa." In *The Return of the White Plague: Global Poverty and the "New" Tuberculosis*, edited by M. Gandy and A. Zumla, 112–24. London: Verso, 2003.

Reichman, Lee B., and Janice Hopkins Tanne. *Timebomb: The Global Epidemic of Multi-Drug Resistant Tuberculosis*. New York: McGraw-Hill, 2002.

Rothschild, B., et al. "Mycobacterium Tuberculosis Complex DNA from an Extinct Bison Dated 17,000 Years before the Present." *Clinical Infectious Diseases* 33 (2001): 305–11.

Ryan, Frank. *The Forgotten Plague: How the Battle against Tuberculosis Was Won—and Lost*. Boston: Little, Brown, 1992.

Smith, F. B. *The Retreat of Tuberculosis, 1850–1950*. London: Croom Helm, 1988.

Stern, Vivien. "*The House of the Dead* Revisited: Prisons, Tuberculosis and Public Health in the Former Soviet Bloc." In *The Return of the White Plague: Global Poverty and the "New" Tuberculosis*, edited by M. Gandy and A. Zumla, 178–91. London: Verso, 2003.

Wallace, Deborah, and Rodrick Wallace. "The Recent Tuberculosis Epidemic in New York City: Warning from the De-Developing World." In *The Return of the White Plague: Global Poverty and the "New" Tuberculosis*, edited by M. Gandy and A. Zumla, 125–46. London: Verso, 2003.

Cholera

Arnold, David. "Cholera and Colonialism in British India." *Past and Present* 113 (1986): 118–51.

Delaporte, François. *Disease and Civilization: The Cholera in Paris, 1832*. Cambridge, Mass.: MIT Press, 1986.

Durey, Michael. *The Return of the Plague: British Society and the Cholera, 1831–2*. Dublin: Gill and Macmillan, 1979.

Evans, Richard J. *Death in Hamburg: Society and Politics in the Cholera Years, 1830–1910*. Oxford: Oxford University Press, 1987.

———. "Epidemics and Revolutions: Cholera in Nineteenth-Century Europe." In *Epidemics and Ideas: Essays on the Historical Perception of Pestilence*, edited by T. Ranger and P. Slack, 149–73. Cambridge: Cambridge University Press, 1992.

Hamlin, Christopher. *Cholera: The Biography*. Oxford: Oxford University Press, 2009.

Hays, Jo N. "Nineteenth-Century Cholera in Twentieth-Century Historical Writing." Annual meeting of the American Historical Association, Washington, D.C., January 3–6, 2008.

Howard-Jones, Norman. "Cholera Therapy in the Nineteenth Century." *Journal of the History of Medicine and Allied Sciences* 27 (1972): 373–95.

Ileto, Reynaldo C. "Cholera and the Origins of the American Sanitary Order in the Philippines." In *Imperial Medicine and Indigenous Societies*, edited by D. Arnold, 125–48. Manchester, UK: Manchester University Press, 1988.

Kudlick, Catherine J. *Cholera in Post-Revolutionary Paris: A Cultural History*. Berkeley: University of California Press, 1996.

McGrew, Roderick E. *Russia and the Cholera, 1823–1832*. Madison: University of Wisconsin Press, 1965.

Morris, R. J. *Cholera 1832: The Social Response to an Epidemic*. New York: Holmes and Meier, 1976.

Morris, Robert D. *The Blue Death: Disease, Disaster, and the Water We Drink*. New York: HarperCollins, 2007.

Rosenberg, Charles E. *The Cholera Years*. Chicago: University of Chicago Press, 1962.

Snowden, Frank M. *Naples in the Time of Cholera, 1884–1911*. Cambridge: Cambridge University Press, 1995.

Sullivan, Rodney. "Cholera and Colonialism in the Philippines, 1899–1903." In *Disease, Medicine, and Empire: Perspectives on Western Medicine and the Experience of European Expansion*, edited by R. M. MacLeod and M. J. Lewis, 284–300. London: Routledge, 1988.

Influenza

Barry, John M. *The Great Influenza: The Epic Story of the Deadliest Plague in History*. New York: Viking Penguin, 2004.

Beveridge, W. I. B. *Influenza: The Last Great Plague: An Unfinished Story of Discovery*. New York: Prodist, 1977.

Collier, Richard. *The Plague of the Spanish Lady: The Influenza Pandemic of 1918–1919*. New York: Atheneum, 1974.

Crosby, Alfred W. *America's Forgotten Pandemic: The Influenza of 1918*. 2nd ed. Cambridge: Cambridge University Press, 2003.

———. *Epidemic and Peace, 1918*. Westport, Conn.: Greenwood Press, 1976.

Davis, Mike. *The Monster at Our Door: The Global Threat of Avian Flu*. New York: Owl Books, 2005.

Hope-Simpson, R. Edgar. *The Transmission of Epidemic Influenza*. New York: Plenum, 1992.

Kilbourne, Edwin D. *Influenza*. New York: Plenum Medical Book, 1987.

Kolata, Gina. *Flu: The Story of the Great Influenza Pandemic of 1918 and the Search for the Virus that Caused It*. New York: Farrar, Straus and Giroux, 1999.

Mercola, Joseph, and Pam Killeen. *The Great Bird Flu Hoax: The Truth They Don't Want You to Know about the "Next Big Pandemic."* Nashville: Nelson Books, 2006.

Mills, I. D. "The 1918–1919 Influenza Pandemic: The Indian Experience." *Indian Economic and Social History Review* 23 (1986): 1–40.

Osborn, June E., ed. *History, Science and Politics: Influenza in America, 1918–1976*. New York: Prodist, 1977.

Patterson, K. David. *Pandemic Influenza, 1700–1900: A Study in Historical Epidemiology*. Totowa, N.J.: Rowman & Littlefield, 1986.

Pettit, Dorothy A., and Janice Bailie. *A Cruel Wind: Pandemic Flu in America, 1918–1920.* Murfreesboro, Tenn.: Timberland Books, 2008.

Phillips, Howard, and David Killingray, eds. *The Spanish Influenza Pandemic of 1918–19: New Perspectives.* New York: Routledge, 2003.

Quinn, Tom. *Flu: A Social History of Influenza.* London: New Holland Publishers, 2008.

Tambyah, Paul, and Ping-Chung Leung, eds. *Bird Flu: A Rising Pandemic in Asia and Beyond?* Singapore: World Scientific Publishing, 2006.

Wenzel, Richard. "What We Learned from H1N1's First Year." *New York Times,* April 13, 2010.

AIDS

Abdool Karim, S. S., and Q. Abdool Karim, eds. *HIV/AIDS in South Africa.* Cambridge: Cambridge University Press, 2005.

Adeyi, Olusoji, ed. *Averting AIDS Crises in Eastern Europe and Central Asia: A Regional Support Strategy.* Washington, D.C.: World Bank, 2003.

Aggleton, Peter, Peter Davies, and Graham Hart, eds. *AIDS: Individual, Cultural and Policy Dimensions.* Basingstoke, UK: Falmer Press, 1990.

Alcamo, I. Edward. *AIDS: The Biological Basis.* 3rd ed. Sudbury, Mass.: Jones and Bartlett, 2003.

Alexandrova, Anna, ed. *AIDS, Drugs and Society.* Rev. ed. New York: International Debate Education Association, 2004.

Almond, Brenda, ed. *AIDS: A Moral Issue—The Ethical, Legal and Social Aspects.* 2nd ed. New York: St. Martin's Press, 1996.

Barnett, Tony, and Piers Blaikie. *AIDS in Africa: Its Present and Future Impact.* New York: Guilford Press, 1992.

Barnett, Tony, and Alan Whiteside. *AIDS in the Twenty-First Century: Disease and Globalization.* Basingstoke, UK: Palgrave Macmillan, 2002.

Batsell, Jake. "AIDS, Politics, and NGOs in Zimbabwe." In *The African State and the AIDS Crisis,* edited by A. S. Patterson, 59–77. Burlington, Vt.: Ashgate, 2005.

Baylies, Carolyn, Janet Bujra, et al. *AIDS, Sexuality and Gender in Africa: Collective Strategies and Struggles in Tanzania and Zambia.* London: Routledge, 2000.

Berridge, Virginia, and Philip Strong, eds. *AIDS and Contemporary History.* Cambridge: Cambridge University Press, 1993.

Bethel, Elizabeth Rauh. *AIDS: Readings on a Global Crisis.* Boston: Allyn and Bacon, 1995.

Bond, George, John Kreniske, Ida Susser, and Joan Vincent, eds. *AIDS in Africa and the Caribbean.* Boulder, Colo.: Westview, 1997.

Brandt, Allan M. "AIDS and Metaphor: Toward the Social Meaning of Epidemic Disease." In *In Time of Plague: The History and Social Consequences of Lethal Epidemic Disease,* edited by A. Mack, 91–110. New York: New York University Press, 1991.

Buzy, Jeanine M., and Helene D. Gayle. "The Epidemiology of HIV and AIDS in Women." In *Women's Experiences with HIV/AIDS: An International Perspective,* edited by L. D. Long and E. M. Ankrah, 181–204. New York: Columbia University Press, 1996.

Cerullo, Margaret, and Evelynn Hammonds. "AIDS in Africa: The Western Imagination and the Dark Continent." In *AIDS: Readings on a Global Crisis*, edited by E. R. Bethel, 45–54. Boston: Allyn and Bacon, 1995.

Chin, James. *The AIDS Pandemic: The Collision of Epidemiology with Political Correctness.* Oxford, UK: Radcliffe, 2007.

Chirimuuta, Richard, and Rosalind Chirimuuta. *AIDS, Africa, and Racism.* 2nd ed. London: Free Association Books, 1989.

Choi, Susanne Y. P., and Roman David. "Law Enforcement, Public Health, and HIV/AIDS in China," In *The Global Politics of AIDS*, edited by P. G. Harris and P. D. Siplon, 137–54. Boulder, Colo.: Lynne Rienner, 2007.

Cohen, Felissa L, and Jerry D. Durham. *Women, Children, and HIV/AIDS.* New York: Springer, 1993.

Deane, Nawaal. "The Political History of AIDS Treatment." In *HIV/AIDS in South Africa*, edited by S. S. Abdool Karim and Q. Abdool Karim, 538–47. Cambridge: Cambridge University Press, 2005.

Doka, Kenneth J. *AIDS, Fear, and Society: Challenging the Dreaded Disease.* Bristol, Pa.: Taylor and Francis, 1997.

Duh, Samuel V. *Blacks and AIDS: Causes and Origins.* Newbury Park, Calif.: Sage, 1991.

Engel, Jonathan. *The Epidemic: A Global History of AIDS.* New York: HarperCollins, 2006.

Epprecht, Marc. *Heterosexual Africa? The History of an Idea from the Age of Exploration to the Age of AIDS.* Athens: Ohio University Press, 2008.

Epstein, Helen. *The Invisible Cure: Africa, the West, and the Fight against AIDS.* New York: Farrar, Straus and Giroux, 2007.

Essex, Max, Souleymane Mboup, Phyllis Kanki, Richard Marlink, and Sheila Tlou, eds. *AIDS in Africa.* 2nd ed. New York: Kluwer Academic/Plenum Publishers, 2002.

Fan, Hung Y., Ross F. Conner, and Luis P. Villarreal. *AIDS: Science and Society.* 5th ed. Sudbury, Mass.: Jones and Bartlett, 2007.

Farmer, Paul. *AIDS and Accusation: Haiti and the Geography of Blame.* Berkeley: University of California Press, 1992.

———. "AIDS and Accusation: Haiti, Haitians, and the Geography of Blame." In *Culture and AIDS*, edited by D. A. Feldman, 67–91. New York: Praeger, 1990.

Fassin, Didier. *When Bodies Remember: Experiences and Politics of AIDS in South Africa.* Translated by A. Jacobs and G. Varro. Berkeley: University of California Press, 2007.

Fee, Elizabeth, and Daniel M. Fox, eds. *AIDS: The Burdens of History.* Berkeley: University of California Press, 1988.

———, eds. *AIDS: The Making of a Chronic Disease.* Berkeley: University of California Press, 1992.

Feldman, Douglas A., ed. *Culture and AIDS.* New York: Praeger, 1990.

———, ed. *Global AIDS Policy.* Westport, Conn.: Bergin and Garvey, 1994.

Follér, Maj-Lis, and Håkan Thörn, eds. *The Politics of AIDS: Globalization, the State and Civil Society.* New York: Palgrave Macmillan, 2008.

Foster, Geoff, Carol Levine, and John Williamson, eds. *A Generation at Risk: The Global Impact of HIV/AIDS on Orphans and Vulnerable Children*. Cambridge: Cambridge University Press, 2005.

Frasca, Tim. *AIDS in Latin America*. Basingstoke, UK: Palgrave Macmillan, 2005.

Fumento, Michael. *The Myth of Heterosexual AIDS*. New York: Basic Books, 1991.

Furlong, Patrick, and Karen Ball. "The More Things Change: AIDS and the State in South Africa, 1987–2003." In *The African State and the AIDS Crisis*, edited by A. S. Patterson, 127–53. Burlington, Vt.: Ashgate, 2005.

Godinho, Joana, et al. *Reversing the Tide: Priorities for HIV/AIDS Prevention in Central Asia*. Washington, D.C.: World Bank, 2005.

Gostin, Lawrence O. *The AIDS Pandemic: Complacency, Injustice, and Unfulfilled Expectations*. Chapel Hill: University of North Carolina Press, 2004.

Gould, Peter. *The Slow Plague: A Geography of the AIDS Pandemic*. Oxford, UK: Blackwell, 1993.

Gow, Jeff, and Chris Desmond, eds. *Impacts and Interventions: The HIV/AIDS Epidemic and the Children of South Africa*. Pietermaritzburg, South Africa: University of Natal Press, 2002.

Grmek, Mirko D. *History of AIDS: Emergence and Origin of a Modern Pandemic*. Translated by R. C. Maulitz and J. Duffin. Princeton, N.J.: Princeton University Press, 1990.

Guest, Emma. *Children of AIDS: Africa's Orphan Crisis*. 2nd ed. London: Pluto, 2003.

Haacker, Markus, and Mariam Claeson, eds. *HIV and AIDS in South Asia: An Economic Development Risk*. Washington, D.C.: World Bank, 2009.

Harris, Paul G., and Patricia D. Siplon, eds. *The Global Politics of AIDS*. Boulder, Colo.: Lynne Rienner, 2007.

Hoad, Neville. *African Intimacies: Race, Homosexuality, and Globalization*. Minneapolis: University of Minnesota Press, 2007.

Hooper, Edward. *The River: A Journey to the Source of HIV and AIDS*. Boston: Little, Brown, 1999.

Hunter, Susan. *AIDS in America*. New York: Palgrave Macmillan, 2006.

———. *AIDS in Asia: A Continent in Peril*. Basingstoke, UK: Palgrave Macmillan, 2005.

———. *Black Death: AIDS in Africa*. Basingstoke, UK: Palgrave Macmillan, 2003.

Iliffe, John. *The African AIDS Epidemic: A History*. Athens: Ohio University Press, 2006.

Itano, Nicole. *No Place Left to Bury the Dead: Denial, Despair, and Hope in the African AIDS Pandemic*. New York: Atria Books, 2007.

Jenkins, Carol, and David A. Robalino. *HIV/AIDS in the Middle East and North Africa: The Costs of Inaction*. Washington, D.C.: World Bank, 2003.

Jonsen, Albert R., and Jeff Stryker, eds. *The Social Impact of AIDS in the United States*. Washington, D.C.: National Academy Press, 1993.

Kalipeni, Ezekiel, Susan Craddock, and Jayati Ghosh. "Mapping the AIDS Pandemic in Eastern and Southern Africa: A Critical Overview." In *HIV and AIDS in Africa: Beyond Epidemiology*, edited by E. Kalipeni, S. Craddock, J. R. Oppong, and J. Ghosh, 58–69. Oxford, UK: Blackwell, 2004.

Kalipeni, Ezekiel, Susan Craddock, Joseph R. Oppong, and Jayati Ghosh, eds. *HIV and AIDS in Africa: Beyond Epidemiology*. Oxford, UK: Blackwell, 2004.

Kauffman, Kyle D., and David L. Lindauer, eds. *AIDS and South Africa: The Social Expression of a Pandemic*. Basingstoke, UK: Palgrave Macmillan, 2004.

Leclerc-Madlala, Suzanne. "Global Struggles, Local Contexts: Prospects for a Southern African AIDS Feminism." In *The Politics of AIDS: Globalization, the State and Civil Society*, edited by M. Follér and H. Thörn, 141–43. New York: Palgrave Macmillan, 2008.

Levenson, Jacob. *The Secret Epidemic: The Story of AIDS and Black America*. New York: Pantheon Books, 2004.

Levin, Martin A., and Mary Bryna Sanger. *After the Cure: Managing AIDS and Other Public Health Crises*. Lawrence: University Press of Kansas, 2000.

Long, Lynellyn D., and E. Maxine Ankrah, eds. *Women's Experiences with HIV/AIDS: An International Perspective*. New York: Columbia University Press, 1996.

Lyons, Maryinez. "Mobile Populations and HIV/AIDS in East Africa." In *HIV and AIDS in Africa: Beyond Epidemiology*, edited by E. Kalipeni, S. Craddock, J. R. Oppong, and J. Ghosh, 175–90. Oxford, UK: Blackwell, 2004.

———. "The Point of View: Perspectives on AIDS in Uganda." In *AIDS in Africa and the Caribbean*, edited by G. Bond, J. Kreniske, I. Susser, and J. Vincent, 131–46. Boulder, Colo.: Westview, 1997.

Lyttleton, Chris. "AIDS and Civil Belonging: Disease Management and Political Change in Thailand and Laos." In *The Politics of Aids: Globalization, the State and Civil Society*, edited by M. Follér and H. Thörn, 255–73. New York: Palgrave Macmillan, 2008.

Mathews, Catherine. "Reducing Sexual Risk Behaviours: Theory and Research, Successes and Challenges." In *HIV/AIDS in South Africa*, edited by S. S. Abdool Karim and Q. Abdool Karim, 143–65. Cambridge: Cambridge University Press, 2005.

McNeil, Donald G., Jr. "At Front Lines, AIDS War Is Falling Apart." *New York Times*, May 9, 2010.

Mello e Souza, André de. "Defying Globalization: Effective Self-Reliance in Brazil." In *The Global Politics of AIDS*, edited by P. G. Harris and P. D. Siplon, 37–49. Boulder, Colo.: Lynne Rienner, 2007.

Nattrass, Nicoli. *The Moral Economy of AIDS in South Africa*. Cambridge: Cambridge University Press, 2004.

Nelkin, Dorothy, David P. Willis, and Scott V. Parris, eds. *A Disease of Society: Cultural and Institutional Responses to AIDS*. Cambridge: Cambridge University Press, 1991.

Oppong, Joseph R., and Samuel Agyei-Mensah. "HIV/AIDS in West Africa: The Case of Senegal, Ghana, and Nigeria." In *HIV and AIDS in Africa: Beyond Epidemiology*, edited by E. Kalipeni, S. Craddock, J. R. Oppong, and J. Ghosh, 70–82. Oxford, UK: Blackwell, 2004.

Oppong, Joseph R., and Ezekiel Kalipeni. "Perceptions and Misperceptions of AIDS in Africa." In *HIV and AIDS in Africa: Beyond Epidemiology*, edited by E. Kalipeni, S. Craddock, J. R. Oppong, and J. Ghosh, 47–57. Oxford, UK: Blackwell, 2004.

Orubuloye, I. O., John C. Caldwell, and James P. M. Ntozi, eds. *The Continuing HIV/AIDS Epidemic in Africa: Responses and Coping Strategies*. Canberra: Australian National University, 1999.

Ostergard, Robert L., Jr. "Politics in the Hot Zone: AIDS and National Security in Africa." In *Global Health and Governance: HIV/AIDS*, edited by N. K. Poku and A. Whiteside, 143–60. Basingstoke, UK: Palgrave Macmillan, 2004.

Outwater, Anne. "The Socioeconomic Impact of AIDS on Women in Tanzania." In *Women's Experiences with HIV/AIDS: An International Perspective*, edited by L. D. Long and E. M. Ankrah, 112–22. New York: Columbia University Press, 1996.

Patterson, Amy S., ed. *The African State and the AIDS Crisis*. Burlington, Vt.: Ashgate, 2005.

———. *The Politics of AIDS in Africa*. Boulder, Colo.: Lynne Rienner, 2006.

Poku, Nana K. *AIDS in Africa: How the Poor Are Dying*. Cambridge, UK: Polity Press, 2005.

Poku, Nana K., and Alan Whiteside, eds. *Global Health and Governance: HIV/AIDS*. Basingstoke, UK: Palgrave Macmillan, 2004.

Renwick, Neil. "The 'Nameless Fever': The HIV/AIDS Pandemic and China's Women." In *Global Health and Governance: HIV/AIDS*, edited by N. K. Poku and A. Whiteside, 187–203. Basingstoke, UK: Palgrave Macmillan, 2004.

Richardson, Diane. "AIDS Education and Women: Sexual and Reproductive Issues." In *AIDS: Individual, Cultural and Policy Dimensions*, edited by P. Aggleton, P. Davies, and G. Hart, 169–79. Basingstoke, UK: Falmer Press, 1990.

Rushing, William A. *The AIDS Epidemic: Social Dimensions of an Infectious Disease*. Boulder, Colo.: Westview, 1995.

Shannon, Gary, Gerald Pyle, and Rashid Bashshur. *The Geography of AIDS: Origins and Course of an Epidemic*. New York: Guilford Press, 1991.

Shepard, Benjamin Heim. "Shifting Priorities in US AIDS Policy." In *The Global Politics of AIDS*, edited by P. G. Harris and P. D. Siplon, 171–99. Boulder, Colo.: Lynne Rienner, 2007.

Shilts, Randy. *And the Band Played On: Politics, People, and the AIDS Epidemic*. New York: St. Martin's Press, 1987.

Siplon, Patricia D., and Kristin M. Novotny. "Overcoming the Contradictions: Women, Autonomy, and AIDS in Tanzania." In *The Global Politics of AIDS*, edited by P. G. Harris and P. D. Siplon, 87–107. Boulder, Colo.: Lynne Rienner, 2007.

Smallman, Shawn. *The AIDS Pandemic in Latin America*. Chapel Hill: University of North Carolina Press, 2007.

Sontag, Susan. *AIDS and Its Metaphors*. New York: Picador/Farrar, Straus and Giroux, 1989.

Stillwaggon, Eileen. *AIDS and the Ecology of Poverty*. Oxford: Oxford University Press, 2006.

van der Vliet, Virginia. "South Africa Divided against AIDS: A Crisis of Leadership." In *AIDS and South Africa: The Social Expression of a Pandemic*, edited by K. D. Kauffman and D. L. Lindauer, 48–96. Basingstoke, UK: Palgrave Macmillan, 2004.

Van Niekerk, Anton A., and Loretta M. Kopelman, eds. *Ethics and AIDS in Africa: The Challenge to Our Thinking*. Walnut Creek, Calif.: Left Coast Press, 2006.

Vicziany, Marika. "The Political Economy of HIV/AIDS in India." In *The Global Politics of AIDS*, edited by P. G. Harris and P. D. Siplon, 109–36. Boulder, Colo.: Lynne Rienner, 2007.

Whiteside, Alan. "Poverty and HIV/AIDS in Africa." In *Global Health and Governance: HIV/AIDS*, edited by N. K. Poku and A. Whiteside, 123–42. Basingstoke, UK: Palgrave Macmillan, 2004.

Williams, Al Olufemi, ed. *AIDS: An African Perspective*. Boca Raton, Fla.: CRC Press, 1992.

Wilson, David, and Mariam Claeson. "Dynamics of the HIV Epidemic in South Asia." In *HIV and AIDS in South Asia: An Economic Development Risk*, edited by M. Haacker and M. Claeson, 3–40. Washington, D.C.: World Bank, 2009.

Worth, Dooley. "Minority Women and AIDS: Culture, Race, and Gender." In *Culture and AIDS*, edited by D. A. Feldman, 111–35. New York: Praeger, 1990.

Index

Abbott, 172

Achmat, Zackie, 164

acquired immune deficiency syndrome (AIDS), 135–77; biology and origins of, 135–36; cancers occurring with, 137–38; in Caribbean, 166–70; causes of, 74, 156–59; conceptions of, 16; controversies over, 146–49 (*see also* dissidence concerning); course of, 137–38; death rates from, 150, 155, 174; dissidence concerning, 142–44, 163; drug use and, 138–39, 143, 146, 149, 151–53, 156, 174–75; emergence of, 137; gay community and, 145–50, 152–53; geographical origins of, 141–42, 144; history of, 144–50, 155, 160–61; in Latin America, 170–73; and morality, 152–53; opportunistic infections occurring with, 137–38, 157–58; as pandemic, 11; in Pattern I countries, 135, 138, 139, 140, 144, 156; in Pattern II countries, 135, 137, 156, 160, 166; in Pattern III countries, 135, 139, 173–75; policies on, 147–49, 153, 159, 161–64, 168–71; positive aspects of, 12–13; race and, 151–52, 168; sexuality and, 16, 139, 146, 151–57; social aspects of, 10; societal factors in, 135, 146–54, 159–67, 175–77, 183; spread of, 161; in sub-Saharan Africa, 141, 144, 155–66; surveillance and control related to, 153–54; symptoms of, 137–38; TB and, 96, 158; tests for, 146; treatment of, 147–49, 163–65, 171; uniqueness of, 144, 176–77; in the United States, 144–55. *See also* human immunodeficiency virus

acute infection syndrome, 137

acute respiratory distress syndrome (ARDS), 119

Africa. *See* sub-Saharan Africa

afterlife, conceptions of, 58–59

Agramont, Jacme d', 43

Agreement on Trade-Related Aspects of Intellectual Property Rights (TRIPS), 171, 173

❋

About the Author

John Aberth received his PhD in medieval history from the University of Cambridge in England and has taught at various universities and colleges throughout Vermont, where he lives with his wife, horses, and cats. He specializes in the Black Death or plague of the late Middle Ages and is the author of *The Black Death: The Great Mortality of 1348–1350: A Brief History with Documents*, published with Bedford/St. Martin's Press; *The First Horseman: Disease in Human History*, with Pearson/Prentice Hall; and *From the Brink of the Apocalypse: Confronting Famine, War, Plague and Death in the Later Middle Ages*, with Routledge Press. He is currently working on a new book, *Doctoring the Black Death: The Late Medieval Medical Response to Epidemic Disease*, also to be published with Rowman & Littlefield.